17 May 1978

Who's too old for yoga?
Not you!

Health specialists recommend this non-stress method of keeping in shape and restoring flexibility to neglected muscles. Students in Eve Diskin's yoga class, shown in the photographs that dot this book, demonstrate that they can perform the exercises with ease and that they are fun, too. Even the partially invalided who must exercise in chair or bed are invigorated by yoga.

Start now to enjoy yoga and its benefits. Begin with the simple exercises at the beginning of the book. Follow each step as illustrated, and you'll discover how much better you feel. Gradually you will find yourself able to do more advanced exercises. You will be able to establish your own personalized routine from among the mini-programs to suit your body's needs. You will sleep more soundly and enjoy your waking hours to the fullest with YOGA FOR YOUR LEISURE YEARS.

Books By
Eve Diskin

Joy of Life Through Yoga
with Eugene Rawls

Yoga For Beauty and Health
with Eugene Rawls

Yoga For Children

Published By
Warner Books

YOGA FOR YOUR LEISURE YEARS

by
EVE DISKIN

WARNER BOOKS

A Warner Communications Company

WARNER BOOKS EDITION

Copyright © 1978 by Eve Diskin
All rights reserved

ISBN 0-446-82152-7

Back cover photo by Kenn Duncan

Warner Books, Inc., 75 Rockefeller Plaza, New York, N.Y. 10019

Printed in the United States of America

Not associated with Warner Press, Inc., of Anderson, Indiana

First Printing: May, 1978

10 9 8 7 6 5 4 3 2 1

CONTENTS

DEDICATION

I dedicate this book to Wayne L. Pruitt, whose steadfastness and support have been a continuing comfort to me.

ACKNOWLEDGMENTS

I thank my son, Steven Diskin, for the technical assistance, the consistently good quality of his photographs, and the artistic insight he brought to his work.

I am grateful to Jose Perez, who prepared all the illustrations.

I am thankful to Sylvia Shubert for her many excellent ideas and her long hours of help during the writing of the manuscript.

I appreciate the information given to me by Terri Francis Brower, R.N., FNP, whose years of work with geriatric patients has made her knowledgeable in the field.

I also appreciate the help given me by my friend John Stepanick, who is a librarian. He spent considerable time in locating suitable material for my purposes.

I thank the older adults and senior citizens who posed for individual pictures. Their unfailing enthusiasm and good humor brought much fun to the picture-taking sessions. They are: Raymond Abrams, Barbara Adelman, Lisa Adelman, Al Appelbaum, Kay Appelbaum, Geraldine Bellins, Ben Belluards, Libby Belluards, Eva Brock, Ken Brock, Kay Broday, Dorothy Bunes, Shirley

Campbell, Ruth Coblentz, Anna Davida Cram, Fred Cram, Emily Dohre, Freda Dreyer, Morris Dreyer, Edgar Ehlen, Jack Ensink, Hank Feld, Lillian Feldman, Rose Feinstein, Sam Fink, Alice Fink, Hy Fried, Dorothy Gallagher, Ali Moore, Cheryl Moore, Mary Gardner, Clara Greenberg, Martin Greif, Miriam Greif, Frances Hanashewski, Minni Hants, Sam Hants, Maria Harmande, Edna F. Haynes, Kitty Henig, Louis Henig, Helen Hickey, Abe Jacobs, Harry Jacobs, Ruth S. Jeans, Esther Kahan, Anne Kapiloff, Rositta Kennedy, Augie King, Harper Klein, Sonny Klein, Spencer Klein, Ruth and Michael Levine, Henry Levy, Irene Levy, Bea Lippman, Albert Longetta, John Luciw, Charles McLaughlin, Gertrude Novin, Ann Porras, Wayne Pruitt, Adele Roso, Jan Russell, Ruth Siebel, Alfonso Spirig, Rosalyn Starr, Jack Stelzer, Amelia Stepanick, Bernice Sullivan, Dianne Weaver, Mae Wecksler, Phil Weldon, Eleanor Winhold, Natalie Winhold.

The contributions made by the following organizations and clubs have been most helpful to me: American Round Dance Club—Director Nate Sirota; Beau Rivage Hotel—Jony Fernans, Cabana Manager; Doral Country Club—Al Burnes, Golf Professional and Beverly Wheeler, Social Director; Justine Associates—Ralph Surrency, President; Kenko Judo Karate Club—Koji Sugiomoto (black belt); Miami Jewish Home and Hospital for the Aged; Miami Park and Recreation Center—Wilfred Canales.

COMMENTS FROM SEVERAL MEMBERS OF THE HEALTH PROFESSIONS

TERRI FRANCIS BROWER, R.N., FNP

Assistant Professor of Nursing, University of Miami, School of Nursing; Project Director of the Geriatric Nurse Practitioner Project, University of Miami, School of Nursing; Member of the State Ombudsman Committee for Long Term Care

I was excited when Eve first approached me to discuss her plans for this book. An avid follower of yoga myself, I was sure she had a winner.

To me, yoga is the perfect form of exercise for the older adult. As a philosophy of the mind and body, it teaches moderation of effort.

Unlike many other forms of exercise—jogging, for instance—yoga nags at seldom-used muscles that tend to shorten and fall asleep from disuse. I can say as a nurse conversant with geriatrics that its slow, gentle stretches can be done even by people who are somewhat incapacitated. Yoga is easy to do, easier, in fact, than any other form of exercise, and should be carried out by older adults no matter how stiff they feel, and even though the aches that result from degenerative changes make them think, "not for me," they should not give in to their desire to cheat on exercise. They will find that by practicing yoga faithfully, their sluggish bowels will function more normally, and their appetites will increase.

I can cite countless reports and studies on the benefits of exercise for health. The President himself urges physical fitness. More and more older adults are becoming aware of their health needs and are flocking to health food stores, spending a great deal of money on aids that promise youthfulness and vigor, but their efforts may well come to naught if they fail to support their nutritional needs with exercise.

Yoga gives the individual the opportunity to proceed at his own pace, since, unlike calisthenics, its techniques are adaptable to anybody at any age. Yoga can take all of the physical alterations of an aging body in stride.

Terri Francis Brower, R.N.

NORMAN C. SPITZER, M.D.

Postdoctoral Fellow in Neurology (E.E.G.) University of Miami School of Medicine.

I am in regular contact with senior citizens and their problems. I find that many of them are doing less and less and having more and more "empty" time. They lack stimulating activity for their minds and bodies.

A number of senior citizens have allowed their muscles to atrophy and their joints to stiffen unnecessarily. The result is growing physical rigidity and the tendency to lose their balance and fall. As their bodies are immobilized, their minds suffer. Among other things, they are afraid to go out. A program of yoga exercises, even if they are performed sitting in a chair or lying in bed, can counteract physical rigidity and improve the oxygen circulation in the system. It can, at the same time, ease emotional insecurity.

Yoga can also provide a group activity that leads to new social interests. For people with too much free time, it can offer many hours of all-purpose enjoyment. By keeping older citizens occupied and making it possible for them to move their bodies around with confidence, yoga can give them the desire for achievement. It should not be too long thereafter before their comment, "See, I can do this," reflects their pride of accomplishment and their sense of well-being.

Norman C. Spitzer, M.D.

MARSHALL F. GILULA, M.D.

Psychiatric Director, Life Energies Research Institute, Miami, Florida

Director of Medical Education, Anna State Hospital, Anna, Illinois

The process of aging does not necessarily lead to losing body flexibility and mental adaptability. One of the best antidotes I am aware of for the negative effects of aging is yoga. Yoga requires the individual to be active rather than passive. It has a rejuvenating effect because it is gentle in its application, it reaches the main organs of the body, and it soothes the mind. It removes the need to depend on outside influences for inner

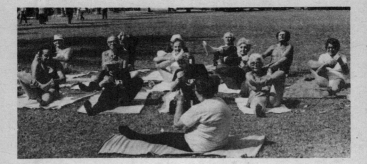

tranquility by helping one learn how to let the body serve as its own tranquilizer. Yoga is a medically effective technique for releasing stress.

Controlled scientific research at Harvard and other universities shows that meditation definitely enhances the release of stress that may be stored within. And each yoga asana is a meditation in itself when properly done.

I have found that yoga is experiential and a way of getting back to being in touch with myself. Yoga makes it more and more evident to me that mind and body are firmly stuck together. What I do for my mind influences my physical structure and vice versa. The same relationship is evident in my patients whose lives I am temporarily sharing via the psychotherapy relationship.

In its broadest sense, psychotherapy may facilitate harmony between mind and body, thought and feelings. If a patient of mine seems open to the idea, I, as a psychiatrist, often advise using yoga. Many of my patients who have engaged in yoga have shown some unlocking of structural rigidity and the development of somewhat more flexible mental attitudes. Other people who have become at least a little practiced in yoga have commented on how their day-to-day energy grows. Nurses at the Marion, Illinois, Veterans Administration Hospital, where I was employing yoga as a form of treatment, sat with patients and learned to do the yoga exercises. They subsequently reported that they had lost weight, were more positive about their physical structures, and had found more energy for their husbands. Both the nurses and the patients remarked about the youthfulness they felt within themselves and also saw in others taking part in the program.

There are times when the gentle, noncompetitive movements of yoga actually seem to reverse the aging process for a while. Gloria Swanson, Bob Cummings, and Yehudi Menuhin, to name just a few, have demonstrated the rejuvenating effects of yoga in their lives. They have shown that resiliency of the physical structure always parallels resiliency of the mind. And resiliency—or the lack of it—often determines how skillfully a person adapts to the aging process.

Many people become sedentary and stiff long before their sixties and seventies. Those who use yoga often find that there is no need to become sedentary and stiff at any age. Actually, it is almost never too late to reverse the slow-down process of the bodily functions. Individuals can reject the concept that the consequences of aging have to be mainly negative.

The rediscovery of yoga in our culture during the '70s probably indicates a re-emphasis of the inner self and appropriate return to the conservation of cultural energy. We have been wasting our elderly, and the elderly have been wasting themselves. Now there apparently is a movement toward the recycling of experience and wisdom. Growing older with yoga can truly be marked by the development of genuine wisdom and superior adaptive abilities.

Marshall F. Gilula, M.D.

A MESSAGE TO THE HEALTH PROFESSIONS

Many students in my classes during the last fifteen years began the course with various complaints: backache, nervous tension, overweight, poor digestion, poor circulation, shallow breathing, arthritis, constipation, inability to fall asleep. After a few weeks of taking part in a series of properly planned yoga exercises, I could observe that they had strengthened their weakened organs, improved their state of mind, upgraded their general health and had fewer complaints.

I began to realize that yoga could play an important part in improving people's health, that yoga could be a useful adjunct to all the healing professions. More and more doctors were coming to class for their own relaxation, and were becoming increasingly aware of the cumulative mental and physical benefits for everyone in the yoga postures. Many of them now recommend yoga to their patients, and in some instances, give special instructions to yoga teachers for particular patients.

Yoga is adaptable to all ages and is interesting and psychologically satisfying. Its slow-moving stretching and breathing exercises can be adjusted to fit a variety of needs. Its postures can be implemented at any time: while sitting, standing, or lying in bed. A few can even be done while walking. Most of the exercises take no longer than a minute to perform and do not require a great amount of energy.

In sustaining the health of the public, yoga can be an excellent source of help to the healing professions.

Eve Diskin

WHAT THE PRESIDENT'S COUNCIL ON PHYSICAL FITNESS AND SPORTS SAYS ABOUT EXERCISE

In the pamphlet issued by the U.S. Government Printing Office: 1973 0-507-872, the foreword on **More Awareness Than Action** and the section called **Why Fitness?** make a number of points that are well worth repeating. Some of them are listed below for your reflection:

More Awareness Than Action
Foreword

To look your best, to feel your best, and to be able to do your best, you must exercise regularly. That is man's nature, and modern technology can't change it.

When the activity required of you by your job and other duties falls below the level necessary to support good health, you must supplement it with planned activity. Your sense of well-being, your ability to perform, and even your survival depend on it.

You already know that regular, vigorous exercise increases muscle strength and endurance. It also improves the functioning of the lungs, heart, and blood vessels; promotes flexibility of the joints, releases mental and physical tensions, and aids in weight control or reduction.

In short, exercise can make the difference. The options are mere existence or a full life. The choice is yours.

WHY FITNESS?:

Why do we worry about strength and endurance in a pushbutton age? These are some of the reasons why exercise and fitness are of value even when the physical demands of living are minimal:

1. *Strength and endurance developed through regular exercise enable you to perform daily tasks with relative ease. You use only a small part of your physical reserve in routine activity.*

2. *Skill and agility gained through practice provide for economy of movement. This is another factor in minimizing physical effort required for routine tasks.*

3. *Poise and grace are by-products of efficient movement. They help you to feel at ease in social situations and are factors in good appearance.*

4. *Good muscle tone and posture can protect you from certain back problems caused by sedentary living.*

5. *Enjoyable exercise can provide relief from tension and nerves as a safe and natural tranquilizer.*

6. *Feeling physically fit helps you to build a desirable self-concept. You need to see yourself at your optimum physically as well as in other ways.*

Dear Students,

If you consider yourselves senior citizens or older adults, this book is for you. You now have the leisure time to look after yourselves. Why not do it with yoga?

Senior citizens and older adults need moderate exercise. Yoga permits you to exercise moderately; that is, without the expenditure of too much effort. Yoga postures are carried out in a smooth and rhythmic manner. They help your heart and lungs work efficiently. They gently stretch away tension. They never exhaust you. They actually increase your energy. Because they serve your special time of life so admirably, they are an ideal form of physical activity for you.

I have no hesitation whatever in saying that you will be delighted with the results of your yoga practice. The exercises in this book can give you a new and eminently young approach to living.

Welcome to the yoga club.

Eve Diskin

WHAT YOGA CAN DO FOR YOU

Yoga is a highly developed system of meditation and exercise that originated in India many thousands of years ago. Its two major forms are *raja* yoga and *hatha* yoga.* *Raja* yoga pertains to

---

*Throughout this book, the term in use is the one-word form YOGA. Every time yoga is used, it means *hatha* yoga. When it is necessary to make a distnction, *raja* yoga is specified.

meditation, and *hatha* yoga to exercise. Each of these forms has its followers. Some people choose to perform both kinds of yoga. Although this book deals with *hatha* yoga, it introduces you to one *raja* yoga exercise to help you experience the kind of peacefulness that accompanies the practice of *raja* yoga.

Hatha yoga involves stretching exercises and inversion postures, breathing techniques, and special cleansing movements. The stretching exercises relieve tension throughout your body and keep it flexible. They also improve your circulation and your posture. The breathing techniques bring oxygen to your system. They also strengthen your lungs and help you to sleep well. The cleansing movements clear your nasal passages and remove impurities from your lungs, aiding your respiratory functions. All the yoga exercises contribute to your physical and mental energy.

In the process of involving you in a natural form of relaxation, yoga brings new insights into your life. With these insights can come the peace that makes for a harmonious existence.

To the superior man
Time is no longer a hindrance
But the means of making actual
That which is potential

Pantanjali—yoga philosopher
300 B.C.

OLDER ADULTS AND SENIOR CITIZENS, YOU CAN ENJOY YOUR LEISURE YEARS!

If you are an older adult, or a senior citizen, 50 years of age or over, you will no doubt notice that more people are, like you, retiring earlier and living longer. You now have the time to look after yourselves. If you take care of your health, you can enjoy your leisure years. A good way to take care of your health is to exercise. Yoga is a convenient, "outgoing," practical form of exercise for you.

You can engage in yoga, first as a student, then, as you become more proficient at it, as a leader of a neighborhood group. As a leader, you can lecture and give demonstrations. You can become a teacher and instruct classes at a resort, hotel, or condominium. You can also teach at the "Y" and in adult education centers. You can even give immeasurable service in nursing homes and hospitals by supplementing activities there.

And why not bring the benefits of yoga to your

family? Yoga is more than a way to exercise. It is an enjoyable recreation source. You can help your children and grandchildren to fun and good health by exercising together the yoga way.

By being constantly active, you can ward off the ailments that beset advancing age. As a matter of fact, if you practice your yoga regularly, you may some day be able to share the attitudes of citizens of such faraway places as Hunza in Kashmir-Pakistan and Abkhazia in the Georgian Soviet Socialist Republic. In those countries, individuals do not regard themselves as senior citizens until they reach the magic demarcation line of age one hundred. Many of them face the first quarter of the second century physically and mentally alert and hardy. You can be as active and as sturdy as they are.

A number of the people shown doing yoga in this book are in their seventies and eighties. Join them in yoga exercise that will keep not only your muscles from atrophying, but your brain and spirit as well.

RULES FOR THE PRACTICE OF YOGA

1. Work out a weekly schedule. You do not have to practice every day. You can, for example, practice three days in succession, then take the fourth day off.

2. Try to set aside the same time of the day or evening for practice.

3. You can practice indoors or outdoors, but exercise in a place that is free from noise and interruption. If you practice indoors, make sure the room is well ventilated.

4. Wear loose, comfortable clothing. Avoid wearing jewelry that impedes your movements.

5. Do not exercise on a full stomach. Wait about a half-hour after a snack, and about two hours after a complete meal.

6. Practice on a firm, but not a hard surface. Never practice directly on a wood or cement floor. Be sure you use a pad that is thick enough for comfort.

7. Never rush your yoga practice. Take your time. Rest five or ten seconds between techniques. The more difficult the exercise, the longer you need to rest. In the miniprograms, be sure to rest for twenty to thirty seconds after you do the standing exercises.

8. Try to concentrate on what you are doing. Do not allow your mind to wander.

9. Remember that some exercises must be done for both sides of the body; that is, if you start on the left, repeat the exercise on the right. If you start on the right, repeat the exercise on the left. By the same token, some techniques such as the eye and neck exercises can be done more comfortably while sitting in the Tailor or Half Lotus position. Whenever you are requested to sit cross-legged, select one of those positions.

10. The majority of the yoga exercises have a holding position that is shown by a photograph. The holding position is the peak position of the exercise. A few of the exercises have continuous movements that you do not hold. Those movements are, however, the main part of the exercise and are also shown by photographs.

Never pull, tug, or strain when you are holding the postures. Never stretch beyond the limits of your ability. You do not have to perfect the exercise to benefit from it. Relax and breathe rhythmically as you do them.

11. The longer you hold an exercise, the more stretch you get. Keep to the counts given.

12. When you are asked to hold a position for a given number of seconds, count softly like this: one hundred and one, one hundred and two, and so on. To repeat aloud the expression "one hundred and one" takes one second.

HOW TO USE THIS BOOK

1. This book is divided into four sections:

Section I.
LEARNING THE EXERCISES

Section II.
MINIPROGRAMS FOR THE CARE AND DEVELOPMENT OF THE TOTAL BODY

Section III.
MINIPROGRAMS FOR THE CARE AND DEVELOPMENT OF PARTICULAR BODY PARTS

Section IV.
MINIPROGRAMS FOR COMMON PROBLEMS

2. The postures in Section I, Learning the Exercises, are arranged in six chapters. Each succeeding chapter is somewhat more advanced than the chapter before it.

Section II takes the exercises from Section I and divides them into a number of miniprograms to develop and strengthen your *entire body*.

Section III takes the exercises from Section I and divides them into a series of miniprograms to develop and strengthen such *specific body parts* as your abdomen, arms, back, chest, head, legs, neck, and shoulders.

The miniprograms in Section IV are concerned with such *common problems* as balance, constipation, posture, sleep, and tension. They utilize the exercises in Section I that are best designed to aid you with these problems.

3. The best method to follow in working your way

two to learn each chapter and familiarize yourself with the exercises.

If, after you have finished all six chapters, you feel the need for greater confidence and control, you may repeat Section I. Do not expect to perfect the exercises yet.

4. Go on to the miniprograms. They have been arranged to give you variety. Each miniprogram takes about ten minutes. Use the miniprograms for the total body as the *foundation* of your exercise program. Add the miniprograms for particular body parts (e.g., arms, legs) and/or those dealing with common problems (e.g., sleep, posture), when you feel you need them.

A sample program* might consist of:

First day   total body
particular body parts (arms)
common problems (sleep)

Second day   total body

Third day   total body
common problems (posture)

Fourth day   rest**

*If you favor certain miniprograms, do them more often than others.
**See item one in Rules for the Practice of Yoga.

Fifth day   common problems (sleep)

Sixth day   total body
common problems (sleep)

Seventh day   total body
common problems (tension)

Eighth day   rest**

5. The exercises consist of drawings, photographs, and instructions. The drawings lead you to the holding positions of the exercises, which are distinguished by the photographs. Drawings then lead you out of the exercises. Occasionally, an exercise does not have any drawings, and the photographs show you all the steps.

6. Every miniprogram gives you the names of the exercises to be practiced and provides you with the drawings that represent those exercises. It also gives you the original page number of each exercise and takes you a step further: It gives you an advanced count to use. When you feel that you have reached the level of flexibility that will permit you to hold the exercise comfortably for an even greater length of time than required by the advanced count, a potential count is suggested. Note that every exercise does not have an advanced or a potential count. If an exercise in the miniprograms does not have an advanced count, continue to use the last count given in Section I.

In some exercises you will be able to advance the count sooner than in others. Do not at any time exceed the potential count.

7. Several blank pages have been provided for your use at the end of each miniprogram section, should you wish to jot down any notes.

8. At the end of the book you will find three appendices and a general index. The exercises in appendix A can be performed in bed. The exercises in appendix B can be done in a chair. These two appendices are included for the benefit of people whose bodies and legs are too stiff to permit them to lower themselves to and raise themselves from the floor. Appendix C provides an alphabetic list of all the exercises together with the beginning, the advanced, and the potential counts.

You should have no difficulty reading the book, as the print throughout is large and clear, and the instructions represent the photographs and drawings precisely.

Section I.

LEARNING THE EXERCISES

CHAPTER I

TAILOR

FINGER CLASP

BACK OF LEG STRETCH

CAT

REFRESHING BREATH

COW

COMPLETE BREATH

TAILOR

In olden days, the tailor sat on a large platform with his legs crossed. He learned to sit for hours without a sign of fatigue. Once your legs acquire a measure of flexibility, you, too, can assume this relaxed way of sitting. Do so whenever you have an opportunity. Among other things, you can watch your favorite television program while practicing the Tailor position.

DO THE EXERCISE TWICE.

1. Sit on the floor with your legs extended and together. Place your hands on your knees.

2. Place your hands on the floor beside you. Bend your knees. Cross your left ankle over your right ankle.

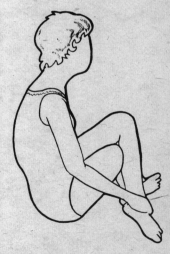

3. Hold on to your toes and bring your feet in toward your thighs.

4. Lower your knees. Rest
your hands on them. Hold for
10 seconds.

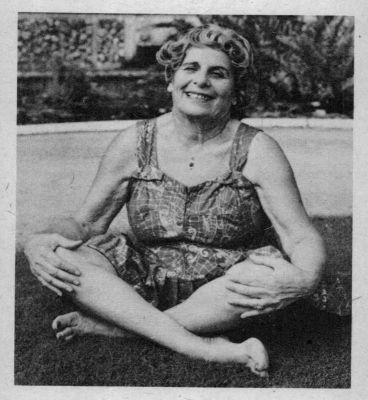

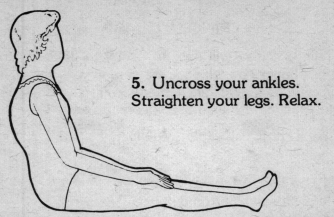

5. Uncross your ankles. Straighten your legs. Relax.

REPEAT THE STEPS ON THE OPPOSITE SIDE, WITH YOUR RIGHT ANKLE CROSSED OVER YOUR LEFT ANKLE. YOU HAVE COMPLETED THE EXERCISE.

HOW TO PRACTICE THE EXERCISE:
After you cross your legs, bring your feet as close to your body as possible. Lower your knees as much as you can. This is the easiest of all the yoga sitting positions, and should not present much difficulty even when you start.

WHAT THE EXERCISE DOES FOR YOU:
It permits you to expand your rib cage, allowing for improved breathing.

It enables you to move your diaphragm freely.

It stretches your legs, and keeps your hips, knees, and ankles flexible.

It quiets your mind.

It serves as a standard sitting position for many other exercises.

FINGER CLASP

This exercise will help to promote flexibility in your fingers by relieving stiffness in your joints. If you tend to have stiff, aching hands, take a minute to practice the exercise several times a day.

DO THE EXERCISE TWICE.

1. Sit comfortably with your legs crossed.* Extend your arms in front of you. Cross your right wrist over your left.

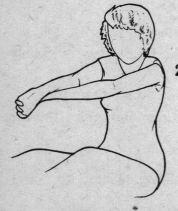

2. Interlock your fingers.

*The Tailor position.

3. Bend your elbows and draw your hands to your chest.

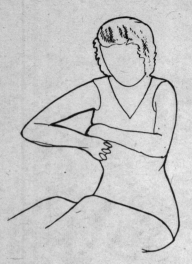

4. Slide your hands up your chest to your chin.

5. Slowly straighten your elbows as you extend your arms forward. Hold for 5 seconds.

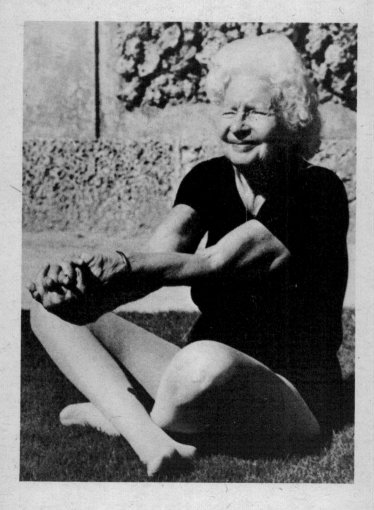

6. Return your hands to your chin; then slide them down your chest.

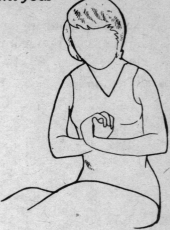

7. Lower your hands to your knees. Straighten your elbows.

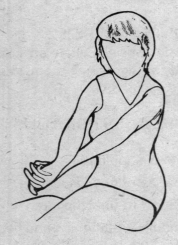

8. Unclasp your fingers. Rest your hands on your knees. Relax.

REPEAT THE STEPS ON THE OPPOSITE SIDE, BY CROSSING YOUR LEFT WRIST OVER YOUR RIGHT. YOU HAVE COMPLETED THE EXERCISE.

HOW TO PRACTICE THE EXERCISE:
Be careful. Do not force your elbows to straighten. If you have difficulty straightening them, keep your hands less tightly clasped.

WHAT THE EXERCISE DOES FOR YOU:

It relieves tension in your shoulders.

It strengthens the muscles of your forearms.

It improves the circulation to your fingers.

It keeps your fingers mobile, your wrists and your elbows limber.

BACK OF LEG STRETCH

This is a simple but important exercise. It exerts a stretch over the backs of your legs from your heels to your upper thighs. It increases your ability to walk long distances.

DO THE EXERCISE TWICE.

1. Sit on the floor. Bend your knees. Hold your toes.

2. Straighten your legs without releasing your toes. Lower your head forward. Hold for 5 seconds.

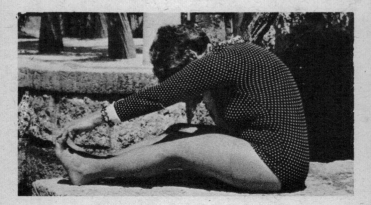

3. Release your toes. Slide your hands slowly up your legs to your thighs. Keep your head down.

4. Raise your head and sit up straight.

5. Relax.

HOW TO PRACTICE THE EXERCISE:

It may take months before you are able to straighten your legs completely. Practicing in a tub of warm water can help the process of relaxing the tight ligaments and tendons of your legs.

WHAT THE EXERCISE DOES FOR YOU:

It keeps your neck and shoulders supple.

It stretches your entire back, particularly your lower back.

It stretches the backs of your legs, especially the area behind your knees.

It gives your toes flexibility.

It helps you stand erect.

CAT

An easy back exercise that offers considerable benefit is the Cat stretch. It gently tones the muscles of your back and keeps your spine limber. The catlike and graceful movements you achieve can make you feel so good, you will want to purr like a contented cat.

DO THE EXERCISE TWICE.

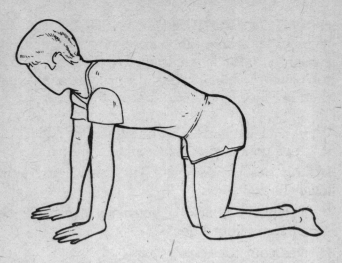

1. Kneel on the floor. Place your hands, palms down, in front of you. Look straight ahead.

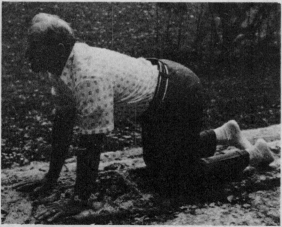

2. Raise your head and look up. Lower your back. Hold for 5 seconds.

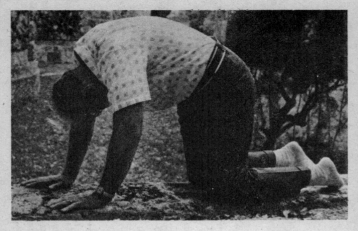

3. Drop your head and arch your spine up. Hold for 5 seconds.

4. Sit back on your feet. Put your hands on your thighs. Relax.

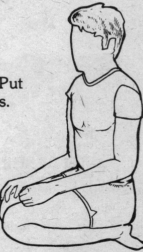

HOW TO PRACTICE THE EXERCISE:
Be sure to keep your head back when you lower your spine. As you arch your spine up, press your hands against the floor. This will give your spine a

greater stretch. As you progress in the exercise, add another dimension to it: Inhale as you raise your head and lower your back, and exhale as you lower your head and raise your back.

WHAT THE EXERCISE DOES FOR YOU:

It relieves tension in your neck and spine.

It strengthens your shoulders, arms, and wrists.

It keeps your knees flexible.

It massages your visceral organs.

It exercises your pelvic region.

REFRESHING BREATH

This is a happy way to start the day. After a long night's sleep, your body needs fresh air—oxygen to wake it up. Take a deep breath, give your body a greater stretch, and you are ready to go. With this technique, it is easy to greet the day with a smile.

DO THE EXERCISE TWICE.

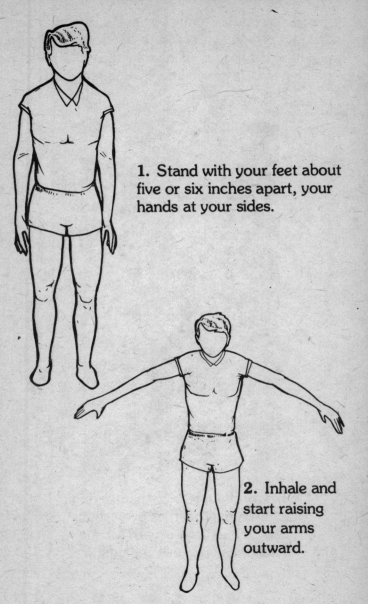

1. Stand with your feet about five or six inches apart, your hands at your sides.

2. Inhale and start raising your arms outward.

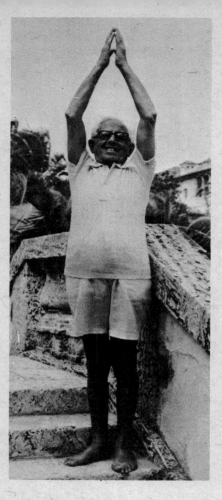

3. Continue to inhale and bring your palms together over your head. Hold your breath for the 3 seconds you hold the posture.

4. "Whistle" the air slowly out
of your mouth as you lower
your arms to your sides.

5. Stand at ease.

HOW TO PRACTICE THE EXERCISE:
You may not be able to continue inhaling to the

hold position at first. You need to increase your lung capacity to do so. After a few weeks of practice, try to do something a little more advanced. Come up on your toes as you raise your arms. Bring your heels to the floor as you lower your arms.

WHAT THE EXERCISE DOES FOR YOU:

It gives your body added oxygen.

It strengthens your lungs.

It stimulates your visceral organs.

It stretches your arms, legs, and sides.

It improves your body alignment.

When you do the exercise on your toes, it strengthens your toes, ankles, and arches and improves your balance.

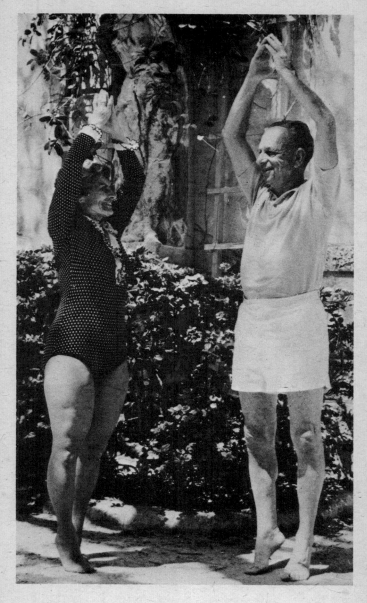

COW

The Cow stretches the tight, aching muscles of your back and neck and improves the circulation to your head. In no time at all, it eliminates nervous fatigue. Do the Cow whenever you need a quick "pick-me-up." The Cow is a favorite technique for most students.

DO THE EXERCISE TWICE.

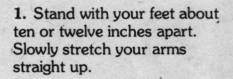

1. Stand with your feet about ten or twelve inches apart. Slowly stretch your arms straight up.

2. Bend forward from the waist. Lower your head. Relax your arms.

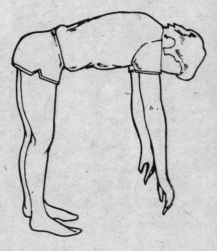

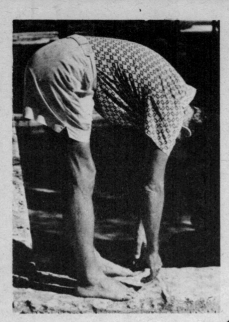

3. Try to touch your fingers to the floor. Hold for 5 seconds.

4. Keeping your chin close to your chest and your shoulders rounded, straighten up slowly, starting with your lower back.

53

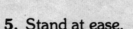

5. Stand at ease.

HOW TO PRACTICE THE EXERCISE:

One of the criteria for doing this exercise is that you move slowly going into it and coming out of it. If you cannot touch your fingers to the floor, simply let your arms hang loose at the point they reach. Each time you maintain this position, the weight from your waist up will gradually stretch the tight muscles of your back increasing the flexibility of your back. Be certain that your neck is fully relaxed, and your head is down. Breathe freely.

WHAT THE EXERCISE DOES FOR YOU:

It nourishes your brain.

It improves the circulation to your face and scalp.

It soothes your neck and shoulder muscles.

It relaxes tight muscles in your back.

It stretches the backs of your legs.

COMPLETE BREATH

Slow, deep breathing is an important factor in relaxation. By practicing the Complete Breath exercise, which involves slow, deep breathing, you can shed accumulated tension in minutes. You can do the exercise anywhere at any time. The beauty of it is that it works. You really relax. You do not need pills or any other artificial device to soothe you.

DO THE
EXERCISE TWICE.

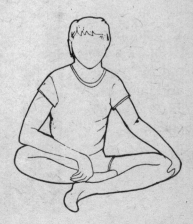

1. Sit comfortably, with your legs crossed* and rest your hands on your knees.

*The Tailor posture.

2. Inhale slowly through your nose and push your abdomen out at the same time.

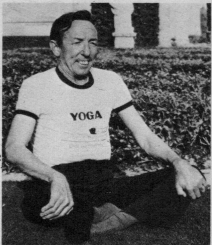

3. Continue to inhale slowly but pull your abdomen in and expand your chest.

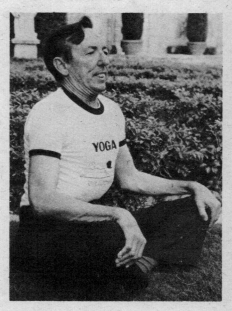

4. Continue inhaling slowly, and raise your shoulders. Hold your breath for 3 seconds as you hold the position.

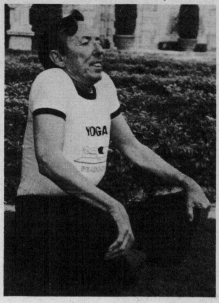

5. Exhale through your nose and lower your shoulders.

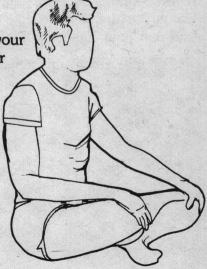

6. Relax.

57

HOW TO PRACTICE THE EXERCISE:

Before you begin the exercise, practice pushing your abdomen out and pulling it in, breathing as usual. When you start to do the exercise, try to allow ten seconds for inhaling and ten seconds for exhaling.

Figure 2 is the most difficult part of the exercise to coordinate because it causes you to breathe in an unfamiliar way. You must learn to push your abdomen out when you breathe in. The movement gives the lower part of your lungs the room they need to receive additional oxygen.

Do not be surprised if at first you are unable to continue inhaling as you raise your shoulders. When you have more control over your breathing, and your lung capacity increases, you will be able to inhale more completely.

If you cannot sit comfortably in the Tailor or Half Lotus posture, extend your legs in front of you, and rest your hands on the floor behind you.

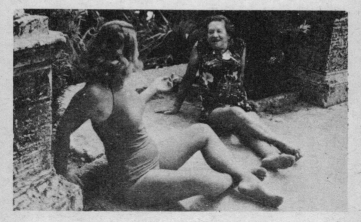

You can also do the exercise sitting in a chair. If you have difficulty falling asleep, you can do the exercise in bed.

WHAT THE EXERCISE DOES FOR YOU:

It increases the oxygen supply to your brain and improves your thinking ability.

It brings increased oxygen to all the cells of your body.

It calms your nerves.

It improves your coordination.

It encourages restful sleep.

It strengthens your upper chest muscles and your diaphragm.

It enables you to use your lungs to their fullest capacity.

It relaxes you to the point where your sleep will be restful.

CHAPTER II

CLEANSING BREATH

STANDING TWIST

SQUAT

ROCK-A-BYE-BABY

SPREAD LEG STRETCH

CURL

SLOW NECK ROLL

CLEANSING BREATH

This is a well-thought-out exercise. The movement of your abdominal muscles forces the air out of your lungs, shaking loose many impurities lodged in them. The rapid in-and-out movement of air stimulates the circulation to your lungs and hastens the oxygen flow through your entire system.

DO THE EXERCISE TWICE.

1. Sit comfortably with your legs crossed and your hands on your knees.*

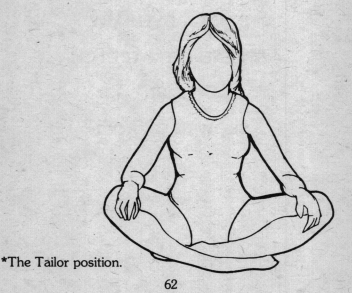

*The Tailor position.

2. Inhale slowly through your nose as you push your abdomen out.

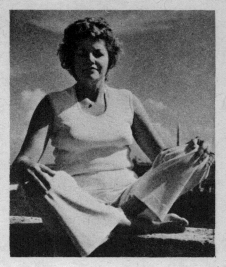

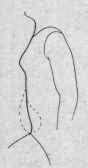

3. Pull your abdomen in quickly and exhale through your nose.

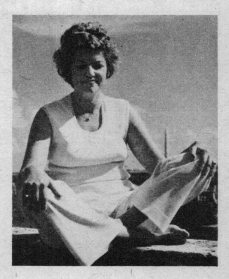

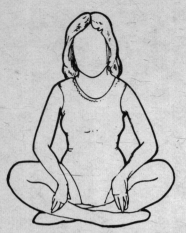

4. Relax.

DO FIVE CLEANSING BREATHS.

HOW TO PRACTICE THE EXERCISE:
It is important that you establish a rhythm when you do this exercise. Inhale to the count of three and exhale to the count of one. When you feel that you are proficient in doing the exercise, inhale to the count of one and exhale to the count of one. Do not do this exercise before you go to bed. It will stimulate you and keep you from falling asleep.

WHAT THE EXERCISE DOES FOR YOU:
It opens your sinus passages.

It brings increased amounts of oxygen into your body.

It makes your lungs resilient.

It warms your body.

It wakes you up.

STANDING TWIST

There are very few exercises that stretch the spine in a spiral motion. Indeed, most of the yoga postures move the spine concavely or convexly. This exercise is especially important because it excercises a rarely used body movement.

DO THE EXERCISE TWICE.

1. Stand with your feet five or six inches apart. Raise your arms forward at shoulder level.

2. Twist your upper body to your left, moving your head and arms around slowly. Hold for 5 seconds.

3. Return your upper body to the forward position, again moving your head and arms slowly.

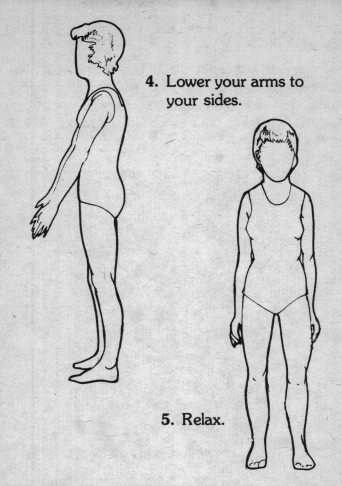

4. Lower your arms to your sides.

5. Relax.

REPEAT THE MOVEMENTS IN THE OPPO-
SITE DIRECTION. YOU HAVE COMPLETED
THE EXERCISE.

HOW TO PRACTICE THE EXERCISE:
Try not to move your hips when you twist your

arms and trunk to the side. Do not move your feet. Keep them in place.

When you have perfected this stance—it may take many weeks—do the movement on your toes: Go up on your toes as you raise your arms (figure 1). Bring your heels to the floor as you lower your arms (figure 4).

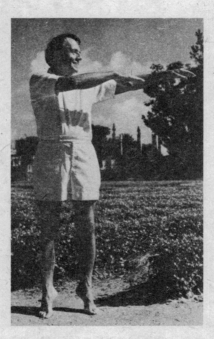

WHAT THE EXERCISE DOES FOR YOU:
It keeps your neck limber.

It strengthens your shoulder muscles.

It relieves stiffness in the muscles of your back and promotes the flexibility of your spine.

It helps to firm your waistline.

When you perform it on your toes, it improves your balance and increases the flexibility of your feet. At the same time, it strengthens your toes, ankles, and arches, and firms the calves of your legs.

SQUAT

Consistent practice of the Squat position encourages regularity in your daily biological function.

DO THE EXERCISE TWICE.

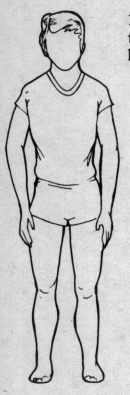

1. Stand with your feet about twelve inches apart, and your hands at your sides.

2. Bend your knees and slowly lower your body into a squatting position. Keep your heels on the floor.

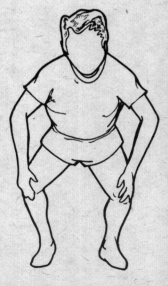

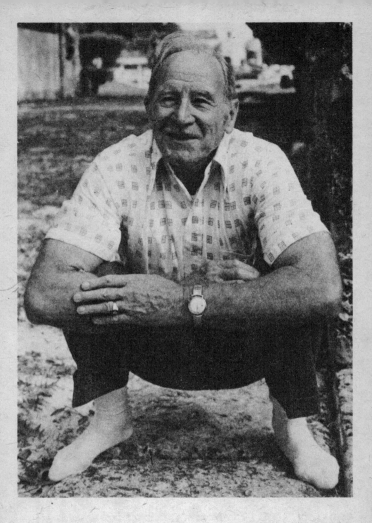

3. Squat. Fold your arms and rest your elbows against your knees. Hold for 10 seconds.

4. Straighten up slowly.

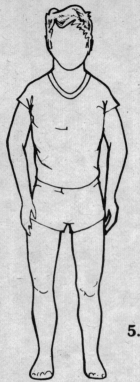

5. Relax.

HOW TO PRACTICE THE EXERCISE:
You will probably be unable to keep your heels on the floor at first. Keep practicing until you can. If you need support, hold on to a chair or a table. Try to practice regularly.

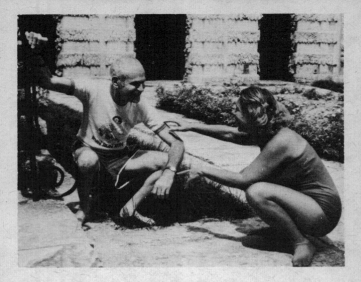

WHAT THE EXERCISE DOES FOR YOU:

It improves the mobility of your hips.

It stretches your legs.

It improves the flexibility of your knees.

It strengthens your ankles.

It helps your equilibrium.

It helps you overcome constipation difficulties.

ROCK-A-BYE-BABY

This is a unique way to exercise your hip joints. The rocking motion you perform is designed to keep your hips flexible. There are few exercises that so well manipulate the area of your hips. The raised position in which you hold each leg is easy to maintain. If you sing the song "Rock-a-bye-Baby" as you rock each leg back and forth with your arms, you will establish the correct rhythm for the exercise.

DO THE EXERCISE TWICE.

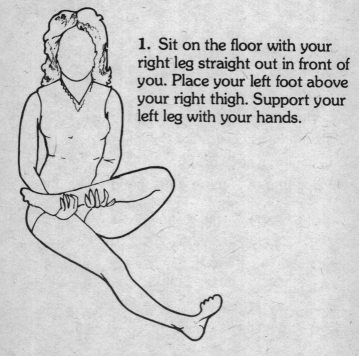

1. Sit on the floor with your right leg straight out in front of you. Place your left foot above your right thigh. Support your left leg with your hands.

2. Bring your foot to your chest and raise it toward your chin, as high as you can. Rock your leg from side to side 5 times.

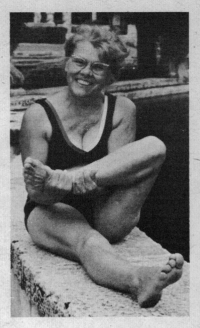

3. Straighten your left leg.

4. Relax.

REPEAT THE STEPS FOR THE OTHER SIDE.
YOU HAVE COMPLETED THE EXERCISE.

HOW TO PRACTICE THE EXERCISE:
Rock each leg from side to side with as wide a movement as you can.

WHAT THE EXERCISE DOES FOR YOU:
It strengthens the muscles in your arms, chest, and upper back.

It maintains the flexibility of your hips.

It promotes the flexibility of your knees and ankles.

It stretches your legs.

It strengthens your lower back.

SPREAD LEG STRETCH

The Spread Leg Stretch brings considerable flexibility to your spine and makes the insides of your legs elastic. By practicing the Spread Leg Stretch regularly, you will acquire a welcome new freedom of movement in an "out-of-the-way" area of your body, where the muscles and tendons are seldom put to use.

DO THE EXERCISE TWICE.

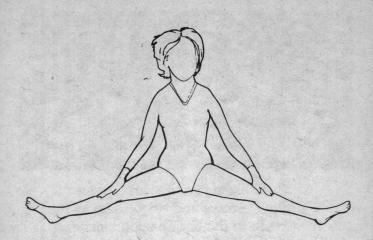

1. Sit on the floor with your legs apart. Rest your hands on your knees.

2. Drop your chin toward your chest and slide your hands down your legs to your ankles.

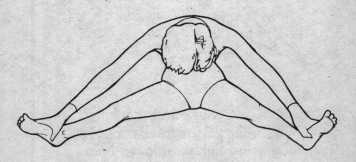

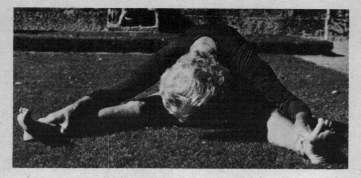

3. Clasping your ankles, bend your elbows and bring them as close to the floor as you can. Also bring your forehead as close to the floor as you can. Hold for 5 seconds.

4. Slide your hands back up your legs. Straighten up slowly, starting with your lower back.

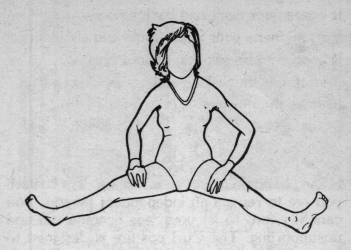

5. Sit with your hands on your thighs and relax.

HOW TO PRACTICE THE EXERCISE:
Do not be surprised if your hands fail to slide below the calves of your legs. It may take you many months before the ligaments on the insides of your thighs stretch sufficiently to give you the flexibility you need. Do not force the exercise. Pull yourself down carefully and slowly. If necessary, keep your knees bent at first.

WHAT THE EXERCISE DOES FOR YOU:
It increases the flow of blood to your head.

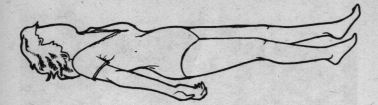

4. Lie down.

5. Relax.

HOW TO PRACTICE THE EXERCISE:
You can do this exercise in bed the first thing upon arising or in the evening before you go to sleep.

Do not struggle to accomplish the posture. Let the muscles and ligaments of your back and legs limber up gradually. Grip your hands tightly over your knees when you raise your head from the floor. The more tightly you grip your knees the higher you will be able to raise your shoulders.

WHAT THE EXERCISE DOES FOR YOU:
It keeps your back and neck flexible.

It stretches your spinal column.

It massages your digestive organs and helps them to function.

It tightens your abdominal muscles.

It keeps your knee and hip joints limber.

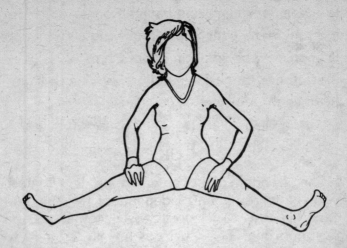

5. Sit with your hands on your thighs and relax.

HOW TO PRACTICE THE EXERCISE:
Do not be surprised if your hands fail to slide below the calves of your legs. It may take you many months before the ligaments on the insides of your thighs stretch sufficiently to give you the flexibility you need. Do not force the exercise. Pull yourself down carefully and slowly. If necessary, keep your knees bent at first.

WHAT THE EXERCISE DOES FOR YOU:
It increases the flow of blood to your head.

It keeps your neck and back limber.

It strengthens your upper arms and shoulders.

It improves the rotation of your hips.

It stretches the insides and backs of your legs.

It tones the muscles of your legs.

CURL

Having freedom of movement in your legs is vital if you are to remain an independent person. You cannot afford to let your legs become stiff and unsupporting. The Curl posture is designed to keep your legs in good working condition. You will want to do this exercise fairly regularly to be sure you give your legs the treatment they deserve.

DO THE EXERCISE TWICE.

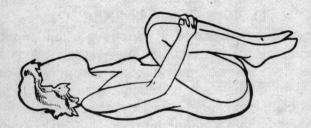

1. Lie down. Bend your knees and put your hands around your knees. Pull your knees as close to your chest as you can.

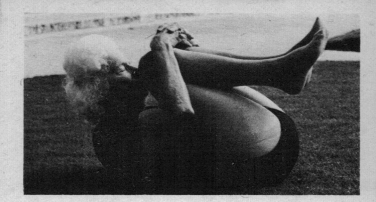

2. Raise your head and shoulders from the floor, and bring your chin to your knees. Hold for 5 seconds.

3. Release the grip on your knees, and lower your back and your head to the floor.

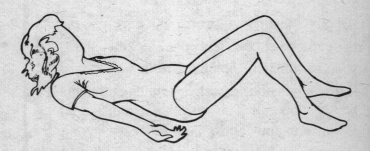

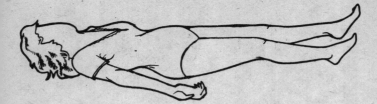

4. Lie down.

5. Relax.

HOW TO PRACTICE THE EXERCISE:

You can do this exercise in bed the first thing upon arising or in the evening before you go to sleep.

Do not struggle to accomplish the posture. Let the muscles and ligaments of your back and legs limber up gradually. Grip your hands tightly over your knees when you raise your head from the floor. The more tightly you grip your knees the higher you will be able to raise your shoulders.

WHAT THE EXERCISE DOES FOR YOU:

It keeps your back and neck flexible.

It stretches your spinal column.

It massages your digestive organs and helps them to function.

It tightens your abdominal muscles.

It keeps your knee and hip joints limber.

SLOW NECK ROLL

Many people roll their heads instinctively when their neck muscles feel tight, but their movements are usually too rapid and casual for beneficial results. The Slow Neck Roll, which calls for a gentle swivel of the neck while the face is held in repose, quickly and efficiently relieves the discomfort of tension buildup.

DO THE EXERCISE TWICE.

1. Sit comfortably with your hands on your knees and your knees crossed.* Keep your back straight.

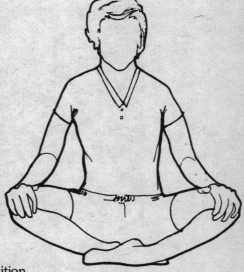

*The Tailor position.

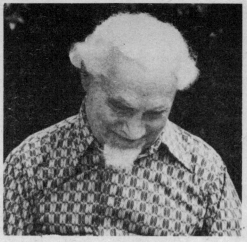

2. In a continuous rolling movement, lower your chin to your chest.

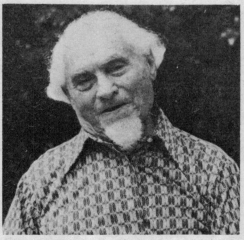

3. Continue to roll your head slowly to your right shoulder.

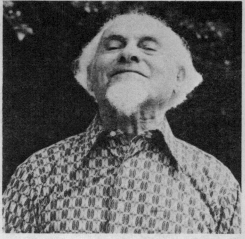

4. Continue rolling your head back.

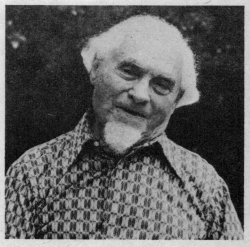

5. Continue to roll your head to your left shoulder.

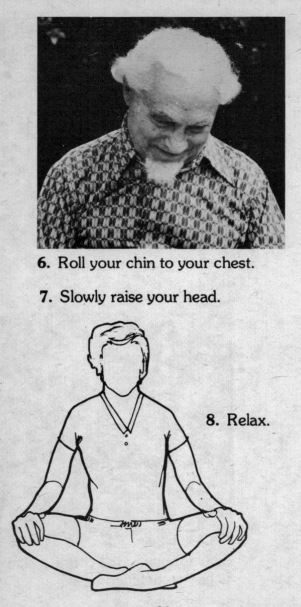

6. Roll your chin to your chest.

7. Slowly raise your head.

8. Relax.

**REPEAT IN THE OPPOSITE DIRECTION.
YOU HAVE COMPLETED THE EXERCISE.**

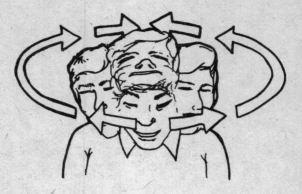

WHAT THE EXERCISE DOES FOR YOU:

It keeps your neck and shoulders supple.

It calms your nerves and quiets your mind.

It contributes to restful sleep.

HOW TO PRACTICE THE EXERCISE:

Try to sit erectly. Do not slump. Keep your mouth lax and your eyes either partially or completely closed throughout the exercise. Take approximately 15 to 20 seconds to roll your head once around. Make as wide a circle as possible. Breathe in a relaxed manner. Concentrate on the free feeling you get in your neck as you roll your head.

CHAPTER III

ARM AND LEG

SLOW HIP ROLL

TWIST IN THE CHAIR

EYE MOVEMENTS

PRELIMINARY BACK AND LEG STRETCH

KNEE AND THIGH

FOUR-WAY NECK STRETCH

COBRA

ARM AND LEG

This exercise is especially good for you if you have poor posture. It relieves backache and accumulated tension in back muscles. Practiced for as little as half a minute regularly, it can prevent hours of discomfort.

DO THE EXERCISE TWICE.

1. Stand comfortably with your feet about five or six inches apart. Raise your left arm to the side of your head.

2. Bend your right leg back and grasp your foot with your right hand.

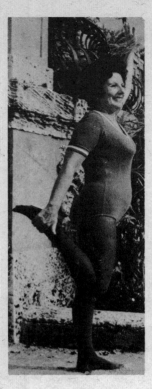

3. Pull your right leg up and try to touch your heel to your buttocks. Hold for 5 seconds.

4. Release your leg. Slowly lower your arm and leg simultaneously.

5. Relax.

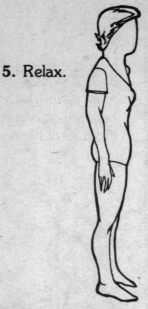

REPEAT THE STEPS ON THE OPPOSITE SIDE. YOU HAVE COMPLETED THE EXERCISE.

HOW TO PRACTICE THE EXERCISE:

Focus your eyes on a stationary object when you hold your position. If you cannot maintain your balance, stand close to the wall and lean your arm against it for support.

After a few weeks of practice, try to pull the leg you are holding as far back as you can so that your lower spine gets more of a stretch. Also, drop your head and your arm back slightly so that your upper spine gets a stretch. Try to balance yourself without the wall.

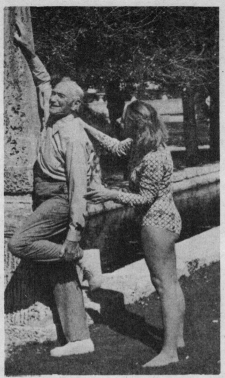

WHAT THE EXERCISE DOES FOR YOU:
It develops your sense of balance.

It improves your posture and gives you added poise in walking.

It firms the backs of your upper arms.

It stretches your lower back.

It stretches and firms your thighs and keeps your legs limber.

It gives your knee joints elasticity.

It improves your ability to concentrate.

SLOW HIP ROLL

This exercise has a gentle, controlled, rolling movement. You will enjoy doing it. It will give your hips an easy, youthful swing when you walk.

DO THE EXERCISE TWICE.

1. Stand with your hands on your hips and your feet about ten to twelve inches apart.

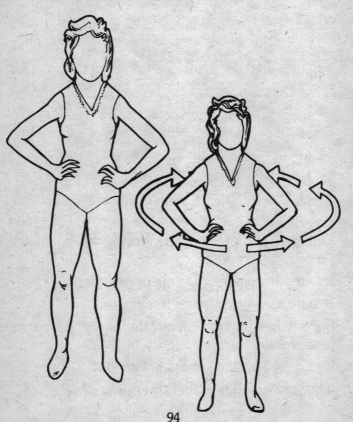

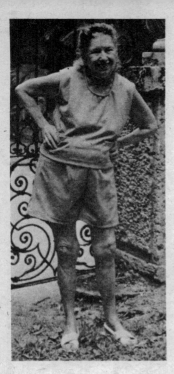

2. Roll your hips around to your right.

3. Continue the rolling motion, and rotate your hips to the rear.

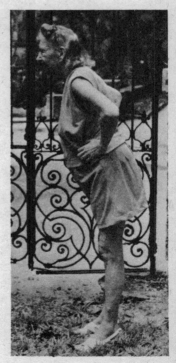

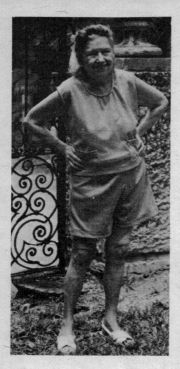

4. Go on with the rolling motion, and move your hips to your left.

5. Complete the movement by rolling your hips forward.

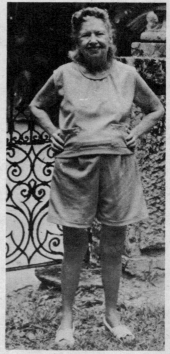

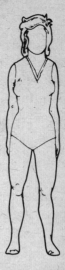

6. Straighten up. Lower your hands to your sides. Relax.

REPEAT THE STEPS FOR THE OTHER SIDE. YOU HAVE COMPLETED THE EXERCISE.

HOW TO PRACTICE THE EXERCISE:
Roll your hips around slowly and rhythmically without pausing. Be sure that your feet are a comfortable distance apart so that you have proper balance while doing the exercise.

WHAT THE EXERCISE DOES FOR YOU:
It keeps your spine flexible.

It gives your hip joints freedom of movement, allowing for greater ease in walking.

It stretches your legs and hips and helps you to stand erectly.

It promotes general elasticity in your hips and waist.

TWIST IN THE CHAIR

This exercise, done sitting in a chair, is a modified version of the Twist done sitting on the floor. With little effort, you can put it to use whenever you wish. It will help your spine stay flexible.

DO THE EXERCISE TWICE.

1. Sit in a chair. Cross your left knee over your right knee.

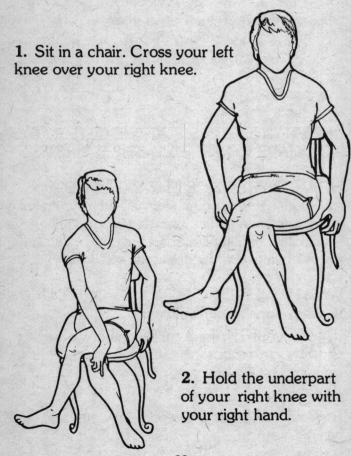

2. Hold the underpart of your right knee with your right hand.

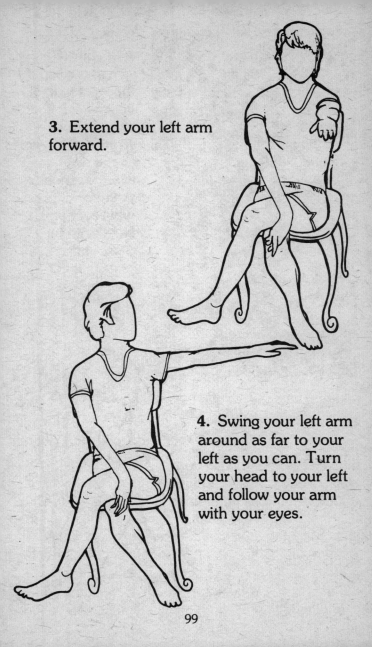

3. Extend your left arm forward.

4. Swing your left arm around as far to your left as you can. Turn your head to your left and follow your arm with your eyes.

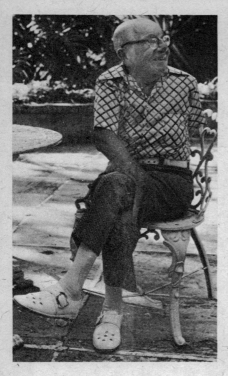

5. Reach over with your left arm and clasp the right side of your waist. If you cannot stretch your arm all the way around, anchor your hand wherever you can. Hold for 5 seconds.

6. Release the grip on your waist. Face forward. Lower your left hand to your side.

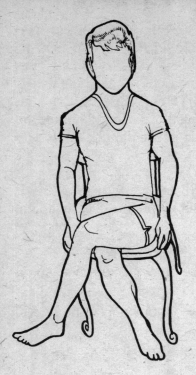

7. Release the grip on your knee. Lower your hand to your side.

8. Uncross your legs. Put your hands on your knees. Relax.

REPEAT THE STEPS FOR THE OPPOSITE SIDE. YOU HAVE COMPLETED THE EXERCISE.

HOW TO PRACTICE THE EXERCISE:

Twist only from the waist. Your head should be turned as far as possible in the direction in which you are twisting.

WHAT THE EXERCISE DOES FOR YOU:

It stimulates the nerves throughout your spinal column.

It tones the vertical muscles of your torso.

It stretches your entire upper back in a spiral manner.

It improves the mobility of your neck, shoulders, and elbows.

It firms your waist.

EYE MOVEMENTS

Your eyes are a rarely exercised part of your body. Although you use them constantly during your waking hours, you do not give them the exercise they need because you do not operate them independently of your head movements. To give them proper stimulation, you must move them around in their sockets. Here is a series of movements designed to strengthen them.

Sit comfortably with your legs crossed.* Pretend that a large clock is directly in front of you. Keep your eyes open.

FIRST EYE MOVEMENT:

DO THE EXERCISE THREE TIMES.

You are going to move your eyes clockwise, then counterclockwise, pausing *momentarily* at each number.

Look up at 12 o'clock. Move your eyes from 12 to 1. Continue moving them clockwise from number to number until you come back to 12 o'clock. Close your eyes tightly. Open your eyes.

REPEAT THE PROCEDURE COUNTER-CLOCKWISE. YOU HAVE COMPLETED THE EXERCISE.

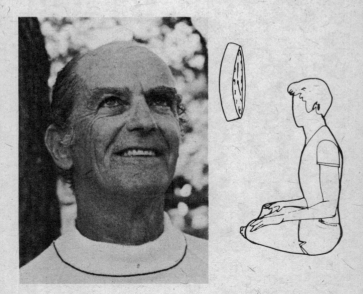

SECOND EYE MOVEMENT:

DO THE EXERCISE THREE TIMES.

Now you are going to move your eyes diagonally.

Look at 2 o'clock. Shift your gaze diagonally across to 7 o'clock.

Look at 11 o'clock. Shift your gaze diagonally across to 5 o'clock.

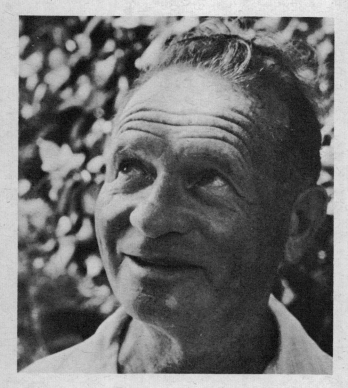

YOU HAVE COMPLETED THE EXERCISE.

THIRD EYE MOVEMENT:

DO THE EXERCISE THREE TIMES.

You are going to *roll* your eyes clockwise and then counterclockwise.

Look up at 12 o'clock. Roll your eyes to 1 o'clock. Continue rolling them clockwise. Come back to 12 o'clock. Close your eyes tightly. Open your eyes.

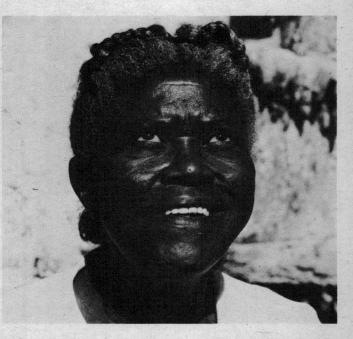

REPEAT THE POSTURE COUNTERCLOCK-WISE. YOU HAVE COMPLETED THE EXER-CISE.

FOURTH EYE MOVEMENT:

DO THE EXERCISE THREE TIMES.

You are going to move your eyes horizontally.

Look at 3 o'clock. Pause briefly. Shift your gaze to 9 o'clock. Pause briefly.

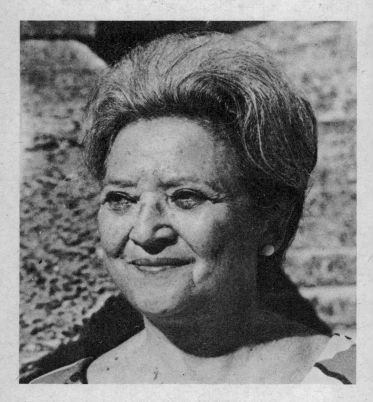

YOU HAVE COMPLETED THE EXERCISE.

FIFTH EYE MOVEMENT:

DO THE EXERCISE THREE TIMES.

You are now going to focus your eyes near and far.

Raise your hand and place it about twelve inches from your face. Focus your eyes on your hand. Hold them there for 5 seconds.

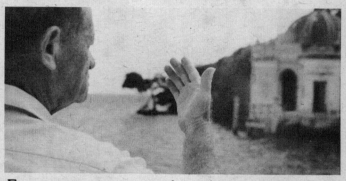

Focus your eyes on an object far away from you— in the distance. Hold your gaze there for 5 seconds.

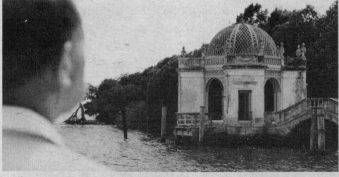

YOU HAVE COMPLETED THE EXERCISE.

SIXTH EYE MOVEMENT:

DO THE EXERCISE ONCE.

Rub your hands together for about five seconds, until they feel warm. You are going to rest your hands over your eyes.

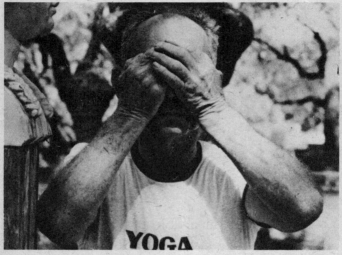

Place your hands over your eyes so that the fingers of one hand cross over the fingers of your other hand. Be sure that you are not pressing on your eyeballs. Keep your eyes closed. Count 10 seconds. Open your eyes. Lower your hands to your sides. Relax.

YOU HAVE COMPLETED THE EXERCISE.

HOW TO DO THE EXERCISE:
Do not wear glasses when you perform the eye movements.

WHAT THE EXERCISE DOES FOR YOU:

It relaxes your eyes when they are tired.

It keeps your eye muscles strong, preventing your eyes from receding in their sockets.

It promotes the flexibility of the lenses of your eyes.

It decreases the loss of visual acuity due to cellular aging.

PRELIMINARY BACK AND LEG STRETCH

The Preliminary Back and Leg Stretch is a basic yoga posture. You can perform it at any time. When you do it in the morning, in bed, it helps you start the day free from stiffness in your back.

DO THE EXERCISE TWICE.

1. Sit on the floor with your legs together and your hands on your knees. Try to keep your back straight and your knees flat.

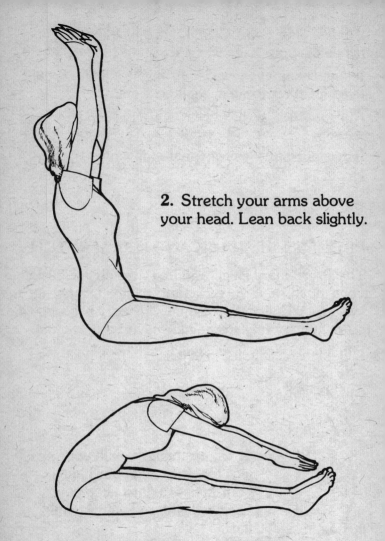

2. Stretch your arms above your head. Lean back slightly.

3. Stretch forward, lowering your chin toward your chest, and extending your arms in front of you.

4. Grasp your ankles (your feet, if you can reach them). Keep your head lowered and your legs together.

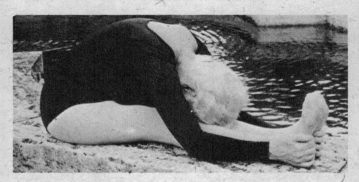

5. Bend your elbows and place them as close to the floor as you can. Draw your forehead down to your legs. Hold for 5 seconds.

6. Relax the grip on your ankles, and slide your hands up to your thighs. Start to straighten your back, keeping your head down.

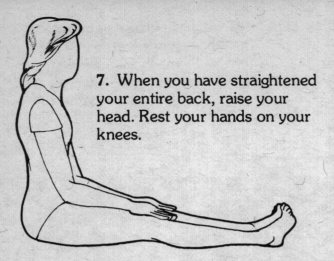

7. When you have straightened your entire back, raise your head. Rest your hands on your knees.

8. Relax.

HOW TO PRACTICE THE EXERCISE:

Do not stretch beyond your comfortable limit. Few people can reach their ankles on the first try. If your hands reach only halfway down your legs, stop at that point. It may take many weeks or even months before you achieve the flexibility that will permit your hands to reach your ankles. It may also take many months for your forehead to touch your legs, and if your legs are stiff, it may take weeks before you can do the exercise with your legs straight. As with all forward stretches, the way to come out of the position is to uncurl your body slowly, starting with your lower back and moving gradually upward.

WHAT THE EXERCISE DOES FOR YOU:

It improves the circulation of blood to your face.

It stretches your vertebrae from your neck to the base of your spine, promoting flexibility.

It tones the muscles of your arms and shoulders.

It stretches the muscles and tendons in the backs of your legs.

KNEE AND THIGH

Walking is a therapeutic activity for both your body and your mind. If you want to get full pleasure and benefit out of your daily walks, you must keep your legs in the best possible condition. The Knee and Thigh stretch can help you keep your legs flexible and can increase your walking endurance.

DO THE EXERCISE TWICE.

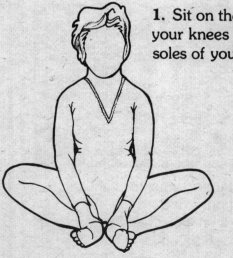

1. Sit on the floor. Bend your knees and draw the soles of your feet together.

2. Clasp your hands around your toes and pull your feet in toward your body.

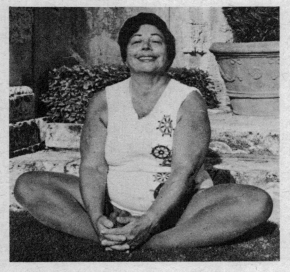

3. Pull up on your toes and lower your knees to the floor. Try to keep your back straight. Hold for 5 seconds.

114

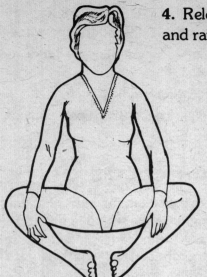

4. Release your feet, and raise your knees.

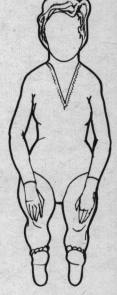

5. Straighten your legs. Place your hands on your knees. Relax.

HOW TO PRACTICE THE EXERCISE:

It takes months to perfect this posture because the inside of your legs and thighs becomes stiff with the passing years. Do not force the stretch. Pulling up on your toes helps you lower your knees to the floor. Persevere. This stretch is highly beneficial for your legs.

WHAT THE EXERCISE DOES FOR YOU:

It firms the muscles in your shoulders and arms.

It stretches the muscles, ligaments, and tendons of your legs.

It improves the circulation in your legs.

It stretches your ankles, knees, and hips and gives them flexibility.

FOUR-WAY NECK STRETCH

You can literally do this exercise anywhere. It can be carried out whether you are sitting or standing, and it takes less than a minute to perform. The slow manipulation of your neck soothes your nervous system and dissipates tension. In less than sixty seconds, you can begin to relax.

DO THE EXERCISE TWICE.

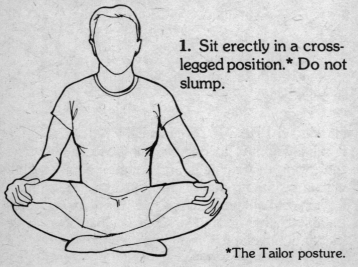

1. Sit erectly in a cross-legged position.* Do not slump.

*The Tailor posture.

116

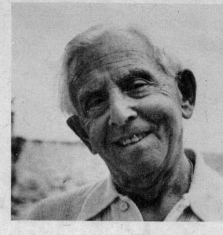

2. Incline your head to your right. Hold for 5 seconds.

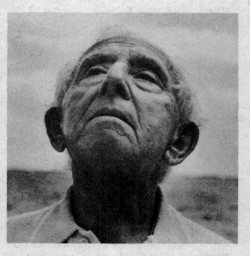

3. Drop your head back. Hold for 5 seconds.

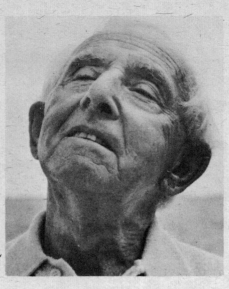

4. Incline your head to your left. Hold for 5 seconds.

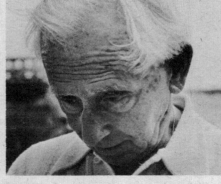

5. Drop your head forward. Relax your mouth. Hold for 5 seconds.

6. Raise your head. Relax.

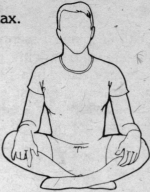

REPEAT THE EXERCISE IN THE OPPOSITE DIRECTION. YOU HAVE COMPLETED THE EXERCISE.

HOW TO PRACTICE THE EXERCISE:
If you prefer, you may close your eyes while you are sitting. The straighter you keep your back, the more stretch you will get in your neck. Do not move your shoulders. When you stretch your head to your side, try to keep your ear directly above your shoulder. The exercise will be less relaxing if you perform it in a standing position. Do it in a standing position only when the circumstances make it more convenient that way.

WHAT THE EXERCISE DOES FOR YOU:
It relieves tension in your neck and shoulders.

It gives your neck freedom of movement.

It calms your nerves.

It improves your ability to concentrate.

It helps you sleep.

119

COBRA

A healthy spine is essential to your well-being. The snake-like movements of the Cobra keep your spine flexible and healthy. They manipulate every vertebra in your spinal column slowly and methodically, and they nourish your entire nervous system.

DO THE EXERCISE TWICE.

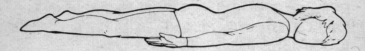

1. Lie on your abdomen. Rest your cheek on the floor. Place your hands at your sides, palms up.

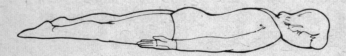

2. Lay your forehead on the floor.

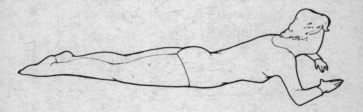

3. Raise your head and chest from the floor.

4. Bend your elbows and place your hands, palms down, on the floor, about eight inches in front of your face. Keep your hands about three inches from each other.

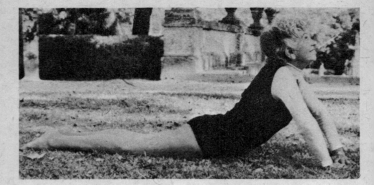

5. Push your hands down against the floor and try to straighten your arms. Drop your head back and keep your chin raised high. Hold for 5 seconds.

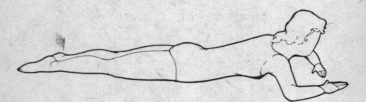

6. Bend your elbows and lower your chest to the floor slowly.

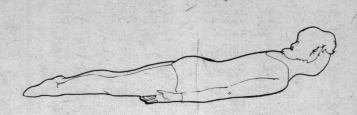

7. Place your arms at your sides and lower your shoulders.

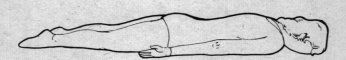

8. Put your forehead on the floor.

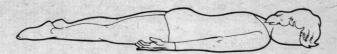

9. Place your cheek on the floor.

10. Relax.

HOW TO PRACTICE THE EXERCISE:

The placement of your hands is especially important. It determines how much your back will stretch. The closer your hands are to your face, the more stretch your back will get. If your spine is particularly stiff, put your hands on the floor about twelve inches ahead of your face. As your spine becomes more limber, move your arms closer to your face. Try not to raise your abdomen from the floor when you hold the position.

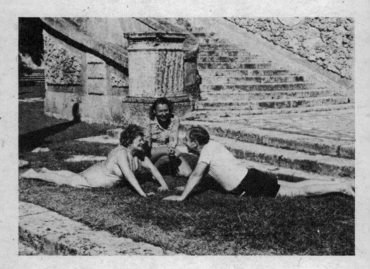

When you feel comfortable with this technique, you can add a supplementary benefit for your neck. Rotate your head once to your right and once to your left as you hold the position.

WHAT THE EXERCISE DOES FOR YOU:

It relaxes your neck.

It develops strength in your upper back.

It improves the flexibility of your spine.

It makes your arms strong.

It promotes flexibility in your fingers and wrists.

It develops your chest muscles.

It expands your rib cage.

It massages your visceral organs.

It strengthens your lower back and keeps it flexible.

It firms your hips, thighs, and buttocks.

CHAPTER IV

TREE

TWIST ON THE FLOOR

BACKWARD BEND

LEG STRETCHES

LION

SHOULDER STRETCH

LOCUST

NINETY-SECOND RELAXER

TREE

A tree is lovely to look at. It stands tall, straight, and strong. This exercise helps you to stand tall, straight, and strong. It helps you to achieve balance and poise. It is simple to do. It should be a regular part of your yoga routine.

DO THE EXERCISE TWICE.

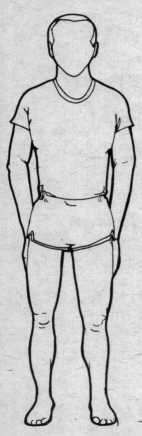

1. Stand with your feet a comfortable distance apart, your hands at your sides.

2. Bend your left leg. Grasp your leg near the ankle, and place the sole of your foot against your inner right thigh as high as possible.

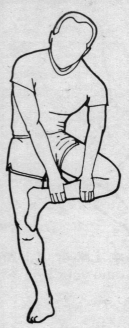

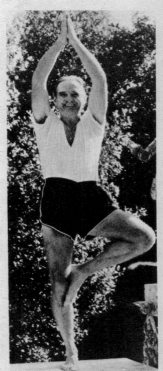

3. Slowly raise your arms above your head. Put the palms of your hands together. Balance yourself. Hold for 5 seconds.

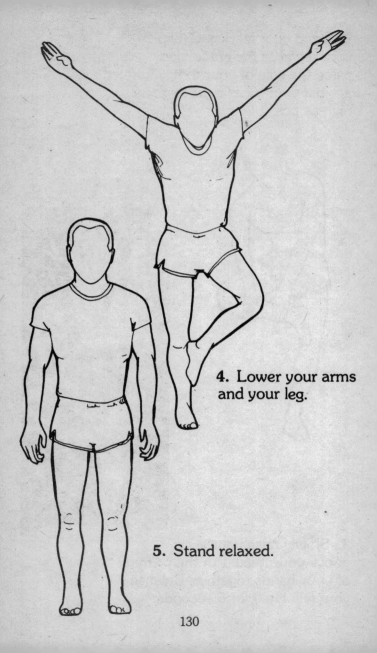

4. Lower your arms and your leg.

5. Stand relaxed.

REPEAT FOR THE OPPOSITE SIDE. YOU HAVE COMPLETED THE EXERCISE.

HOW TO PRACTICE THE EXERCISE:

Many people—young and old—have difficulty balancing. If you have difficulty balancing yourself, use a wall for support. Place your heel two or three inches away from the wall and lean your back against the wall. When you feel that you can steady yourself, move your body away from the wall.

Do not force the position of your foot against your thigh. The more flexible your leg gets, the higher you will be able to rest your foot on the inside of your thigh.

WHAT THE EXERCISE DOES FOR YOU:

It improves your posture and your balance.

It helps you to walk gracefully.

It stretches your torso vertically.

It keeps your hip joints and your knees flexible.

It helps you to concentrate.

TWIST ON THE FLOOR

The Twist on the Floor is one of the rare exercises that provide you with a spiral stretch. It is quite advanced. In doing the Twist, you improve the circulation to your spine, which aids all of your organs in their functions, and gives you a general feeling of well-being. The Twist is an excellent technique for keeping your body in good form.

DO THE EXERCISE TWICE.

1. Sit on the floor. Place your right foot against the inside of your upper left thigh.

2. Bend your left leg, and place your hands around your ankle. Gently pull your left heel to your thigh.

3. Lift your left leg over your right knee. Rest your foot flat on the floor.

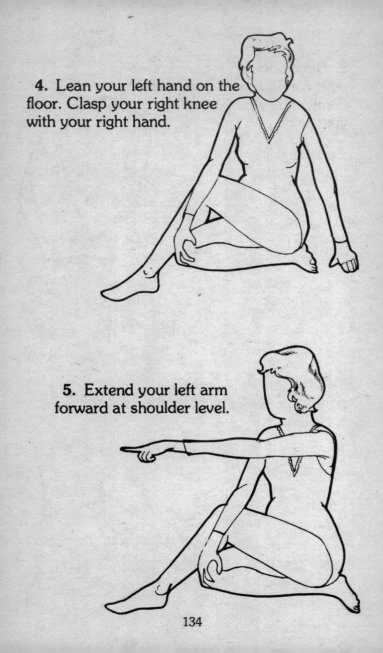

4. Lean your left hand on the floor. Clasp your right knee with your right hand.

5. Extend your left arm forward at shoulder level.

6. Swing your arm around to your left as far as it will go. Turn your head to your left and follow your arm with your eyes.

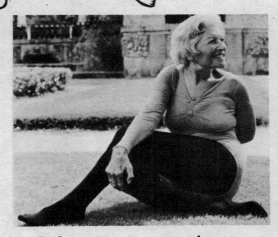

7. Lower your arm and try to grasp the right side of your waist. If you cannot stretch your arm all the way around, anchor your hand wherever you can. Hold for 5 seconds.

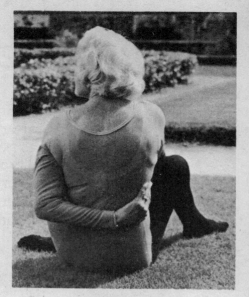

8. Figure 8 is the Twist as seen from the rear.

9. Lean your left hand on the floor, and face forward.

10. Clasp your left ankle with both hands.

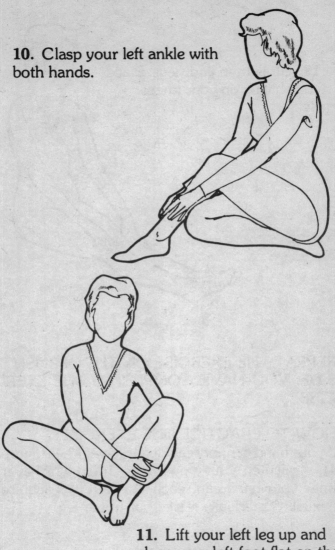

11. Lift your left leg up and place your left foot flat on the floor beside your right foot.

12. Straighten your legs. Place your hands on your knees. Relax.

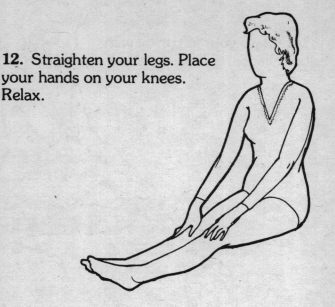

REPEAT THE EXERCISE ON THE OPPOSITE SIDE. YOU HAVE COMPLETED THE EXERCISE.

HOW TO PRACTICE THE EXERCISE:
If your hand cannot reach your lower knee (figure 4), straighten your upper leg. Grasp whichever knee your hand can reach. As your legs acquire flexibility, gradually raise your upper leg.

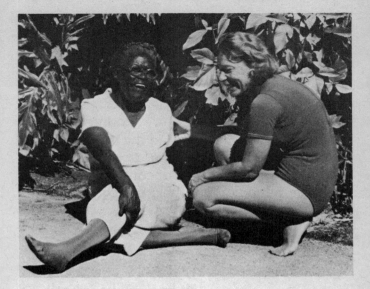

WHAT THE EXERCISE DOES FOR YOU:

It relieves tension in your neck, shoulders, and back.

It promotes the flexibility of your neck, shoulders, waist, hips, and legs.

It firms your waist.

It gives your spine a spiral stretch.

It exercises your arms, keeping your elbows and wrists limber.

BACKWARD BEND

If you learn to sit on your feet as the Japanese do, you will probably find that you have stronger, healthier feet. When you sit on them, you put gentle pressure on your feet and keep them flexible. The sitting posture counteracts the effects of confining shoes and the lack of suitable exercise for this neglected part of your body. You should also keep your feet unconfined and should flex them periodically to help strengthen them.

DO THE EXERCISE TWICE.

1. Kneel on the floor, and sit back on your heels. Place your hands on the floor behind you. Do not spread your hands too far apart. They should approximate the width of your body and be about ten to twelve inches from your feet.

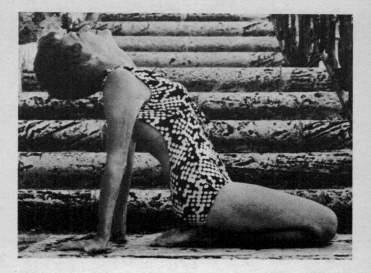

2. Drop your head back. Relax your mouth. Push your chest up. Do not raise yourself off your feet. Hold for 5 seconds.

3. Raise your head. Move your hands toward your feet.

141

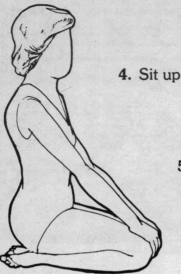

4. Sit up straight.

5. Relax.

HOW TO PRACTICE THE EXERCISE:

If at first you cannot sit all the way back on your heels, place your hands on the floor near your knees and sit back as far as you can. Keep practicing until you are able to sit on your heels.

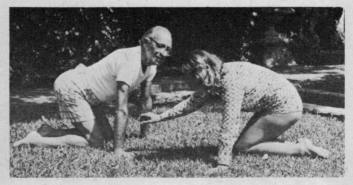

Even when you achieve a comfortable sitting position, you may not be able to reach the floor with your hands. Find a high object on which to rest your hands until your back is flexible enough for your hands to reach the floor.

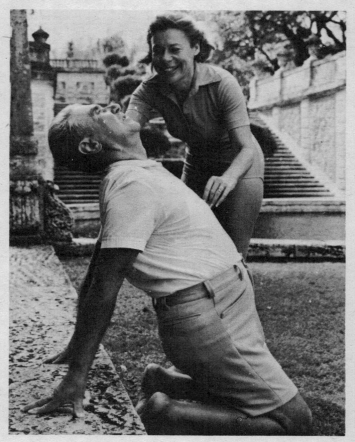

After a while, you may be able to lean on a lower object. Your goal, of course, is to rest your palms on the floor.

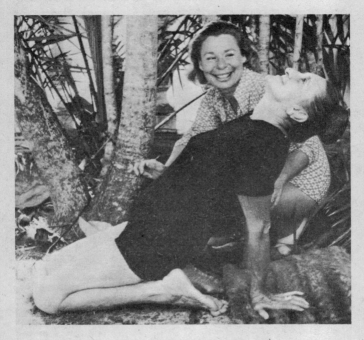

Constant repetition of this posture will gradually stretch the tight areas of your feet and your legs. In time, you will be able to sit completely back on your feet. Once you feel fairly comfortable sitting on your feet—even if you cannot complete the exercise by stretching your spine backward—try to do the exercise on your toes. Turn your toes forward and allow them to rest on the floor; that is, let the cushioned underpart of your toes touch the floor.

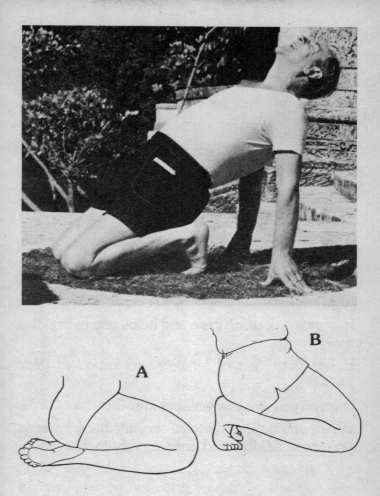

A

B

You can also practice a simple form of the exercise, alternating the position of your toes. Turn your toes backward and sit on your heels;

then turn your toes forward and sit on your heels; that is, practice with your toes pointed backward (illustration a), your insteps resting on the floor, then practice with your toes pointed forward, the cushions of your toes resting flat on the floor (illustration b).

WHAT THE EXERCISE DOES FOR YOU:

It brings increased circulation to your scalp.

It strengthens your neck and helps your neck and spine maintain their flexibility.

It improves your posture.

It firms your upper arms.

It develops the flexibility of your hands.

It stretches your chest and abdomen.

It expands your rib cage and helps you to breathe more freely.

It rids your feet of tension and improves their flexibility.

It gives you greater walking stability.

When you do the exercise on your toes, it keeps your toes flexible and improves their circulation.

LEG STRETCHES

The Leg Stretches are a combination of easy leg postures. They give your legs the kind of movement they need for good health but do not ordinarily receive. With this exercise you have the opportunity to stretch your legs in many directions, thus avoiding the stiff, cramped sensation that frequently accompanies advancing age. If you practice regularly, the movements should be of considerable help to you not only in retaining whatever elasticity you have in your legs, but in making them even more pliant.

Lie flat on your back. Legs apart. Arms relaxed.

FIRST LEG STRETCH:

DO THE EXERCISE TWICE.

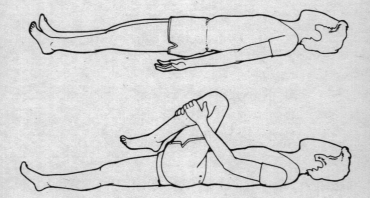

1. Bend your left leg, and grasp your left knee with both hands.

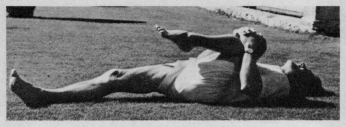

2. Pull your knee as close to your chest as you can. Rotate your ankle three times to your right and three times to your left. Hold for 5 seconds.

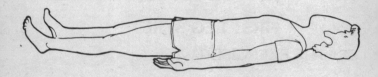

3. Straighten your leg.

4. Relax.

REPEAT FOR THE OPPOSITE SIDE. YOU HAVE COMPLETED THE EXERCISE.

SECOND LEG STRETCH:

DO THE EXERCISE TWICE.

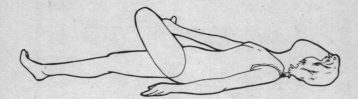

1. Bend your left leg. Place your foot on your right thigh, and grasp your foot with your right hand.

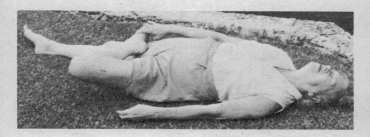

2. Lower your knee toward the floor. Hold for 5 seconds.

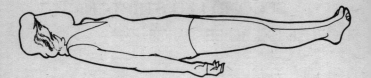

3. Straighten your leg.

4. Relax.

REPEAT ON THE OPPOSITE SIDE. YOU HAVE COMPLETED THE EXERCISE.

THIRD LEG STRETCH:

DO THE EXERCISE TWICE.

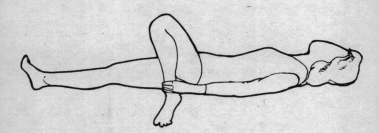

1. Raise your left knee, and grasp your ankle.

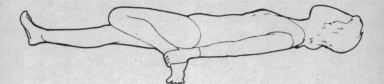

2. Moving your foot slowly, draw it as close as you can to the side of your buttocks.

3. Lower your knee to the floor. Hold for 5 seconds.

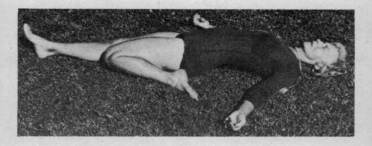

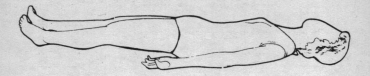

4. Straighten your leg. Relax.

REPEAT ON THE OPPOSITE SIDE. YOU HAVE COMPLETED THE EXERCISE.

HOW TO PRACTICE THE EXERCISE:
Be careful not to force your legs into any of the positions. If you exercise them gently but regularly, you will see results in a very short time.

Once you are familiar with the movements, you can vary the procedure by practicing all three stretches first on your left side and then on your right side. It takes a little less time. You may do the exercise in bed if you wish.

WHAT THE EXERCISE DOES FOR YOU:
It massages your visceral organs.

It keeps your hip joints flexible.

It rotates your pelvic structure.

It rotates your knees inward and outward.

It relieves gas.

It stretches your knees and thighs.

It alleviates stiffness in your legs.

LION

The Lion posture tones the muscles of your face and gives your cheeks a rosy glow. It also benefits your throat. Growl like a lion, if you wish, and when you finish, purr with pleasure at the results.

DO THE EXERCISE TWICE.

1. Kneel on the floor, and sit back on your heels. Rest your hands on your knees.

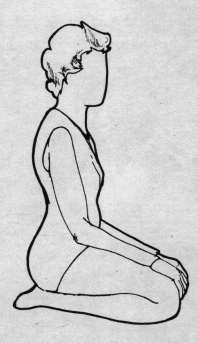

2. Open your eyes wide. Extend your tongue down toward your chin. Spread your fingers far apart. Lean slightly forward. Tense your body. Hold for 5 seconds.

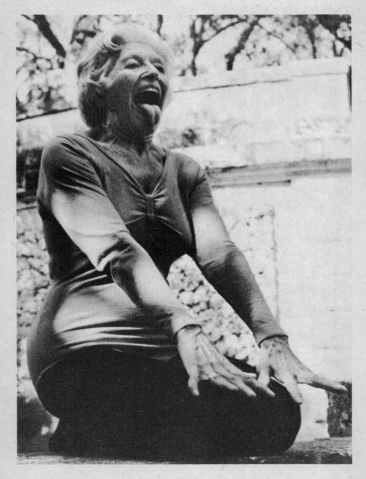

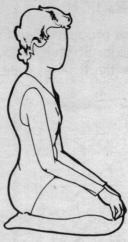

3. Relax your face and your hands. Sit back comfortably.

4. Rest.

HOW TO PRACTICE THE EXERCISE:

You may also do the Lion posture sitting in the Tailor or the Half Lotus position. Extend your tongue as far as you can. Do not force the stretch. Do not hold your breath.

WHAT THE EXERCISE DOES FOR YOU:

It improves the circulation to your face.

It opens your nasal passages.

It increases the blood supply to your throat.

It stimulates the facial muscles around your mouth.

It clears your bronchial tubes.

When you lean forward, it strengthens the muscles of your upper body.

When you perform it with the roaring sound, it improves the tonal quality of your voice.

SHOULDER STRETCH

You can help to overcome the problem of round shoulders by adding the Shoulder Stretch to your repertoire. Perform it frequently. It takes only a few seconds to do.

DO THE EXERCISE TWICE.

1. Sit comfortably with your legs crossed.* Bring your left arm around to the middle of your back with your fingers pointing up.

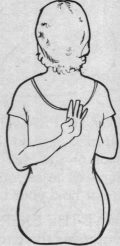

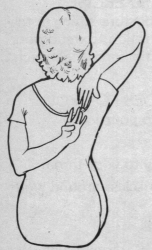

2. Raise your right arm and touch your upper back with your hand.

*The Tailor posture.

3. Inch your fingers toward each other and interlock them. Hold for 5 seconds.

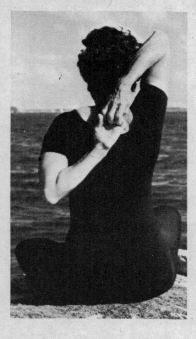

4. Lower your hands to your sides. Relax.

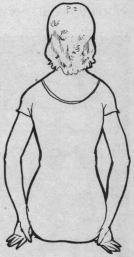

PERFORM THE MOVEMENT BEGINNING ON THE OPPOSITE SIDE. YOU HAVE COMPLETED THE EXERCISE.

HOW TO PRACTICE THE EXERCISE:

If you cannot clasp your fingers because your upper back muscles are tight, hold on to the ends of a scarf. Gradually inch your hands closer together. It may be several weeks before you can discard the scarf.

You can also do the exercise standing.

WHAT THE EXERCISE DOES FOR YOU:

It improves your posture and your coordination.

It improves your breathing ability.

It expands your rib cage.

It promotes the flexibility of your shoulders, elbows, wrists, and fingers.

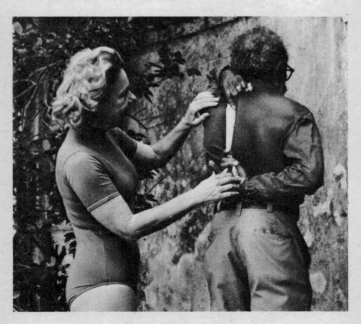

LOCUST

Many people are plagued by lower back trouble.
You can strengthen your lower back muscles and
ligaments with exercises like the Locust. The
repetitive movement of your legs as they are
raised in this posture increases the mobility of
your hip joints, and gives you greater ease in
walking. Practice the Locust regularly. Take pride
in fitness.

DO THE EXERCISE TWICE.

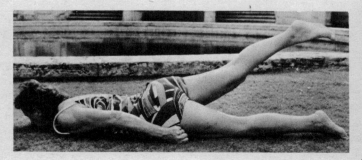

1. Lie on your abdomen. Rest
your chin on the floor. Clench
your hands into fists. Turn your
fists thumbs down on the floor.

2. Press your hands against the
floor and raise your right leg
very slowly. Hold for 3 seconds.

3. Lower your leg slowly.

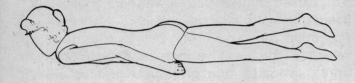

4. Rest your cheek on the floor.
Open your hands. Relax.

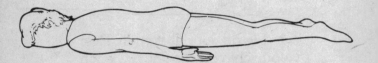

REPEAT FOR THE OPPOSITE SIDE. YOU
HAVE COMPLETED THE EXERCISE.

HOW TO PRACTICE THE EXERCISE:
Raise your leg slowly and carefully to avoid
straining your back. Try to keep your knee
straight. Pressing your fists against the floor
makes it easier for you to raise your leg. Be sure
that you do not shift your hip to the side when you
raise your leg. Keep your chin on the floor as you
raise your leg.

WHAT THE EXERCISE DOES FOR YOU:

It strengthens your upper arms and shoulders.

It tones the muscles of your back.

It stimulates your visceral organs.

It firms your abdomen, thighs, hips, and buttocks.

It exercises your pelvic area.

It improves the circulation of your legs.

NINETY-SECOND RELAXER

You can be a new person—a fully relaxed person. All you have to do is move your upper body in a specified time sequence. By the simple act of lowering your head, rounding your shoulders, and leaning forward, you can achieve a state of repose in ninety seconds.

DO THE EXERCISE ONCE.

1. Sit in a cross-legged position.* Turn your head slightly to your right. Close your eyes partially. Drop your lower jaw. Breathe slowly and evenly.

*The Tailor posture.

2. Take 30 seconds to lower your chin to your chest, round your shoulders, and lean forward.

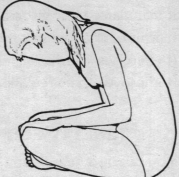

3. Leaning as far forward as you comfortably can, allow your body to go limp. Hold for 30 seconds.

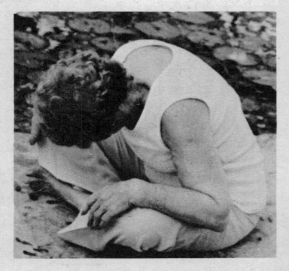

4. Take 30 seconds to come up, keeping your chin close to your chest. Straighten your lower back first, then your middle back, then your shoulders, and finally your neck.

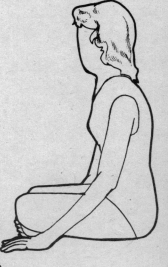

5. Sit quietly. Relax.

HOW TO PRACTICE THE EXERCISE:

The specified counts are 30 seconds each to lower your body, hold the posture, and raise your body. One performance is sufficient to achieve the benefits. Count silently. Breathe slowly and evenly throughout the exercise.

You may use the exercise for falling asleep if you vary it slightly: Hold the posture (figure 3) until you feel sleepy. Then let your upper body lower itself to your sleeping position.

WHAT THE EXERCISE DOES FOR YOU:

It dispels nervous tension.

It keeps your neck and spine limber.

It improves the circulation to your face and scalp.

It helps you sleep.

CHAPTER V

ABDOMINAL LIFT

HALF LOTUS

SIDE STRETCH

CHEST EXPANSION

BOW

ALTERNATE LEG STRETCH

SHOULDER STAND

NETI

ABDOMINAL LIFT

This exercise massages your body internally. It promotes peristaltic action in your intestines and helps to overcome constipation. There are no other techniques that duplicate its effects.

DO THE EXERCISE TWICE.

LYING POSITION:

1. Lie on your back with your hands at your sides, palms down. Bend your knees. Exhale the air slowly through your mouth.

2. Without taking in more air, pull your abdomen in and up slowly. Hold for 2 or 3 seconds. (This is one lift.)

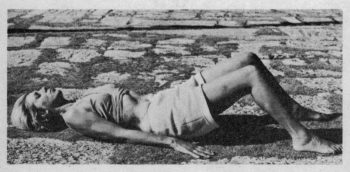

3. Push your abdomen out
quickly. Inhale.

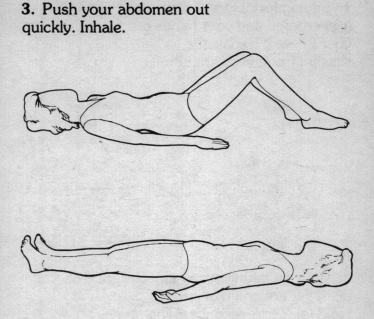

4. Straighten your legs. Turn
your palms up. Relax.

SITTING POSITION:

DO FIVE LIFTS.
WHEN YOU FEEL THAT YOU ARE READY
FOR A MORE ADVANCED VERSION OF THE
EXERCISE, DO TWO LIFTS AFTER EACH
EXHALATION.

DO THE EXERCISE TWICE.

1. Sit comfortably with your legs crossed and your hands on your knees.* Exhale the air slowly through your mouth.

*The Tailor position.

2. Without taking in any air, pull your abdomen in and up. Hold for 2 or 3 seconds. (This is one lift.)

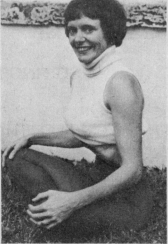

3. Push your abdomen out quickly. Inhale.

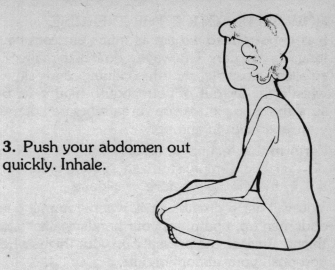

4. Relax.

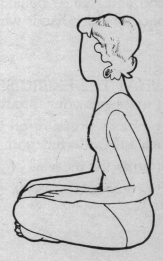

HOW TO PRACTICE THE EXERCISE:

It is important to exhale as much air from your lungs as you can. The way to do it is to make the smallest possible mouth opening and slowly whistle the air out of your mouth (figure 1). Be sure that you exhale your breath *before* you pull your abdomen in and up.

Perform this technique on an empty stomach or on a relatively empty stomach. A good time to try it is in the morning before breakfast.

You will get a greater lift if, when you pull your abdomen up, you press your hands against your thighs. Release the pressure on your thighs when you push your abdomen out.

If your legs are too stiff to assume a cross-legged position when you are doing the exercise sitting up, simply sit with your legs extended before you and your hands behind you on the floor. Lean back on your hands when you do the lifts.

WHAT THE EXERCISE DOES FOR YOU:

It massages your throat area.

It creates pressure on your visceral organs and helps them to function.

It firms the muscles of your abdomen.

It promotes regularity.

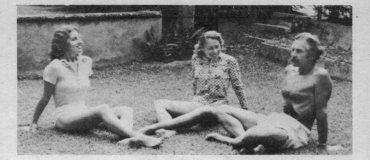

HALF LOTUS

The Half Lotus is a comfortable sitting position in yoga. It stretches your legs and increases their mobility. At the same time, it provides you with an ideal position for meditation.

DO THE EXERCISE TWICE.

1. Sit on the floor with your right leg extended in front of you, your left foot touching the inside of your right thigh.

171

2. Bend your right leg and place your right foot on your left leg between your calf and your thigh. Place your hands on your knees. Hold for 10 seconds.

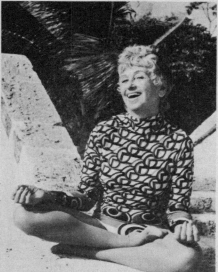

3. Straighten your right leg, then your left leg. Rest your hands on your knees.

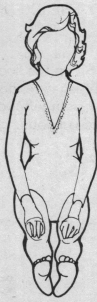

REPEAT THE STEPS FOR THE OPPOSITE SIDE. YOU HAVE COMPLETED THE EXERCISE.

HOW TO PRACTICE THE EXERCISE:
You will not be able to accomplish this technique for a while if your legs are stiff. To help your legs gain the flexibility they need, sit with your hand on your knee as your foot rests on the thigh of your outstretched leg. By applying the weight of your hand on your knee, you will gradually loosen your ankle and your hip joint.

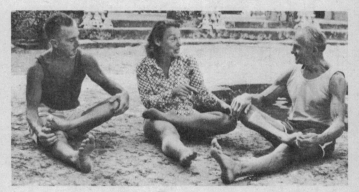

WHAT THE EXERCISE DOES FOR YOU:
It expands your rib cage and gives your lungs more room to breathe.

It keeps your hips, knees, and ankles flexible.

It stretches the tendons on the inside of your upper thighs.

It has a calming effect upon your mind.

It helps you to avoid slumping when you sit.

SIDE STRETCH

You seldom stretch your spine to the side in your daily activities. The Side Stretch exercise gives you an opportunity to accomplish a lateral stretch. The stretch takes little time and effort, yet offers you an effective way to keep your spine supple.

DO THE EXERCISE TWICE.

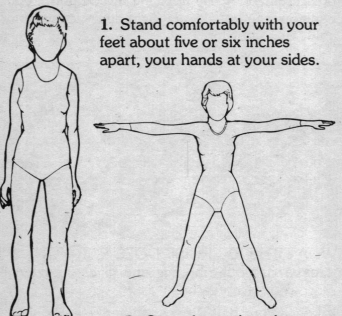

1. Stand comfortably with your feet about five or six inches apart, your hands at your sides.

2. Spread your feet about twenty-four inches apart, and extend your arms sideways at shoulder level. Keep them straight.

3. Lean to your right, lowering your head to the right at the same time.

4. Grasp your right ankle with your right hand. Keep your left arm straight up on a line with your right arm. Hold for 5 seconds.

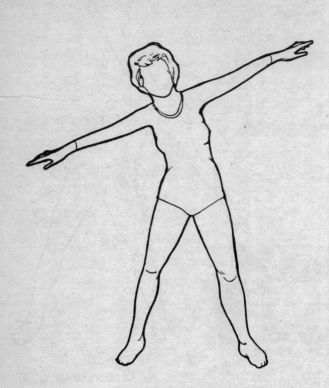

5. Release your ankle, and gradually raise your right arm to shoulder height. Gradually lower your left arm to shoulder height.

6. Stand with both arms extended sideways at shoulder height.

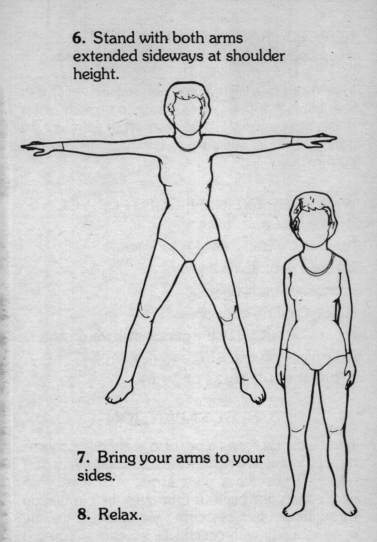

7. Bring your arms to your sides.

8. Relax.

REPEAT THE STEPS FOR THE OPPOSITE SIDE. YOU HAVE COMPLETED THE EXERCISE.

HOW TO PRACTICE THE EXERCISE:

Keep your eyes open. Try not to lean forward as you bend to the side. Relax your neck as you lower your head in the direction toward which you are leaning. If you are not able to stretch as far down as your ankle, hold any part of your leg you can reach. Do not stretch farther than you find comfortable.

WHAT THE EXERCISE DOES FOR YOU:

It improves your balance.

It tones the muscles of your back.

It keeps your spine flexible.

It expands your rib cage.

It helps to firm your waist.

It brings elasticity to the muscles on the outside of your hips and thighs.

It stretches the backs of your legs.

CHEST EXPANSION

The Chest Expansion posture is almost a course by itself because it manipulates virtually every part of you. It stretches your arms, your legs, your neck, and your back. It improves the circulation throughout your system. This exercise can be done in a jiffy with practically no effort. You will feel good immediately.

DO THE EXERCISE TWICE.

1. Stand relaxed with your hands at your sides and your feet about ten or twelve inches apart.

2. Raise your arms to shoulder level, and place your hands against your chest, palms facing out.

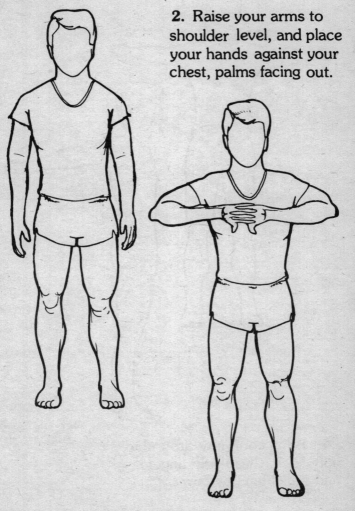

3. Push your hands away from your chest and out to your sides. Keep them high.

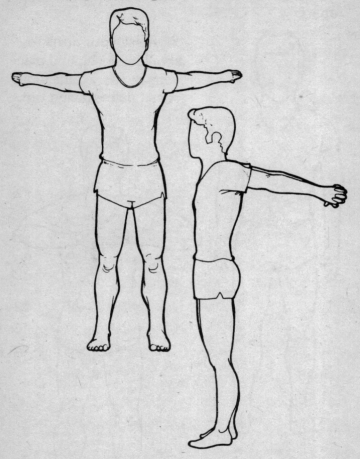

4. Bring your arms around to your back. Clasp your fingers and straighten your arms.

5. Lower your head to the rear as you bend back. Keeping your fingers clasped, raise your arms as high as they will go. Hold for 3 seconds.

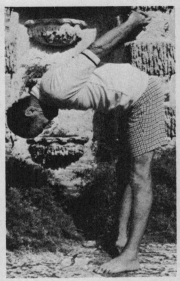

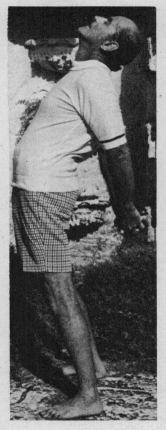

6. Straighten up slowly and bend forward as far as possible, lowering your chin toward your chest. Raise your arms behind you as high as they will go. Hold for 5 seconds.

7. Straighten up slowly—take about 10 seconds. Start with your lower back. Straighten your neck last.

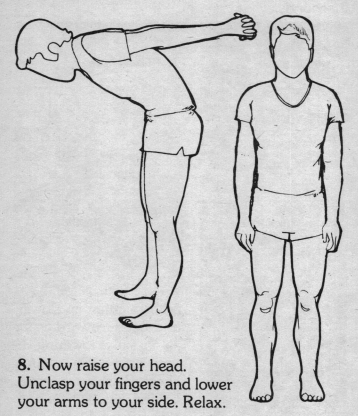

8. Now raise your head. Unclasp your fingers and lower your arms to your side. Relax.

HOW TO PRACTICE THE EXERCISE:
Do not force the stretch. It is a strong one. To maintain proper balance, be sure that you keep your feet a comfortable distance apart, and hold

your eyes open. Bend your knees slightly as you stretch backward. Try not to bend your knees when you stretch forward.

You may do the exercise sitting on the floor.* When you put your head back, move your clasped fingers as far back from your body as you can.

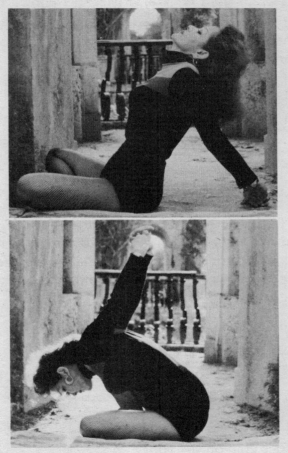

*The Tailor or Half Lotus position.

WHAT THE EXERCISE DOES FOR YOU:

It increases the circulation of blood to your brain.

It relieves tension and keeps your neck, shoulders, and back flexible.

It improves the circulation to your hands.

It keeps your fingers, wrists, and elbows flexible.

If done in a standing position, it stretches the backs of your legs and strengthens your toes and ankles.

If performed in a sitting position, it promotes flexibility in your legs.

It benefits your total posture.

BOW

This is an advanced yoga posture. Do not expect to perfect it immediately. Develop the technique slowly and carefully. Your back and legs will derive considerable benefit throughout the process.

DO THE EXERCISE TWICE.

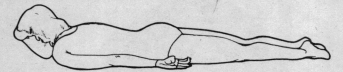

1. Lie on your abdomen. Place your chin on the floor.

2. Bend your right leg. Reach back with your right hand, and grasp your right foot.

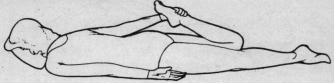

3. Bend your left leg. Reach back with your left hand, and grasp your left foot.

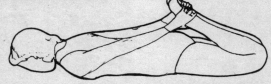

4. Let your legs pull your arms back and slowly raise both your chest and your knees from the floor. Keep your head back. Hold for 3 seconds.

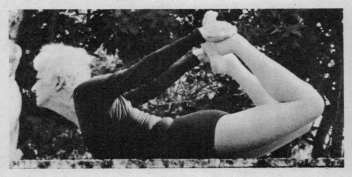

5. Lower your knees, chest, and chin to the floor.

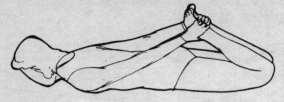

6. Release your feet, and lower your legs to the floor.

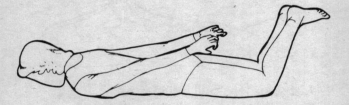

7. Turn your cheek to the floor.

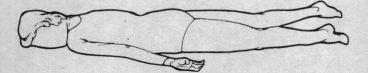

8. Relax.

HOW TO PRACTICE THE EXERCISE:

The ultimate goal is to raise your knees from the floor. To do this, you must let your legs do the work while your arms remain still and straight. Instead of trying to raise your knees by tugging your feet with your hands, allow your feet to pull away from your hands. Pull your legs back very slowly and carefully to avoid straining your leg and back muscles.

If at first you cannot reach your feet with your hands, tie a scarf to each ankle and hold one end. Keep practicing, inching your hands steadily toward your ankles until you can grasp your feet.

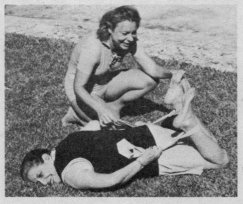

WHAT THE EXERCISE DOES FOR YOU:

It improves the strength of your shoulders, arms, thighs, and back.

It keeps your spine elastic.

It stimulates your pelvic region.

It stretches your thighs.

It keeps your legs flexible.

ALTERNATE LEG STRETCH

It is not your chronological age, but the condition of your mind and your body that determines the way you feel. A good feeling can be induced by good circulation and mobility in your joints. The Alternate Leg Stretch—which focuses on your back and legs, the two areas of your body that must be kept limber if you are to function freely—contributes to the healthy condition of your mind and your body by stimulating your circulation and loosening up your limbs.

DO THE EXERCISE TWICE.

1. Sit on the floor with your left leg extended in front of you, your right foot touching the inside of your left thigh. Place your hands on your knees.

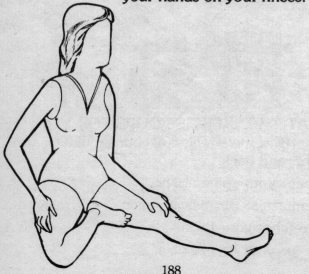

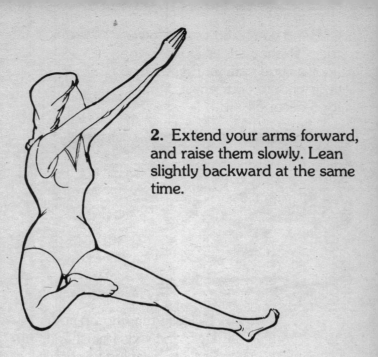

2. Extend your arms forward, and raise them slowly. Lean slightly backward at the same time.

3. Stretch forward as far as you can, and grasp your leg as close to your ankle as possible.

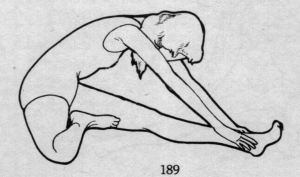

4. Bend your elbows and lower them so they are as close to the floor as you can get them. Drop your chin to your chest. Hold for 5 seconds.

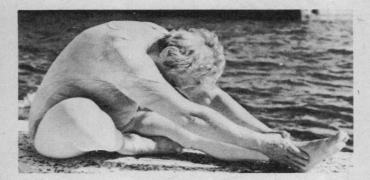

5. Release the grip on your ankles, and slide your hands up your legs. Keeping your chin down, straighten up, starting from your lower back.

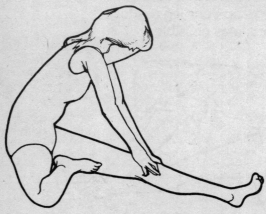

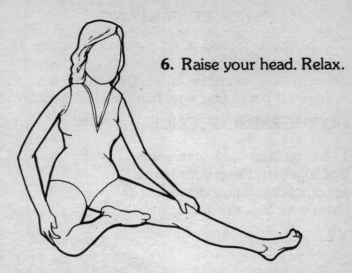

6. Raise your head. Relax.

REPEAT THE STEPS FOR THE OPPOSITE SIDE. YOU HAVE COMPLETED THE EXERCISE.

HOW TO PRACTICE THE EXERCISE:
Muscles get stiff from lack of use. If you cannot reach your ankle, grasp your calf or your knee. It may take many months before you can stretch as far as your ankle. Your goal is to get your elbows to touch the floor and your forehead to touch your knee.

WHAT THE EXERCISE DOES FOR YOU:
It helps your neck move freely.

It stretches the outside areas of your back.

It massages your abdominal wall and promotes regularity.

It keeps your hip joints, knees, and legs flexible.

191

SHOULDER STAND

The Shoulder Stand is an inversion posture. It helps to normalize your weight. A good time to perform the exercise is in the afternoon or evening. It perks you up when you feel fatigued.

DO THE EXERCISE ONCE.

1. Lie on your back with your legs together. Keep your hands at your sides, palms down. Raise your legs slowly.

2. When your legs are straight up in the air, push your hands against the floor, and begin to raise your hips.

3. Raise your hips as high as you can. Bend your elbows, and place your hands on your lower back. Straighten your back. Hold for 30 seconds.

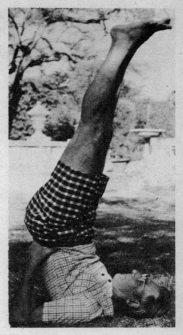

4. Bend your knees, and lower them as close to your forehead as you can.

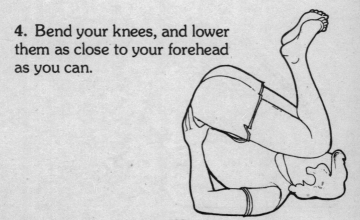

5. Bring your arms, one at a time, to the floor, palms down. Begin to lower your hips to the floor. Keep your knees bent.

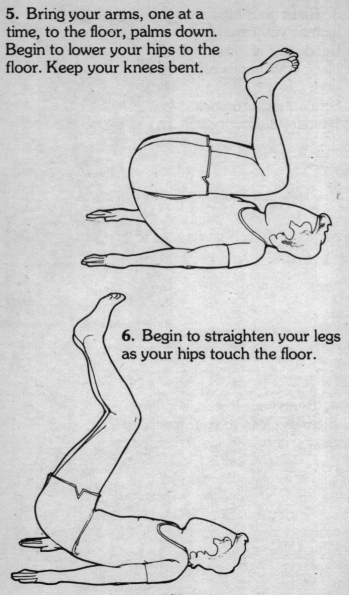

6. Begin to straighten your legs as your hips touch the floor.

7. Straighten your legs, and lower them to the floor.

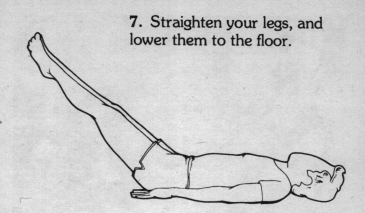

8. Lie flat on the floor with your legs apart and your hands at your sides, palms up. Relax.

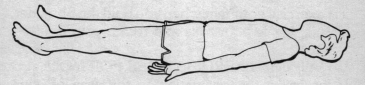

HOW TO PRACTICE THE EXERCISE:
Keep a rug or a mat under you. Do not lie on a hard surface. You will have more strength in your arms if you do not spread your elbows too far apart when you support the weight of your body with your hands. If your arms are not yet strong enough to hold your body up, lean your feet against a wall.

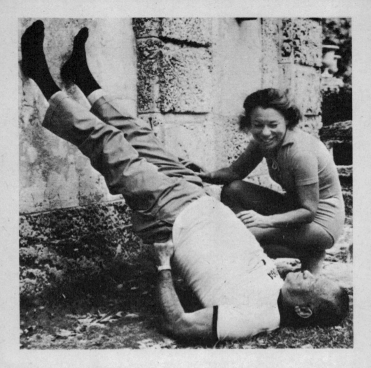

To exercise your feet when you hold the Shoulder Stand, wiggle your toes and rotate your ankles.

WHAT THE EXERCISE DOES FOR YOU:
It increases the circulation to the area of your throat.

It relieves tightness in your neck and shoulders.

It reverses the flow of blood in your body, thereby improving the circulation to your entire system.

It helps to counteract the pull of gravity which causes your abdominal muscles to sag.

It rests your legs.

NETI

This little-known yoga exercise provides you with a natural way to cleanse your nasal passages. All you need do is take several short whiffs of a water-salt preparation, permitting the mixture to filter in and out of your nose several times in succession.

DO THE EXERCISE TWICE.

1. Mix a teaspoon of salt in a glass of warm water. Mix it thoroughly.

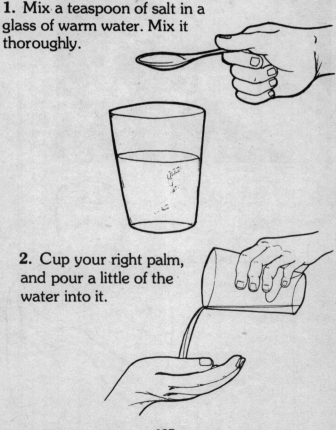

2. Cup your right palm, and pour a little of the water into it.

3. Place your left nostril in the solution. Slowly draw the water into your nostril.

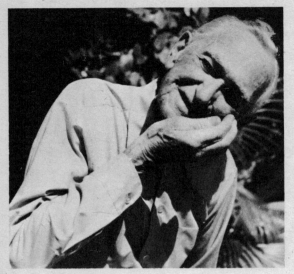

4. Drop your head back.

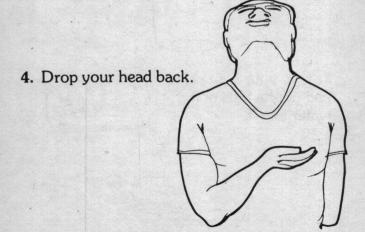

5. Bring your head forward to permit the water to drain out.

6. Raise your head. Relax.

REPEAT THE PROCEDURE ON THE OTHER SIDE. YOU HAVE COMPLETED THE EXERCISE.

HOW TO PRACTICE THE EXERCISE:
Draw the water into your nose slowly.

WHAT THE EXERCISE DOES FOR YOU:
It removes impurities, such as mucus, dust, and dirt, from your nasal passages.

It clears your nasal passages if they are blocked.

CHAPTER VI

STANDING BREATH AND CHEST STRETCH

THREE-WAY NECK STRETCH

ROCK AND ROLL

ARCH

WINGS

PLOW

ALTERNATE NOSTRIL BREATHING

RAJA YOGA

STANDING BREATH AND CHEST STRETCH

This exercise calls for considerable coordination in breathing practice and body activity. It stimulates both your mind and your body. Carry out the movements slowly.

DO THE EXERCISE TWICE.

1. Stand with your feet separated by the approximate width of your shoulders. Place your hands on your hips.

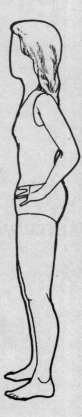

2. Inhale as you stretch the upper part of your body to your right side. Exhale as you straighten up. Rest briefly.

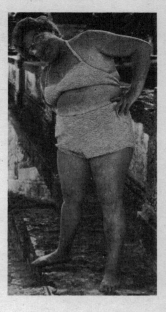

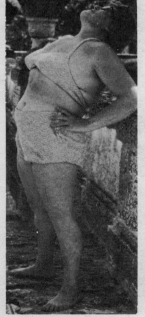

3. Inhale as you bend back. Exhale as you straighten up. Rest briefly.

4. Inhale as you stretch the upper part of your body to your left side. Exhale as you straighten up.

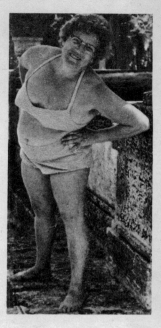

5. Inhale. Exhale as you bend forward. Inhale as you straighten up. Exhale.

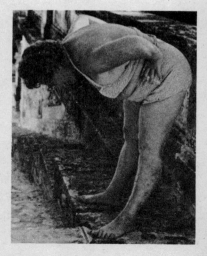

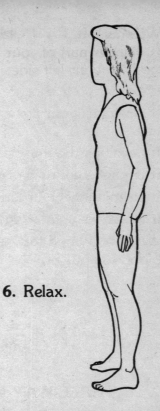

6. Relax.

REPEAT THE STEPS FOR THE OPPOSITE SIDE. YOU HAVE COMPLETED THE EXERCISE.

HOW TO PRACTICE THE EXERCISE:
This is a powerful exercise. Take your time and work carefully in order to do the breathing procedures correctly. Keep your eyes open.

WHAT THE EXERCISE DOES FOR YOU:

It stretches your neck muscles and keeps your neck limber.

It relaxes your shoulder muscles if they are tight.

It stretches your spine concavely, convexly, and laterally.

It develops the muscles of your chest.

It expands your rib cage.

It strengthens your lungs.

It increases your oxygen intake.

When you bend forward, it increases the flow of blood to your brain.

THREE-WAY NECK STRETCH

The Three-Way Neck Stretch provides your neck with a greater stretch than does the Four-Way Neck Stretch because it applies the force of your hands to the stretch. This technique can be performed while you are sitting at a desk or a table. Any time you feel tension building, physical or mental, place your elbows on the nearest table and proceed to do the exercise. It will relax and soothe your nerves.

DO THE EXERCISE TWICE.

1. Put your elbows on the table and rest your head between your hands.

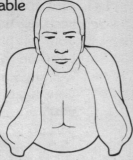

2. Turn your head slowly to your right and place your chin in your right hand. Place your left hand on the back of your head. Using your hands, gently turn your head as far to your right as you can. Hold for 5 seconds.

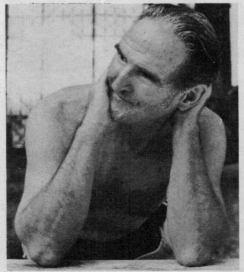

3. Turn your head slowly to your left and place your chin in your left hand. Place your right hand on the back of your head. Using your hands, gently turn your head as far to your left as you can. Hold for 5 seconds.

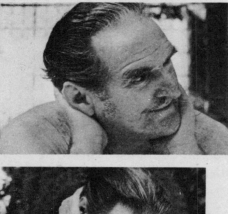

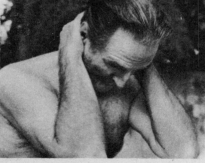

4. Turn your head slowly forward. Drop your head. Put your hands on the back of your head. Gently push your chin down toward your chest. Hold for 5 seconds.

5. Raise your head, and place it between your hands. Relax.

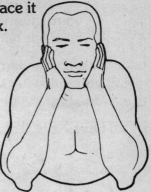

REPEAT THE STEPS IN THE OPPOSITE DIRECTION. YOU HAVE COMPLETED THE EXERCISE.

HOW TO PRACTICE THE EXERCISE:
Be sure that your elbows are not too far apart when they rest on the table. The distance between them should be approximately the width of your head. Do not move them throughout the exercise. When your head is down (figure 4), do not slump forward. The straighter you hold your back, the more stretch your neck will receive.

You can also do this exercise lying on your abdomen.

WHAT THE EXERCISE DOES FOR YOU:
It relaxes the tight muscles of your neck and upper back.

It gives your neck mobility.

It helps you sleep.

ROCK AND ROLL

This is a good exercise for cold nights. It keeps your blood circulating quickly from your head to your toes, and it warms every inch of your body, giving you a glowing sensation. It gently increases the circulation in your spine.

DO THE EXERCISE TWICE.

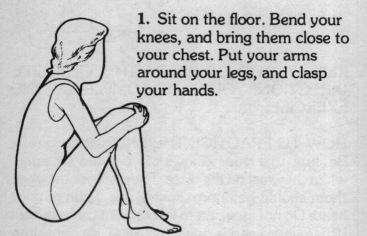

1. Sit on the floor. Bend your knees, and bring them close to your chest. Put your arms around your legs, and clasp your hands.

2. Move forward and back 3 times simulating the movement of a rocking horse.

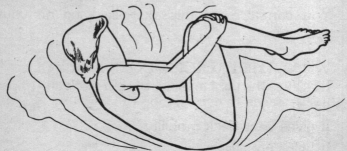

3. Sit up.

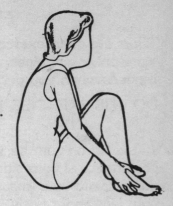

4. Relax.

HOW TO PRACTICE THE EXERCISE:
Be sure to do the exercise on a well-padded surface. Try to roll back far enough so that your head touches the floor. Increase the tempo of the rocking movements gradually, but do not rock so fast or so hard that you exhaust yourself. If you wish, you may lie down and rest each time you do the exercise.

WHAT THE EXERCISE DOES FOR YOU:
It stimulates the nerves emanating from your spinal column.

It flexes your vertebrae.

It tones the muscles of your back.

It relieves tension in your neck, shoulders, and back.

It increases the circulation of your entire body.

It warms your body.

It wakes you up.

ARCH

There are a few yoga stretches for the pelvic area. Your pelvic girdle gets a good part of the exercise it needs when you perform this posture.

DO THE EXERCISE TWICE.

1. Lie flat on your back, with your hands at your sides, palms down. Bend your knees. Keep your legs about twelve inches apart.

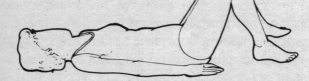

2. Push your feet down hard against the floor and begin to raise your hips off the floor.

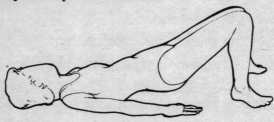

3. Bring your hips up as high as you can. Hold for 5 seconds.

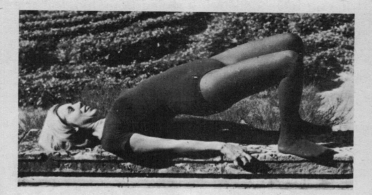

4. Lower your hips to the floor.

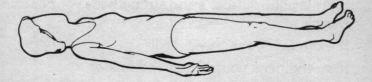

5. Straighten your legs. Turn your palms up.

6. Relax.

HOW TO PRACTICE THE EXERCISE:
If you have difficulty keeping your hips off the ground, you may place your hands under your hips for support.

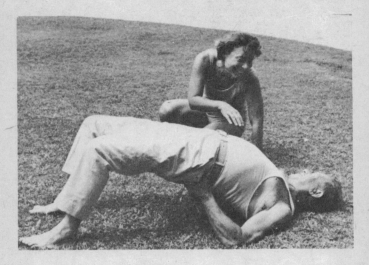

WHAT THE EXERCISE DOES FOR YOU:
It strengthens the frontal portion of your body from your shoulders to your thighs.

It improves the alignment of your spine.

It firms your buttocks and strengthens your back muscles.

It exercises your pelvic girdle.

It strengthens your knees and ankles.

WINGS

Do this exercise frequently for the comfort it can give you. It will relieve tension in your upper back and eliminate stiffness in your neck and shoulders. It will also soothe your nervous system.

DO THE EXERCISE TWICE.

1. Sit in a cross-legged position.* Bend your elbows, and draw your arms back so that your hands are on either side of your upper chest.

*The Tailor or the Half Lotus position.

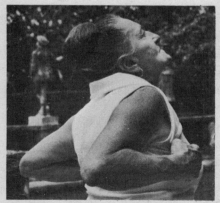

2. Drop your head back, close your eyes, and relax your mouth. Bring your elbows as close together behind you as you can. Hold for 5 seconds.

3. Lower your arms and raise your head.

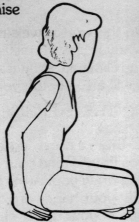

4. Relax.

HOW TO PRACTICE THE EXERCISE:
Try to keep your elbows high. Breathe in a relaxed manner.

WHAT THE EXERCISE DOES FOR YOU:
It makes your neck, shoulders, and upper back limber.

It keeps the joints of your elbows loose.

It calms your nerves.

It helps you sleep.

PLOW

The Plow is a well-known exercise. It stretches your spine along its entire length. The three movements that occur in the Plow put the emphasis of the stretch on a different part of your back each time, giving you results that you might otherwise have to seek with three separate exercises.

DO THE EXERCISE TWICE.

1. Lie flat on your back, arms at your sides. Turn your palms down. Legs together. Raise your legs.

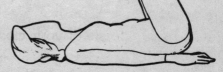

2. Bring your legs straight up in the air.

3. Push your hands down hard against the floor. Raise your hips, and move your legs toward your head.

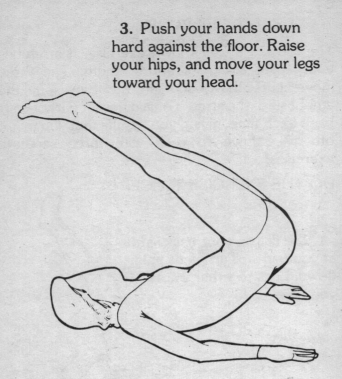

4. Touch your toes to the floor behind your head. Hold for 5 seconds.

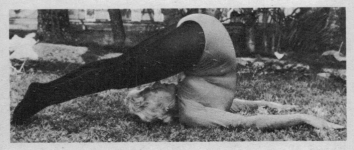

5. Place your hands on top of your head, and rest your arms on the floor. Move your feet as far back as they will go. Let the bottoms of your toes touch the floor. Hold for 5 seconds.

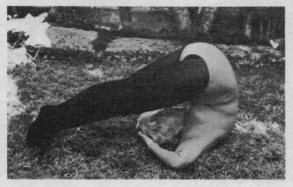

6. Bend your legs, and place your knees next to your ears on either side of your head. Hold for 5 seconds.

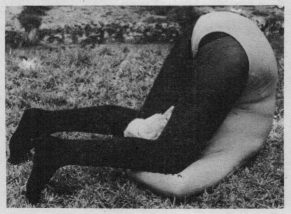

7. Put your hands under your back for support. Bring your bent knees together, and lean them against your forehead. Draw your heels down close to your buttocks.

8. Return your arms to the floor, palms down. Keeping your knees bent, roll your hips forward toward the floor. Hold your knees as close to your chest as you can when your hips move forward.

9. After your hips touch the floor, bring your legs straight up in the air.

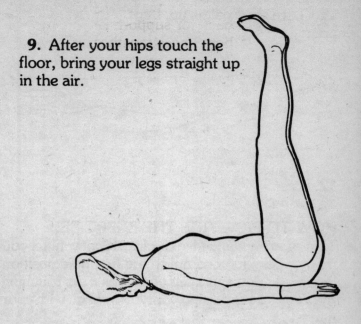

10. Lower your legs to the floor.

11. Turn your palms up. Legs apart.

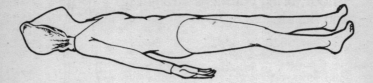

12. Rest.

HOW TO PRACTICE THE EXERCISE:
This is an advanced exercise. It may take you many weeks to accomplish the first hold position (figure 4). You can keep your hips from touching the floor by supporting your lower back with your hands.

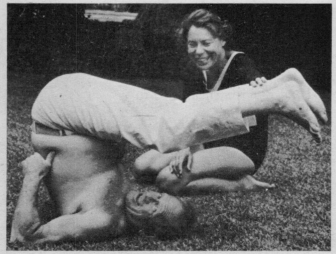

If you are unable to bring your toes to the floor, hold them at whatever point they reach. Figure 4 focuses the stretch on your lower back. Figure 5 focuses the stretch on your middle back. (Do not go on to figure 5 until you have perfected figure 4.) Figure 6 focuses the stretch on your neck and shoulders.

WHAT THE EXERCISE DOES FOR YOU:

It makes your neck, shoulders, and back flexible.

It helps to counteract the pull of gravity which causes your visceral organs to sag.

It massages your abdomen.

It stretches your toes and the backs of your legs.

ALTERNATE NOSTRIL BREATHING

Many senior citizens suffer because their sleep is poor in quality. As a result, they never feel fully rested, and they are nervous and irritable much of the time. Sleeping pills do not solve the problem. The Alternate Nostril Breathing technique can alleviate nocturnal sleeplessness. You are urged to try the technique. It is easy to do, and you can practice it in bed. It will help you to fall asleep quickly and to wake up refreshed.

DO THE EXERCISE FOUR TIMES.

1. Sit comfortably with your legs crossed.*

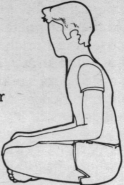

2. Place your right thumb against your right nostril. Press down gently. Rest your first and second fingers between your eyebrows. Straighten your last two fingers. Inhale slowly through your left nostril, counting silently to 4 seconds as you inhale.

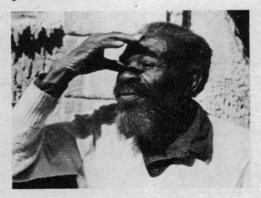

*The Tailor or the Half Lotus posture.

3. With your last two fingers press down on your left nostril. Hold your breath for 4 seconds.

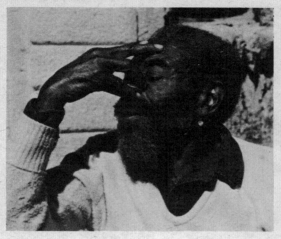

4. Raise your thumb and exhale through your right nostril for 4 seconds.

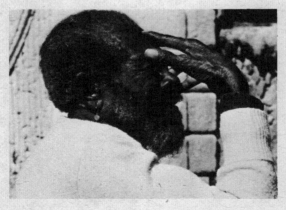

5. Keeping your fingers in the same position, inhale through your right nostril for 4 seconds. Count silently.

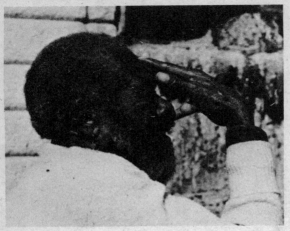

6. Lower your thumb, and press down against your right nostril. Hold your breath for 4 seconds.

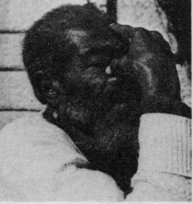

7. Raise your last two fingers, and exhale to the count of 4. Repeat the above steps 3 more times without pausing.

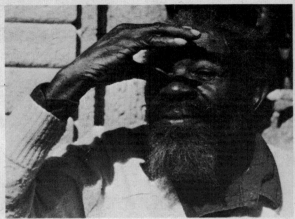

8. Lower your hand. Relax.

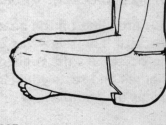

HOW TO PRACTICE THE EXERCISE:

Do this exercise any time you feel nervous or tense. It takes only minutes of your time. Inhale and exhale through your nose. Breathe slowly and rhythmically for maximum effect.

WHAT THE EXERCISE DOES FOR YOU:

It helps to keep your sinuses open.

It increases your oxygen intake.

It strengthens your lungs.

It establishes rhythmic breathing and calms your nervous system.

It helps you to sleep more soundly.

RAJA YOGA

This exercise from *raja* yoga—the yoga of meditation—concentrates on relaxing your body through your mental processes rather than through your physical processes. It helps you to direct your thinking toward positive channels. It gives you an awareness of your own nature and insights into the nature of others. *Raja* yoga is a true avenue to peace.

Lie comfortably on your back and relax. Breathe slowly and deeply. Visualize the following scene:

You are lying on the beach near the water. All is peaceful. There is a tropical breeze rolling in over the ocean. As the breeze caresses your body, it soothes and rests you. Breathe deeply but slowly of the delightful, fragrant ocean air. Relax . . . re-

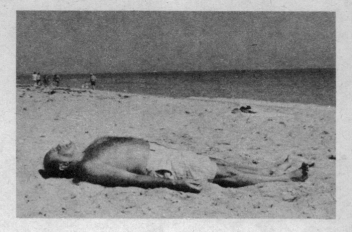

lax . . . relax . . . and listen. . . . Listen to the sounds of the ocean waves as they break upon the shore. . . . Can you hear the bird? He is singing a lovely song. He is happy. . . . He is free. The warmth of the sun is giving him life and strength, just as it is giving you life and strength. Relax . . . relax. . . . Breathe slowly. Feel yourself relaxing . . . sinking deeply into the warm embrace of the sand. You are tranquil. All is serene. Look up. . . . What do you see? Why, you see the blue of the sky. How restful the color is. And look . . . can you see the clouds? They are soft and white . . . gossamer threads of silk suspended in the air. They are beckoning you to accompany them. Choose a delicate one and recline on it. . . . Relax. . . . Relax, and float happily . . . joyfully. . . . You are tranquil. . . . All is serene . . . tranquil . . . serene . . . tranquil . . . serene. . . . Slumber.

MINIPROGRAMS FOR THE CARE AND DEVELOPMENT OF THE TOTAL BODY

MINIPROGRAMS FOR THE CARE AND
DEVELOPMENT OF THE TOTAL BODY

Name of Exercise	Page Number	Advanced Count	Potential Count
Cleansing Breath	62	Do 5 breaths Do the exercise five times	Do 10 breaths Do the exercise five times
Chest Expansion	178	Hold for 5 seconds backward and 10 seconds forward Do the exercise twice	Hold for 5 seconds backward and 20 seconds forward Do the exercise twice
Standing Twist	65	Hold for 10 seconds Do the exercise twice	Hold for 20 seconds Do the exercise twice
Eye Movements	102	There is no advanced	—

count for this exercise;
repeat the last count:

First		Do the exercise 3 times	
Second		Do the exercise 3 times	
Third		Do the exercise 3 times	
Fourth		Do the exercise 3 times	
Fifth		Do the exercise 3 times	
Sixth		Do the exercise once	
Knee and Thigh	113	Hold for 10 seconds / Do the exercise twice	Hold for 20 seconds / Do the exercise twice
Preliminary Back and Leg Stretch	109	Hold for 10 seconds / Do the exercise twice	Hold for 20 seconds / Do the exercise twice
Finger Clasp	36	Hold for 10 seconds / Do the exercise twice	Hold for 20 seconds / Do the exercise twice
Raja Yoga	226	—	—

* * *

Name of Exercise	Page Number	Advanced Count	Potential Count
Side Stretch	174	Hold for 10 seconds Do the exercise twice	Hold for 20 seconds Do the exercise twice
Arm and Leg	90	Hold for 10 seconds Do the exercise twice	Hold for 20 seconds Do the exercise twice
Squat	70	Hold for 20 seconds Do the exercise twice	Hold for 30 seconds Do the exercise twice
Spread Leg Stretch	76	Hold for 10 seconds Do the exercise twice	Hold for 20 seconds Do the exercise twice
Alternate Leg Stretch	188	Hold for 10 seconds Do the exercise twice	Hold for 20 seconds Do the exercise twice
Eye Movements	102	There is no advanced count for this exercise; repeat the last count:	—

First   Do the exercise 3 times
Second   Do the exercise 3 times
Third   Do the exercise 3 times
Fourth   Do the exercise 3 times
Fifth   Do the exercise 3 times
Sixth   Do the exercise once

Slow Neck Roll	83	Roll your head twice to your right and twice to your left Do the exercise twice	Roll your head 3 times to your right and 3 times to your left Do the exercise twice

* * *

Standing Breath and Chest Stretch	202	Roll your torso twice to your right and twice to your left Do the exercise twice	Roll your torso 3 times to your right and 3 times to your left Do the exercise twice
Preliminary Back and Leg Stretch	109	Hold for 10 seconds Do the exercise twice	Hold for 20 seconds Do the exercise twice

Name of Exercise	Page Number	Advanced Count	Potential Count
Rock-A-Bye-Baby	74	Rock your leg from side to side 10 times. Do the exercise twice	—
Cobra	120	Hold for 10 seconds. Do the exercise twice	Hold for 20 seconds. Do the exercise twice
Alternate Nostril Breathing	223	Inhale for the count of 6, hold your breath for the count of 6, and exhale for the count of 6. Do the exercise six times	Inhale for the count of 8, hold your breath for the count of 8, and exhale for the count of 8. Do the exercise eight times
		* * *	
Slow Hip Roll	94	Roll your hips twice to your right and	Roll your hips 3 times to your right and 3

		twice to your left	times to your left
Refreshing Breath	46	Hold for 5 seconds Do the exercise twice	Hold for 10 seconds Do the exercise twice
Squat	70	Hold for 20 seconds Do the exercise twice	Hold for 30 seconds Do the exercise twice
Half Lotus*	171	Hold for 30 seconds Do the exercise twice	Hold for 60 seconds Do the exercise twice
Backward Bend	140	Hold for 10 seconds Do the exercise twice	Hold for 20 seconds Do the exercise twice
Back of Leg Stretch	41	Hold for 10 seconds Do the exercise twice	Hold for 20 seconds Do the exercise twice
Lion	153	Hold for 10 seconds Do the exercise twice	Hold for 20 seconds Do the exercise twice

* If you find the Half Lotus too difficult, do the Tailor posture.

Name of Exercise	Page Number	Advanced Count	Potential Count
Alternate Nostril Breathing	223	Inhale for the count of 6, hold your breath for the count of 6, and exhale for the count of 6 Do the exercise six times	Inhale for the count of 8, hold your breath for the count of 8, and exhale for the count of 8 Do the exercise eight times
		* * *	
Cow	52	Hold for 10 seconds Do the exercise twice	Hold for 20 seconds Do the exercise twice
Tree	128	Hold for 10 seconds Do the exercise twice	Hold for 20 seconds Do the exercise twice
Three-Way Neck Stretch	206	Hold for 10 seconds Do the exercise twice	—

Arch	212	Hold for 10 seconds Do the exercise twice	Hold for 20 seconds Do the exercise twice
Curl	80	Hold for 10 seconds Do the exercise twice	Hold for 20 seconds Do the exercise twice
Rock and Roll	210	Rock back and forth 5 times Do the exercise twice * * *	—
Abdominal Lift*	166	Do 5 lifts Do the exercise five times	Do 10 lifts Do the exercise five times
Twist on the Floor**	132	Hold for 10 seconds Do the exercise twice	Hold for 20 seconds Do the exercise twice
Cat	43	Hold for 10 seconds Do the exercise twice	Hold for 20 seconds Do the exercise twice

*   Do the exercise in the position you prefer, lying or sitting.
** If you find the Twist on the Floor too difficult, do the Twist in the Chair.

239

Name of Exercise	Page Number	Advanced Count	Potential Count
Bow	184	Hold for 5 seconds Do the exercise twice	—
Plow	217	Hold for 10 seconds Do the exercise twice	Hold for 20 seconds Do the exercise twice
Complete Breath	55	Hold your breath for 5 seconds Do the exercise five times	Hold your breath for 10 seconds Do the exercise five times
		* * *	
Neti	197	Do the exercise three times	—
Abdominal Lift*	166	Do 5 lifts Do the exercise five times	Do 10 lifts Do the exercise five times

240

Exercise	Page		
Four-Way Neck Stretch	116	Hold for 10 seconds Do the exercise twice	—
Wings	215	Hold for 10 seconds Do the exercise twice	Hold for 20 seconds Do the exercise twice
Locust	159	Hold for 5 seconds Do the exercise twice	—
Leg Stretches	147	Hold for 10 seconds Do the exercise twice	Hold for 20 seconds Do the exercise twice
Shoulder Stand	192	Hold for 1 minute Do the exercise once	Hold for 2 minutes Do the exercise once
Cleansing Breath	62	Do 5 breaths Do the exercise five times	Do 10 breaths Do the exercise five times
Cow	52	Hold for 10 seconds Do the exercise twice	Hold for 20 seconds Do the exercise twice

* Do the exercise in the position you prefer, lying or sitting.

Name of Exercise	Page Number	Advanced Count	Potential Count
Refreshing Breath	46	Hold for 5 seconds Do the exercise twice	Hold for 10 seconds Do the exercise twice
Chest Expansion	178	Hold for 5 seconds backward and 10 seconds forward Do the exercise twice	Hold for 5 seconds backward and 20 seconds forward Do the exercise twice
Shoulder Stretch	156	Hold for 10 seconds Do the exercise twice	Hold for 20 seconds Do the exercise twice
Knee and Thigh	113	Hold for 10 seconds Do the exercise twice	Hold for 20 seconds Do the exercise twice
Bow	184	Hold for 5 seconds Do the exercise twice	—

Ninety-Second
Relaxer

161   There is no advanced
count for this exercise;
repeat the last count:
Take 30 seconds each
to lower your body,
hold the position,
and raise your body
Do the exercise once   —

*

*

*

MINIPROGRAMS FOR THE CARE AND DEVELOPMENT OF PARTICULAR BODY PARTS

ABDOMEN

Name of Exercise	Page Number	Advanced Count	Potential Count
Abdominal Lift*	166	Do 5 lifts Do the exercise five times	Do 10 lifts Do the exercise five times
Alternate Leg Stretch	188	Hold for 10 seconds Do the exercise twice	Hold for 20 seconds Do the exercise twice
Arch	212	Hold for 10 seconds Do the exercise twice	Hold for 20 seconds Do the exercise twice
Shoulder Stand	192	Hold for 1 minute Do the exercise once	Hold for 2 minutes Do the exercise once

* Do the exercise in the position you prefer, lying or sitting.

*　　　*　　　*

ABDOMEN

Name of Exercise	Page Number	Advanced Count	Potential Count
Abdominal Lift*	166	Do 5 lifts Do the exercise five times	Do 10 lifts Do the exercise five times
Cat	43	Hold for 10 seconds Do the exercise twice	Hold for 20 seconds Do the exercise twice
Curl	80	Hold for 10 seconds Do the exercise twice	Hold for 20 seconds Do the exercise twice
Bow	184	Hold for 5 seconds Do the exercise twice	—

* Do the exercise in the position you prefer, lying or sitting.

* * *

ABDOMEN

Name of Exercise	Page Number	Advanced Count	Potential Count
Chest Expansion	178	Hold for 5 seconds backward and 10 seconds forward Do the exercise twice	Hold for 5 seconds backward and 20 seconds forward Do the exercise twice
Squat	70	Hold for 20 seconds Do the exercise twice	Hold for 30 seconds Do the exercise twice
Twist on the Floor*	132	Hold for 10 seconds Do the exercise twice	Hold for 20 seconds Do the exercise twice
Backward Bend	140	Hold for 10 seconds Do the exercise twice	Hold for 20 seconds Do the exercise twice
Shoulder Stand	192	Hold for 1 minute Do the exercise twice	Hold for 2 minutes Do the exercise twice

* If you find the Twist on the Floor too difficult, do the Twist in the Chair.

* * *

248

ABDOMEN

Name of Exercise	Page Number	Advanced Count	Potential Count
Cow	52	Hold for 10 seconds Do the exercise twice	Hold for 20 seconds Do the exercise twice
Chest Expansion	178	Hold for 5 seconds backward and 10 seconds forward Do the exercise twice	Hold for 5 seconds backward and 20 seconds forward Do the exercise twice
Cobra	120	Hold for 10 seconds Do the exercise twice	Hold for 20 seconds Do the exercise twice
Arch	212	Hold for 10 seconds Do the exercise twice	Hold for 20 seconds Do the exercise twice
Plow	217	Hold for 10 seconds Do the exercise twice	Hold for 20 seconds Do the exercise twice

* * *

ABDOMEN

Name of Exercise	Page Number	Advanced Count	Potential Count
Squat	70	Hold for 20 seconds Do the exercise twice	Hold for 30 seconds Do the exercise twice
Curl	80	Hold for 10 seconds Do the exercise twice	Hold for 20 seconds Do the exercise twice
Abdominal Lift*	166	Do 5 lifts Do the exercise five times	Do 10 lifts Do the exercise five times
Spread Leg Stretch	76	Hold for 10 seconds Do the exercise twice	Hold for 20 seconds Do the exercise twice
Cleansing Breath	62	Do 5 breaths Do the exercise five times	Do 10 breaths Do the exercise five times

Shoulder Stand   192   Hold for 1 minute   Hold for 2 minutes
                         Do the exercise once   Do the exercise once

* Do the exercise in the position you prefer, lying or sitting.

ABDOMEN

Name of Exercise	Page Number	Advanced Count	Potential Count
Squat	70	Hold for 20 seconds Do the exercise twice	Hold for 30 seconds Do the exercise twice
Abdominal Lift*	166	Do 5 lifts Do the exercise five times	Do 10 lifts Do the exercise five times
Preliminary Back and Leg Stretch	109	Hold for 10 seconds Do the exercise twice	Hold for 20 seconds Do the exercise twice
Cobra	120	Hold for 10 seconds Do the exercise twice	Hold for 20 seconds Do the exercise twice
Plow	217	Hold for 10 seconds Do the exercise twice	Hold for 20 seconds Do the exercise twice

* Do the exercise in the position you prefer, lying or sitting

* * *

ARMS

Name of Exercise	Page Number	Advanced Count	Potential Count
Chest Expansion	178	Hold for 5 seconds backward and 10 seconds forward Do the exercise twice	Hold for 5 seconds backward and 20 seconds forward Do the exercise twice
Finger Clasp	36	Hold for 10 seconds Do the exercise twice	Hold for 20 seconds Do the exercise twice
Shoulder Stretch	156	Hold for 10 seconds Do the exercise twice	Hold for 20 seconds Do the exercise twice
Bow	184	Hold for 5 seconds Do the exercise twice	—

* * *

ARMS

Name of Exercise	Page Number	Advanced Count	Potential Count
Arm and Leg	90	Hold for 10 seconds Do the exercise twice	Hold for 20 seconds Do the exercise twice
Chest Expansion	178	Hold for 5 seconds backward and 10 seconds forward Do the exercise twice	Hold for 5 seconds backward and 20 seconds forward Do the exercise twice
Curl	80	Hold for 10 seconds Do the exercise twice	Hold for 20 seconds Do the exercise twice
Finger Clasp	36	Hold for 10 seconds Do the exercise twice	Hold for 20 seconds Do the exercise twice
Cobra	120	Hold for 10 seconds Do the exercise twice	Hold for 20 seconds Do the exercise twice

* * *

ARMS

Name of Exercise	Page Number	Advanced Count	Potential Count
Twist on the Floor*	132	Hold for 10 seconds Do the exercise twice	Hold for 20 seconds Do the exercise twice
Cat	43	Hold for 10 seconds Do the exercise twice	Hold for 20 seconds Do the exercise twice
Finger Clasp	36	Hold for 10 seconds Do the exercise twice	Hold for 20 seconds Do the exercise twice
Wings	215	Hold for 10 seconds Do the exercise twice	Hold for 20 seconds Do the exercise twice
Knee and Thigh	113	Hold for 10 seconds Do the exercise twice	Hold for 20 seconds Do the exercise twice

* * *

* If you find the Twist on the Floor too difficult, do the Twist in the Chair.

ARMS

Name of Exercise	Page Number	Advanced Count	Potential Count
Arm and Leg	90	Hold for 10 seconds Do the exercise twice	Hold for 20 seconds Do the exercise twice
Chest Expansion	178	Hold for 5 seconds backward and 10 seconds forward Do the exercise twice	Hold for 5 seconds backward and 20 seconds forward Do the exercise twice
Finger Clasp	36	Hold for 10 seconds Do the exercise twice	Hold for 20 seconds Do the exercise twice
Backward Bend	140	Hold for 10 seconds Do the exercise twice	Hold for 20 seconds Do the exercise twice
Cobra	120	Hold for 10 seconds Do the exercise twice	Hold for 20 seconds Do the exercise twice

* * *

ARMS

Name of Exercise	Page Number	Advanced Count	Potential Count
Chest Expansion	178	Hold for 5 seconds backward and 10 seconds forward Do the exercise twice	Hold for 5 seconds backward and 20 seconds forward Do the exercise twice
Twist on the Floor*	132	Hold for 10 seconds Do the exercise twice	Hold for 20 seconds Do the exercise twice
Locust	159	Hold for 5 seconds Do the exercise twice	—
Cobra	120	Hold for 10 seconds Do the exercise twice	Hold for 20 seconds Do the exercise twice

* If you find the Twist on the Floor too difficult, do the Twist in the Chair.

*   *   *   *

ARMS

Name of Exercise	Page Number	Advanced Count	Potential Count
Wings	215	Hold for 10 seconds Do the exercise twice	Hold for 20 seconds Do the exercise twice
Finger Clasp	36	Hold for 10 seconds Do the exercise twice	Hold for 20 seconds Do the exercise twice
Shoulder Stretch	156	Hold for 10 seconds Do the exercise twice	Hold for 20 seconds Do the exercise twice
Backward Bend	140	Hold for 10 seconds Do the exercise twice	Hold for 20 seconds Do the exercise twice
Bow	184	Hold for 5 seconds Do the exercise twice	—
Cobra	120	Hold for 10 seconds Do the exercise twice	Hold for 20 seconds Do the exercise twice

* * *

BACK

Name of Exercise	Page Number	Advanced Count	Potential Count
Cow	52	Hold for 10 seconds Do the exercise twice	Hold for 20 seconds Do the exercise twice
Side Stretch	174	Hold for 10 seconds Do the exercise twice	Hold for 20 seconds Do the exercise twice
Chest Expansion	176	Hold for 5 seconds backward and 10 seconds forward Do the exercise twice	Hold for 5 seconds backward and 20 seconds forward Do the exercise twice
Wings	215	Hold for 10 seconds Do the exercise twice	Hold for 20 seconds Do the exercise twice
Preliminary Back and Leg Stretch	109	Hold for 10 seconds Do the exercise twice	Hold for 20 seconds Do the exercise twice

* * *

BACK

Name of Exercise	Page Number	Advanced Count	Potential Count
Standing Twist	65	Hold for 10 seconds Do the exercise twice	Hold for 20 seconds Do the exercise twice
Slow Hip Roll	94	Roll your hips twice to your right and twice to your left Do the exercise twice	Roll your hips 3 times to your right and 3 times to your left Do the exercise twice
Alternate Leg Stretch	188	Hold for 10 seconds Do the exercise twice	Hold for 20 seconds Do the exercise twice
Backward Bend	140	Hold for 10 seconds Do the exercise twice	Hold for 20 seconds Do the exercise twice
Cobra	120	Hold for 10 seconds Do the exercise twice	Hold for 20 seconds Do the exercise twice

* * *

BACK

Name of Exercise	Page Number	Advanced Count	Potential Count
Cow	52	Hold for 10 seconds Do the exercise twice	Hold for 20 seconds Do the exercise twice
Standing Breath and Chest Stretch	202	Roll your torso twice to your right and twice to your left Do the exercise twice	Roll your torso 3 times to your right and 3 times to your left Do the exercise twice
Cat	43	Hold for 10 seconds Do the exercise twice	Hold for 20 seconds Do the exercise twice
Backward Bend	140	Hold for 10 seconds Do the exercise twice	Hold for 20 seconds Do the exercise twice
Twist on the Floor*	132	Hold for 10 seconds Do the exercise twice	Hold for 20 seconds Do the exercise twice

* If you find the Twist on the Floor too difficult, do the Twist in the Chair.

Locust | 159 | Hold for 5 seconds
Do the exercise twice
* * | —

BACK

Name of Exercise	Page Number	Advanced Count	Potential Count
Cow	52	Hold for 10 seconds Do the exercise twice	Hold for 20 seconds Do the exercise twice
Chest Expansion	178	Hold for 5 seconds backward and 10 seconds forward Do the exercise twice	Hold for 5 seconds backward and 20 seconds forward Do the exercise twice
Wings	215	Hold for 10 seconds Do the exercise twice	Hold for 20 seconds Do the exercise twice
Cobra	120	Hold for 10 seconds Do the exercise twice	Hold for 20 seconds Do the exercise twice

* * *

BACK

Name of Exercise	Page Number	Advanced Count	Potential Count
Side Stretch	174	Hold for 10 seconds Do the exercise twice	Hold for 20 seconds Do the exercise twice
Arm and Leg	90	Hold for 10 seconds Do the exercise twice	Hold for 20 seconds Do the exercise twice
Curl	80	Hold for 10 seconds Do the exercise twice	Hold for 20 seconds Do the exercise twice
Twist on the Floor*	132	Hold for 10 seconds Do the exercise twice	Hold for 20 seconds Do the exercise twice
Rock and Roll	210	Rock back and forth 5 times Do the exercise twice	—

* If you find the Twist on the Floor too difficult, do the Twist in the Chair.

* * *

BACK

Name of Exercise	Page Number	Advanced Count	Potential Count
Slow Hip Roll	94	Roll your hips twice to your right and twice to your left Do the exercise twice	Roll your hips 3 times to your right and 3 times to your left Do the exercise twice
Chest Expansion	178	Hold for 5 seconds backward and 10 seconds forward Do the exercise twice	Hold for 5 seconds backward and 20 seconds forward Do the exercise twice
Backward Bend	140	Hold for 10 seconds Do the exercise twice	Hold for 20 seconds Do the exercise twice
Plow	217	Hold for 10 seconds Do the exercise twice	Hold for 20 seconds Do the exercise twice

*   *   *

BACK

Name of Exercise	Page Number	Advanced Count	Potential Count
Cat	43	Hold for 10 seconds Do the exercise twice	Hold for 20 seconds Do the exercise twice
Preliminary Back and Leg Stretch	109	Hold for 10 seconds Do the exercise twice	Hold for 20 seconds Do the exercise twice
Arch	212	Hold for 10 seconds Do the exercise twice	Hold for 20 seconds Do the exercise twice
Twist on the Floor*	132	Hold for 10 seconds Do the exercise twice	Hold for 20 seconds Do the exercise twice
Wings	215	Hold for 10 seconds Do the exercise twice	Hold for 20 seconds Do the exercise twice
Cobra	120	Hold for 10 seconds Do the exercise twice	Hold for 20 seconds Do the exercise twice

Bow

184 Hold for 5 seconds —
Do the exercise twice

* If you find the Twist on the Floor too difficult, do the Twist in the Chair.

* * *

BACK

Name of Exercise	Page Number	Advanced Count	Potential Count
Cow	52	Hold for 10 seconds Do the exercise twice	Hold for 20 seconds Do the exercise twice
Curl	80	Hold for 10 seconds Do the exercise twice	Hold for 20 seconds Do the exercise twice
Alternate Leg Stretch	188	Hold for 10 seconds Do the exercise twice	Hold for 20 seconds Do the exercise twice
Backward Bend	140	Hold for 10 seconds Do the exercise twice	Hold for 20 seconds Do the exercise twice
Wings	215	Hold for 10 seconds Do the exercise twice	Hold for 20 seconds Do the exercise twice
Plow	217	Hold for 10 seconds Do the exercise twice *	Hold for 20 seconds Do the exercise twice

* *

CHEST

Name of Exercise	Page Number	Advanced Count	Potential Count
Refreshing Breath	46	Hold for 5 seconds Do the exercise twice	Hold for 10 seconds Do the exercise twice
Chest Expansion	178	Hold for 5 seconds backward and 10 seconds forward Do the exercise twice	Hold for 5 seconds backward and 20 seconds forward Do the exercise twice
Complete Breath	55	Hold for 5 seconds Do the exercise five times	Hold for 10 seconds Do the exercise five times
Cobra	120	Hold for 10 seconds Do the exercise twice	Hold for 20 seconds Do the exercise twice

* * *

CHEST

Name of Exercise	Page Number	Advanced Count	Potential Count
Standing Breath and Chest Stretch	202	Roll your torso twice to your right and twice to your left Do the exercise twice	Roll your torso 3 times to your right and 3 times to your left Do the exercise twice
Wings	215	Hold for 10 seconds Do the exercise twice	Hold for 20 seconds Do the exercise twice
Twist on the Floor*	132	Hold for 10 seconds Do the exercise twice	Hold for 20 seconds Do the exercise twice
Cat	43	Hold for 10 seconds Do the exercise twice	Hold for 20 seconds Do the exercise twice

* If you find the Twist on the Floor too difficult, do the Twist in the Chair.

*   *   *

CHEST

Name of Exercise	Page Number	Advanced Count	Potential Count
Cleansing Breath	62	Do 5 breaths Do the exercise five times	Do 10 breaths Do the exercise five times
Refreshing Breath	46	Hold for 5 seconds Do the exercise twice	Hold for 10 seconds Do the exercise twice
Chest Expansion	178	Hold for 5 seconds backward and 10 seconds forward Do the exercise twice	Hold for 5 seconds backward and 20 seconds forward Do the exercise twice
Cobra	120	Hold for 10 seconds Do the exercise twice	Hold for 20 seconds Do the exercise twice
Bow	184	Hold for 5 seconds Do the exercise twice	—

| Complete Breath | 55 | Hold for 5 seconds
Do the exercise twice | Hold for 10 seconds
Do the exercise twice |

* *
CHEST
* *

Name of Exercise	Page Number	Advanced Count	Potential Count
Slow Hip Roll	94	Roll your hips twice to your right and twice to your left Do the exercise twice	Roll your hips 3 times to your right and 3 times to your left Do the exercise twice
Refreshing Breath	46	Hold for 5 seconds Do the exercise twice	Hold for 10 seconds Do the exercise twice
Backward Bend	140	Hold for 10 seconds Do the exercise twice	Hold for 20 seconds Do the exercise twice
Arch	212	Hold for 10 seconds Do the exercise twice	Hold for 20 seconds Do the exercise twice
Shoulder Stretch	156	Hold for 10 seconds Do the exercise twice	Hold for 20 seconds Do the exercise twice

* *

CHEST

Name of Exercise	Page Number	Advanced Count	Potential Count
Chest Expansion	178	Hold for 5 seconds backward and 10 seconds forward Do the exercise twice	Hold for 5 seconds backward and 20 seconds forward Do the exercise twice
Cleansing Breath	62	Do 5 breaths Do the exercise five times	Do 10 breaths Do the exercise five times
Wings	215	Hold for 10 seconds Do the exercise twice	Hold for 20 seconds Do the exercise twice
Shoulder Stretch	156	Hold for 10 seconds Do the exercise twice	Hold for 20 seconds Do the exercise twice
Bow	184	Hold for 5 seconds Do the exercise twice	—

* * *

CHEST

Name of Exercise	Page Number	Advanced Count	Potential Count
Wings	215	Hold for 10 seconds Do the exercise twice	Hold for 20 seconds Do the exercise twice
Backward Bend	140	Hold for 10 seconds Do the exercise twice	Hold for 20 seconds Do the exercise twice
Standing Breath and Chest Stretch	202	Roll your torso twice to your right and twice to your left Do the exercise twice	Roll your torso 3 times to your right and 3 times to your left Do the exercise twice
Complete Breath	55	Hold for 5 seconds Do the exercise five times	Hold for 10 seconds Do the exercise five times
Cobra	120	Hold for 10 seconds Do the exercise twice	Hold for 20 seconds Do the exercise twice

* * *

HEAD

Name of Exercise	Page Number	Advanced Count	Potential Count
Chest Expansion	178	Hold for 5 seconds backward and 10 seconds forward Do the exercise twice	Hold for 5 seconds backward and 20 seconds forward Do the exercise twice
Preliminary Back and Leg Stretch	109	Hold for 10 seconds Do the exercise twice	Hold for 20 seconds Do the exercise twice
Eye Movements	102	There is no advanced count for this exercise; repeat the last count:	—
First		Do the exercise 3 times	
Second		Do the exercise 3 times	
Third		Do the exercise 3 times	
Fourth		Do the exercise 3 times	

Fifth		Do the exercise 3 times	
Sixth		Do the exercise once	
Rock and Roll	210	Rock back and forth 5 times	—
		Do the exercise twice	
Neti	197	Do the exercise three times	—

* * *

HEAD

Name of Exercise	Page Number	Advanced Count	Potential Count
Cow	52	Hold for 10 seconds Do the exercise twice	Hold for 20 seconds Do the exercise twice
Backward Bend	140	Hold for 10 seconds Do the exercise twice	Hold for 20 seconds Do the exercise twice
Lion	153	Hold for 10 seconds Do the exercise twice	Hold for 20 seconds Do the exercise twice
Cat	43	Hold for 10 seconds Do the exercise twice	Hold for 20 seconds Do the exercise twice
Locust	159	Hold for 5 seconds Do the exercise twice	—

* * *

HEAD

Name of Exercise	Page Number	Advanced Count	Potential Count
Standing Breath and Chest Stretch	202	Roll your torso twice to your right and twice to your left Do the exercise twice	Roll your torso 3 times to your right and 3 times to your left Do the exercise twice
Chest Expansion	178	Hold for 5 seconds backward and 10 seconds forward Do the exercise twice	Hold for 5 seconds backward and 20 seconds forward Do the exercise twice
Cow	52	Hold for 10 seconds Do the exercise twice	Hold for 20 seconds Do the exercise twice
Eye Movements	102	There is no advanced count for this exercise; repeat the last count:	—

First   Do the exercise 3 times
Second   Do the exercise 3 times
Third   Do the exercise 3 times
Fourth   Do the exercise 3 times
Fifth   Do the exercise 3 times
Sixth   Do the exercise once

Rock and Roll   210   Rock back and forth
5 times   —
Do the exercise twice

*   *   *

HEAD

Name of Exercise	Page Number	Advanced Count	Potential Count
Cow	52	Hold for 10 seconds Do the exercise twice	Hold for 20 seconds Do the exercise twice
Side Stretch	174	Hold for 10 seconds Do the exercise twice	Hold for 20 seconds Do the exercise twice
Cat	43	Hold for 10 seconds Do the exercise twice	Hold for 20 seconds Do the exercise twice
Backward Bend	140	Hold for 10 seconds Do the exercise twice	Hold for 20 seconds Do the exercise twice
Neti	197	Do the exercise three times	—

* * *

HEAD

Name of Exercise	Page Number	Advanced Count	Potential Count
Side Stretch	174	Hold for 10 seconds Do the exercise twice	Hold for 20 seconds Do the exercise twice
Slow Hip Roll	94	Roll your hips twice to your right and twice to your left Do the exericse twice	Roll your hips 3 times to your right and 3 times to your left Do the exercise twice
Eye Movements	102	There is no advanced count for this exercise; repeat the last count:	—
First		Do the exercise 3 times	
Second		Do the exercise 3 times	
Third		Do the exercise 3 times	
Fourth		Do the exercise 3 times	

Fifth		Do the exercise 3 times	Hold for 20 seconds
Sixth		Do the exercise once	Do the exercise twice
Lion	153	Hold for 10 seconds	
		Do the exercise twice	
Rock and Roll	210	Rock back and forth 5 times	
		Do the exercise twice	

*

*

*

HEAD

Name of Exercise	Page Number	Advanced Count	Potential Count
Cow	52	Hold for 10 seconds Do the exercise twice	Hold for 20 seconds Do the exercise twice
Chest Expansion	178	Hold for 5 seconds backward and 10 seconds forward Do the exercise twice	Hold for 5 seconds backward and 20 seconds forward Do the exercise twice
Standing Breath and Chest Stretch	202	Roll your torso twice to your right and twice to your left Do the exercise twice	Roll your torso 3 times to your right and 3 times to your left Do the exercise twice
Cat	43	Hold for 10 seconds Do the exercise twice	Hold for 20 seconds Do the exercise twice

Eye Movements	102	There is no advanced count for this exercise; repeat the last count:	—
First		Do the exercise 3 times	
Second		Do the exercise 3 times	
Third		Do the exercise 3 times	
Fourth		Do the exercise 3 times	
Fifth		Do the exercise 3 times	
Sixth		Do the exercise once	
Backward Bend	140	Hold for 10 seconds Do the exercise twice	Hold for 20 seconds Do the exercise twice
Lion	153	Hold for 10 seconds Do the exercise twice	Hold for 20 seconds Do the exercise twice

*   *   *

LEGS

Name of Exercise	Page Number	Advanced Count	Potential Count
Standing Twist*	65	Hold for 10 seconds Do the exercise twice	Hold for 20 seconds Do the exercise twice
Squat	70	Hold for 20 seconds Do the exercise twice	Hold for 30 seconds Do the exercise twice
Knee and Thigh	113	Hold for 10 seconds Do the exercise twice	Hold for 20 seconds Do the exercise twice
Backward Bend**	140	Hold for 10 seconds Do the exercise twice	Hold for 20 seconds Do the exercise twice
Leg Stretches	147	Hold for 10 seconds Do the exercise twice	Hold for 20 seconds Do the exercise twice

* Do the exercise on your toes. ** After you have completed the exercise with your toes pointed backward, your insteps on the floor, do the exercise twice with your toes pointed forward, the cushions of your toes resting flat on the floor.

*   *   *   *

LEGS

Name of Exercise	Page Number	Advanced Count	Potential Count
Rock-A-Bye-Baby	74	Rock your leg from side to side 10 times Do the exercise twice	—
Back of Leg Stretch	41	Hold for 10 seconds Do the exercise twice	Hold for 20 seconds Do the exercise twice
Knee and Thigh	113	Hold for 10 seconds Do the exercise twice	Hold for 20 seconds Do the exercise twice
Backward Bend*	140	Hold for 10 seconds Do the exercise twice	Hold for 20 seconds Do the exercise twice

* After you have completed the exercise with your toes pointed backward, your insteps on the floor, do the exercise twice with your toes pointed forward, the cushions of your toes resting flat on the floor.

* * *

LEGS

Name of Exercise	Page Number	Advanced Count	Potential Count
Arm and Leg	90	Hold for 10 seconds Do the exercise twice	Hold for 20 seconds Do the exercise twice
Chest Expansion	179	Hold for 5 seconds backward and 10 seconds forward Do the exercise twice	Hold for 5 seconds backward and 20 seconds forward Do the exercise twice
Squat	70	Hold for 10 seconds Do the exercise twice	Hold for 20 seconds Do the exercise twice
Bow	184	Hold for 5 seconds Do the exercise twice	—
Leg Stretches	147	Hold for 10 seconds Do the exercise twice	Hold for 20 seconds Do the exercise twice

* * *

LEGS

Name of Exercise	Page Number	Advanced Count	Potential Count
Half Lotus*	169	Hold for 30 seconds Do the exercise twice	Hold for 60 seconds Do the exercise twice
Rock-A-Bye-Baby	74	Rock your leg from side to side 10 times Do the exercise twice	—
Alternate Leg Stretch	188	Hold for 10 seconds Do the exercise twice	Hold for 20 seconds Do the exercise twice
Backward Bend**	140	Hold for 10 seconds Do the exercise twice	Hold for 20 seconds Do the exercise twice
Back of Leg Stretch	41	Hold for 10 seconds Do the exercise twice	Hold for 20 seconds Do the exercise twice

Name of Exercise	Page Number	Advanced Count		Potential Count	
Leg Stretches	147	Hold for 10 seconds Do the exercise twice		Hold for 20 seconds Do the exercise twice	

* If you find the Half Lotus too difficult, do the Tailor posture.
** After you have completed the exercise with your toes pointed backward, your insteps on the floor, do the exercise twice with your toes pointed forward, the cushions of your toes resting flat on the floor.

* * *

LEGS

Name of Exercise	Page Number	Advanced Count	Potential Count
Arm and Leg	90	Hold for 10 seconds Do the exercise twice	Hold for 20 seconds Do the exercise twice

Squat	70	Hold for 20 seconds Do the exercise twice	Hold for 30 seconds Do the exercise twice
Half Lotus*	171	Hold for 30 seconds Do the exercise twice	Hold for 60 seconds Do the exercise twice
Back of Leg Stretch	41	Hold for 10 seconds Do the exercise twice	Hold for 20 seconds Do the exercise twice
Knee and Thigh	113	Hold for 10 seconds Do the exercise twice	Hold for 20 seconds Do the exercise twice
Curl	80	Hold for 10 seconds Do the exercise twice	Hold for 20 seconds Do the exercise twice

* If you find the Half Lotus too difficult, do the Tailor posture.

*   *   *

LEGS

Name of Exercise	Page Number	Advanced Count	Potential Count
Rock-A-Bye-Baby	74	Rock your leg from side to side 10 times Do the exercise twice	—
Spread Leg Stretch	76	Hold for 10 seconds Do the exercise twice	Hold for 20 seconds Do the exercise twice
Knee and Thigh	113	Hold for 10 seconds Do the exercise twice	Hold for 20 seconds Do the exercise twice
Leg Stretches	147	Hold for 10 seconds Do the exercise twice	Hold for 20 seconds Do the exercise twice

*   *

*

LEGS

Name of Exercise	Page Number	Advanced Count	Potential Count
Standing Twist*	65	Hold for 10 seconds Do the exercise twice	Hold for 20 seconds Do the exercise twice
Squat	70	Hold for 20 seconds Do the exercise twice	Hold for 30 seconds Do the exercise twice
Curl	80	Hold for 10 seconds Do the exercise twice	Hold for 20 seconds Do the exercise twice
Locust	159	Hold for 5 seconds Do the exercise twice	—
Bow	184	Hold for 5 seconds Do the exercise twice	—

* Do the exercise on your toes.

LEGS

Name of Exercise	Page Number	Advanced Count	Potential Count
Rock-A-Bye-Baby	74	Rock your leg from side to side 10 times Do the exercise twice	—
Alternate Leg Stretch	188	Hold for 10 seconds Do the exercise twice	Hold for 20 seconds Do the exercise twice
Spread Leg Stretch	76	Hold for 10 seconds Do the exercise twice	Hold for 20 seconds Do the exercise twice
Backward Bend*	140	Hold for 10 seconds Do the exercise twice	Hold for 20 seconds Do the exercise twice
Back of Leg Stretch	41	Hold for 10 seconds Do the exercise twice	Hold for 20 seconds Do the exercise twice

Bow	184	Hold for 5 seconds Do the exercise twice	—	Hold for 20 seconds Do the exercise twice
Leg Stretches	147	Hold for 10 seconds Do the exercise twice		Hold for 20 seconds Do the exercise twice

* After you have completed the exercise with your toes pointed backward, your insteps on the floor, do the exercise twice with your toes pointed forward, the cushions of your toes resting flat on the floor.

*   *   *

NECK

Name of Exercise	Page Number	Advanced Count	Potential Count
Cow	52	Hold for 10 seconds Do the exercise twice	Hold for 20 seconds Do the exercise twice
Side Stretch	174	Hold for 10 seconds Do the exercise twice	Hold for 20 seconds Do the exercise twice
Arch	212	Hold for 10 seconds Do the exercise twice	Hold for 20 seconds Do the exercise twice
Three-Way Neck Stretch	206	Hold for 10 seconds Do the exercise twice	—
Shoulder Stand	192	Hold for 1 minute Do the exercise twice	Hold for 2 minutes Do the exercise twice

* * *

NECK

Name of Exercise	Page Number	Advanced Count	Potential Count
Slow Neck Roll	83	Roll your head twice to your right and twice to your left Do the exercise twice	Roll your head 3 times to your right and 3 times to your left Do the exercise twice
Backward Bend	140	Hold for 10 seconds Do the exercise twice	Hold for 20 seconds Do the exercise twice
Plow	217	Hold for 10 seconds Do the exercise twice	Hold for 20 seconds Do the exercise twice

Ninety-Second
Relaxer

161 There is no advanced
-count for this exercise;
repeat the last count:
take 30 seconds each to
lower your body, hold
the position, and raise
your body
Do the exercise once

*

*   *

*

NECK

Name of Exercise	Page Number	Advanced Count	Potential Count
Chest Expansion	178	Hold for 5 seconds backward and 10 seconds forward Do the exercise twice	Hold for 5 seconds backward and 20 seconds forward Do the exercise twice
Side Stretch	174	Hold for 10 seconds Do the exercise twice	Hold for 20 seconds Do the exercise twice
Wings	215	Hold for 10 seconds Do the exercise twice	Hold for 20 seconds Do the exercise twice
Four-Way Neck Stretch	116	Hold for 10 seconds Do the exercise twice	—
Cobra	120	Hold for 10 seconds Do the exercise twice * *	Hold for 20 seconds Do the exercise twice

NECK

Name of Exercise	Page Number	Advanced Count	Potential Count
Cow	52	Hold for 10 seconds Do the exercise twice	Hold for 20 seconds Do the exercise twice
Wings	215	Hold for 10 seconds Do the exercise twice	Hold for 20 seconds Do the exercise twice
Cat	43	Hold for 10 seconds Do the exercise twice	Hold for 20 seconds Do the exercise twice
Slow Neck Roll	83	Roll your head twice to your right and twice to your left Do the exercise twice	Roll your head 3 times to your right and 3 times to your left Do the exercise twice

* * *

298

NECK

Name of Exercise	Page Number	Advanced Count	Potential Count
Cow	52	Hold for 10 seconds Do the exercise twice	Hold for 20 seconds Do the exercise twice
Chest Expansion	178	Hold for 5 seconds backward and 10 seconds forward Do the exercise twice	Hold for 5 seconds backward and 20 seconds forward Do the exercise twice
Three-Way Neck Stretch	205	Hold for 10 seconds Do the exercise twice	—
Wings	215	Hold for 10 seconds Do the exercise twice	Hold for 20 seconds Do the exercise twice

*   *   *

NECK

Name of Exercise	Page Number	Advanced Count	Potential Count
Backward Bend	140	Hold for 10 seconds Do the exercise twice	Hold for 20 seconds Do the exercise twice
Curl	80	Hold for 10 seconds Do the exercise twice	Hold for 20 seconds Do the exercise twice
Slow Neck Roll	83	Roll your head twice to your right and twice to your left Do the exercise twice	Roll your head 3 times to your right and 3 times to your left Do the exercise twice
Wings	215	Hold for 10 seconds Do the exercise twice	Hold for 20 seconds Do the exercise twice
	*	*	*

SHOULDERS

Name of Exercise	Page Number	Advanced Count	Potential Count
Chest Expansion	178	Hold for 5 seconds backward and 10 seconds forward Do the exercise twice	Hold for 5 seconds backward and 20 seconds forward Do the exercise twice
Twist on the Floor*	132	Hold for 10 seconds Do the exercise twice	Hold for 20 seconds Do the exercise twice
Wings	215	Hold for 10 seconds Do the exercise twice	Hold for 20 seconds Do the exercise twice
Backward Bend	140	Hold for 10 seconds Do the exercise twice	Hold for 20 seconds Do the exercise twice

* If you find the Twist on the Floor too difficult, do the Twist in the Chair.

*   *   *   *

301

SHOULDERS

Name of Exercise	Page Number	Advanced Count	Potential Count
Chest Expansion	178	Hold for 5 seconds backward and 10 seconds forward Do the exercise twice	Hold for 5 seconds backward and 20 seconds forward Do the exercise twice
Cat	43	Hold for 10 seconds Do the exercise twice	Hold for 20 seconds Do the exercise twice
Wings	215	Hold for 10 seconds Do the exercise twice	Hold for 20 seconds Do the exercise twice
Backward Bend	140	Hold for 10 seconds Do the exercise twice	Hold for 20 seconds Do the exercise twice
Shoulder Stand	192	Hold for 1 minute Do the exercise once	Hold for 2 minutes Do the exercise once

* * *

SHOULDERS

Name of Exercise	Page Number	Advanced Count	Potential Count
Side Stretch	174	Hold for 10 seconds Do the exercise twice	Hold for 20 seconds Do the exercise twice
Arm and Leg	90	Hold for 10 seconds Do the exercise twice	Hold for 20 seconds Do the exercise twice
Backward Bend	140	Hold for 10 seconds Do the exercise twice	Hold for 20 seconds Do the exercise twice
Plow	217	Hold for 10 seconds Do the exercise twice	Hold for 20 seconds Do the exercise twice

* * *

SHOULDERS

Name of Exercise	Page Number	Advanced Count	Potential Count
Wings	215	Hold for 10 seconds Do the exercise twice	Hold for 20 seconds Do the exercise twice
Shoulder Stretch	156	Hold for 10 seconds Do the exercise twice	Hold for 20 seconds Do the exercise twice
Curl	80	Hold for 10 seconds Do the exercise twice	Hold for 20 seconds Do the exercise twice
Bow	184	Hold for 5 seconds Do the exercise twice	—
Cobra	120	Hold for 10 seconds Do the exercise twice	Hold for 20 seconds Do the exercise twice

* * *

SHOULDERS

Name of Exercise	Page Number	Advanced Count	Potential Count
Chest Expansion	178	Hold for 5 seconds backward and 10 seconds forward Do the exercise twice	Hold for 5 seconds backward and 20 seconds forward Do the exercise twice
Twist on the Floor*	132	Hold for 10 seconds Do the exercise twice	Hold for 20 seconds Do the exercise twice
Wings	215	Hold for 10 seconds Do the exercise twice	Hold for 20 seconds Do the exercise twice
Shoulder Stretch	156	Hold for 10 seconds Do the exercise twice	Hold for 20 seconds Do the exercise twice
Rock and Roll	210	Rock back and forth 5 times Do the exercise twice	—

* If you find the Twist on the Floor too difficult, do the Twist in the Chair.

* * *

SHOULDERS

Name of Exercise	Page Number	Advanced Count	Potential Count
Standing Twist	65	Hold for 10 seconds Do the exercise twice	Hold for 20 seconds Do the exercise twice
Chest Expansion	178	Hold for 5 seconds backward and 10 seconds forward Do the exercise twice	Hold for 5 seconds backward and 20 seconds forward Do the exercise twice
Bow	184	Hold for 5 seconds Do the exercise twice	—
Wings	215	Hold for 10 seconds Do the exercise twice	Hold for 20 seconds Do the exercise twice
Plow	217	Hold for 10 seconds Do the exercise twice	Hold for 20 seconds Do the exercise twice

* * *

MINIPROGRAMS FOR COMMON PROBLEMS

BALANCE

Name of Exercise	Page Number	Advanced Count	Potential Count
Refreshing Breath*	46	Hold for 5 seconds Do the exercise twice	Hold for 10 seconds Do the exercise twice
Standing Twist*	65	Hold for 10 seconds Do the exercise twice	Hold for 20 seconds Do the exercise twice
Slow Hip Roll	94	Roll your hips twice to your right and twice to your left Do the exercise twice	Roll your hips 3 times to your right and 3 times to your left Do the exercise twice
Squat	70	Hold for 20 seconds Do the exercise twice	Hold for 30 seconds Do the exercise twice

* Do the exercise on your toes

*   *   *

308

BALANCE

Name of Exercise	Page Number	Advanced Count	Potential Count
Arm and Leg	90	Hold for 10 seconds Do the exercise twice	Hold for 20 seconds Do the exercise twice
Chest Expansion	178	Hold for 5 seconds backward and 10 seconds forward Do the exercise twice	Hold for 5 seconds backward and 20 seconds forward Do the exercise twice
Standing Breath and Chest Stretch	202	Roll your torso twice to your right and twice to your left Do the exercise twice	Roll your torso 3 times to your right and 3 times to your left Do the exercise twice
Squat	70	Hold for 20 seconds Do the exercise twice	Hold for 30 seconds Do the exercise twice

| Leg Stretches | 147 | Hold for 10 seconds
Do the exercise twice | Hold for 20 seconds
Do the exercise twice |

* * *

BALANCE

Name of Exercise	Page Number	Advanced Count	Potential Count
Tree	128	Hold for 10 seconds Do the exercise twice	Hold for 20 seconds Do the exercise twice
Refreshing Breath*	46	Hold for 5 seconds Do the exercise twice	Hold for 10 seconds Do the exercise twice

| Slow Hip Roll | 94 | Roll your hips twice to your right and twice to your left
Do the exercise twice | Roll your hips 3 times to your right and 3 times to your left
Do the exercise twice |
| Leg Stretches | 147 | Hold for 10 seconds
Do the exercise twice | Hold for 20 seconds
Do the exercise twice |

* Do the exercise on your toes.

           *   *   *

BALANCE

Name of Exercise	Page Number	Advanced Count	Potential Count
Arm and Leg	90	Hold for 10 seconds Do the exercise twice	Hold for 20 seconds Do the exercise twice

Standing Breath and Chest Stretch	202	Roll your torso twice to your right and twice to your left Do the exercise twice	Roll your torso 3 times to your right and 3 times to your left Do the exercise twice
Squat	70	Hold for 20 seconds Do the exercise twice	Hold for 30 seconds Do the exercise twice
Backward Bend*	140	Hold for 10 seconds Do the exercise twice	Hold for 20 seconds Do the exercise twice
Knee and Thigh	113	Hold for 10 seconds Do the exercise twice	Hold for 20 seconds Do the exercise twice

* After you have completed the exercise with your toes pointed backward, your insteps on the floor, do the exercise twice with your toes pointed forward, the cushions of your toes resting flat on the floor.

* * * *

BALANCE

Name of Exercise	Page Number	Advanced Count	Potential Count
Tree	128	Hold for 10 seconds Do the exercise twice	Hold for 20 seconds Do the exercise twice
Refreshing Breath*	46	Hold for 5 seconds Do the exercise twice	Hold for 10 seconds Do the exercise twice
Slow Hip Roll	94	Roll your hips twice to your right and twice to your left Do the exercise twice	Roll your hips 3 times to your right and 3 times to your left Do the exercise twice
Spread Leg Stretch	76	Hold for 10 seconds Do the exercise twice	Hold for 20 seconds Do the exercise twice
Back of Leg Stretch	41	Hold for 10 seconds Do the exercise twice	Hold for 20 seconds Do the exercise twice

* Do the exercise on your toes.

* * *

BALANCE

Name of Exercise	Page Number	Advanced Count	Potential Count
Side Stretch	174	Hold for 10 seconds. Do the exercise twice	Hold for 20 seconds. Do the exercise twice
Arm and Leg	90	Hold for 10 seconds. Do the exercise twice	Hold for 20 seconds. Do the exercise twice
Standing Breath and Chest Stretch	202	Roll your torso twice to your right and twice to your left. Do the exercise twice	Roll your torso 3 times to your right and 3 times to your left. Do the exercise twice
Backward Bend*	140	Hold for 10 seconds. Do the exercise twice	Hold for 20 seconds. Do the exercise twice
Rock-A-Bye-Baby	74	Rock your leg from side to side 10 times	—

Do the exercise twice

Back of Leg
Stretch

41 Hold for 10 seconds
Do the exercise twice

Hold for 20 seconds
Do the exercise twice

* After you have completed the exercise with your toes pointed backward, your insteps on the floor, do the exercise twice with your toes pointed forward, the cushions of your toes resting flat on the floor.

*   *   *   *

315

CONSTIPATION

Name of Exercise	Page Number	Advanced Count	Potential Count
Slow Hip Roll	94	Roll your hips twice to your right and twice to your left Do the exercise twice	Roll your hips 3 times to your right and 3 times to your left Do the exercise twice
Squat	70	Hold for 20 seconds Do the exercise twice	Hold for 30 seconds Do the exercise twice
Abdominal Lift*	166	Do 5 lifts Do the exercise five times	Do 10 lifts Do the exercise five times
Leg Stretches	147	Hold for 10 seconds Do the exercise twice	Hold for 20 seconds Do the exercise twice

* Do the exercise in the position you prefer, lying or sitting.

* * *

316

CONSTIPATION

Name of Exercise	Page Number	Advanced Count	Potential Count
Abdominal Lift*	166	Do 5 lifts Do the exercise five times	Do 10 lifts Do the exercise five times
Twist on the Floor**	132	Hold for 10 seconds Do the exercise twice	Hold for 20 seconds Do the exercise twice
Curl	80	Hold for 10 seconds Do the exercise twice	Hold for 20 seconds Do the exercise twice
Shoulder Stand	192	Hold for 1 minute Do the exercise once	Hold for 2 minutes Do the exercise once

* Do the exercise in the position you prefer, lying or sitting.
** If you find the Twist on the Floor too difficult, do the Twist in the Chair.

* * *

CONSTIPATION

Name of Exercise	Page Number	Advanced Count	Potential Count
Slow Hip Roll	94	Roll your hips twice to your right and twice to your left Do the exercise twice	Roll your hips 3 times to your right and 3 times to your left Do the exercise twice
Squat	70	Hold for 20 seconds Do the exercise twice	Hold for 30 seconds Do the exercise twice
Abdominal Lift*	166	Do 5 lifts Do the exercise five times	Do 10 lifts Do the exercise five times
Curl	80	Hold for 10 seconds Do the exercise twice	Hold for 20 seconds Do the exercise twice

Name of Exercise	Page Number	Advanced Count	Potential Count
Bow	184	Hold for 5 seconds Do the exercise twice	—
Rock and Roll	210	Rock back and forth 5 times Do the exercise twice	—

* Do the exercise in the position you prefer, lying or sitting.

* * *

CONSTIPATION

Name of Exercise	Page Number	Advanced Count	Potential Count
Squat	70	Hold for 20 seconds Do the exercise twice	Hold for 30 seconds Do the exercise twice

Abdominal Lift*	166	Do 5 lifts Do the exercise five times	Do 10 lifts Do the exercise five times
Chest Expansion	178	Hold for 5 seconds backward and 10 seconds forward Do the exercise twice	Hold for 5 seconds backward and 20 seconds forward Do the exercise twice
Cobra	120	Hold for 10 seconds Do the exercise twice	Hold for 20 seconds Do the exercise twice
Shoulder Stand	192	Hold for 1 minute Do the exercise once	Hold for 2 minutes Do the exercise once

* Do the exercise in the position you prefer, lying or sitting.

*   *   *

POSTURE

Name of Exercise	Page Number	Advanced Count	Potential Count
Chest Expansion	178	Hold for 5 seconds backward and 10 seconds forward Do the exercise twice	Hold for 5 seconds backward and 20 seconds forward Do the exercise twice
Side Stretch	174	Hold for 10 seconds Do the exercise twice	Hold for 20 seconds Do the exercise twice
Wings	215	Hold for 10 seconds Do the exercise twice	Hold for 20 seconds Do the exercise twice
Backward Bend*	140	Hold for 10 seconds Do the exercise twice	Hold for 20 seconds Do the exercise twice

Rock and Roll   210   Rock back and forth   —
                        5 times
                        Do the exercise twice

* After you have completed the exercise with your toes pointed backward, your
insteps on the floor, do the exercise twice with your toes pointed forward, the
cushions of your toes resting flat on the floor.

*   *   *

POSTURE

Name of Exercise	Page Number	Advanced Count	Potential Count
Wings	215	Hold for 10 seconds Do the exercise twice	Hold for 20 seconds Do the exercise twice
Shoulder Stretch	156	Hold for 10 seconds Do the exercise twice	Hold for 20 seconds Do the exercise twice
Cat	43	Hold for 10 seconds Do the exercise twice	Hold for 20 seconds Do the exercise twice
Cobra	120	Hold for 10 seconds Do the exercise twice	Hold for 20 seconds Do the exercise twice
		*	
	*		
		*	

POSTURE

Name of Exercise	Page Number	Advanced Count	Potential Count
Chest Expansion	178	Hold for 5 seconds backward and 10 seconds forward Do the exercise twice	Hold for 5 seconds backward and 20 seconds forward Do the exercise twice
Cow	52	Hold for 10 seconds Do the exercise twice	Hold for 20 seconds Do the exercise twice
Arch	212	Hold for 10 seconds Do the exercise twice	Hold for 20 seconds Do the exercise twice
Cobra	120	Hold for 10 seconds Do the exercise twice	Hold for 20 seconds Do the exercise twice
Bow	184	Hold for 5 seconds Do the exercise twice	—

Name of Exercise	Page Number	Advanced Count	Potential Count
Shoulder Stand	192	Hold for 1 minute Do the exercise once	Hold for 2 minutes Do the exercise once

* * *

POSTURE

Name of Exercise	Page Number	Advanced Count	Potential Count
Slow Hip Roll	94	Roll your hips twice to your right and twice to your left Do the exercise twice	Roll your hips 3 times to your right and 3 times to your left Do the exercise twice
Arm and Leg	90	Hold for 10 seconds Do the exercise twice	Hold for 20 seconds Do the exercise twice

POSTURE

Name of Exercise	Page Number	Advanced Count	Potential Count
Cat	43	Hold for 10 seconds Do the exercise twice	Hold for 20 seconds Do the exercise twice
Wings	215	Hold for 10 seconds Do the exercise twice	Hold for 20 seconds Do the exercise twice
Rock and Roll	210	Rock back and forth 5 times Do the exercise twice	—
		*	
		*	
		*	

Cow	52	Hold for 10 seconds Do the exercise twice	Hold for 20 seconds Do the exercise twice
Standing Twist*	65	Hold for 10 seconds Do the exercise twice	Hold for 20 seconds Do the exercise twice
Chest Expansion	178	Hold for 5 seconds backward and 10 seconds forward Do the exercise twice	Hold for 5 seconds backward and 20 seconds forward Do the exercise twice
Wings	215	Hold for 10 seconds Do the exercise twice	Hold for 20 seconds Do the exercise twice
Curl	80	Hold for 10 seconds Do the exercise twice	Hold for 20 seconds Do the exercise twice

* Do the exercise on your toes.

* * *

327

POSTURE

Name of Exercise	Page Number	Advanced Count	Potential Count
Standing Breath and Chest Stretch	202	Roll your torso twice to your right and twice to your left Do the exercise twice	Roll your torso 3 times to your right and 3 times to your left Do the exercise twice
Chest Expansion		Hold for 5 seconds backward and 10 seconds forward Do the exercise twice	Hold for 5 seconds backward and 20 seconds forward Do the exercise twice
Shoulder Stretch	178	Hold for 10 seconds Do the exercise twice	Hold for 20 seconds Do the exercise twice
Twist on the Floor*	132	Hold for 10 seconds Do the exercise twice	Hold for 20 seconds Do the exercise twice

Plow   217   Hold for 10 seconds   Hold for 20 seconds
                     Do the exercise twice   Do the exercise twice

* If you find the Twist on the Floor too difficult, do the Twist in the Chair.

           *   *   *

SLEEP

Name of Exercise	Page Number	Advanced Count	Potential Count
Slow Neck Roll	83	Roll your head twice to your right and	Roll your head 3 times to your right and

Exercise			
Wings	215	twice to your left Do the exercise twice	3 times to your left Do the exercise twice
Complete Breath	55	Hold for 10 seconds Do the exercise twice Hold your breath for 5 seconds Do the exercise five times	Hold for 20 seconds Do the exercise twice Hold your breath for 10 seconds Do the exercise five times
Ninety-Second Relaxer	161	There is no advanced count for this exercise, repeat the last count: take 30 seconds each to lower your body, hold the position, and raise your body Do the exercise once	—

Name of Exercise	Page Number	Advanced Count	Potential Count
Cow	52	Hold for 10 seconds. Do the exercise twice	Hold for 20 seconds. Do the exercise twice
Cat	43	Hold for 10 seconds. Do the exercise twice	Hold for 20 seconds. Do the exercise twice
Three-Way Neck Stretch	206	Hold for 10 seconds. Do the exercise twice	—
Alternate Nostril Breathing	223	Inhale for the count of 6, hold your breath for the count of 6, and exhale for the count of 6. Do the exercise six times	Inhale for the count of 8, hold your breath for the count of 8, and exhale for the count of 8. Do the exercise eight times
Raja Yoga	228	— * * *	—

SLEEP

Name of Exercise	Page Number	Advanced Count	Potential Count
Chest Expansion	178	Hold for 5 seconds backward and 10 seconds forward Do the exercise twice	Hold for 5 seconds backward and 20 seconds forward Do the exercise twice
Cobra	120	Hold for 10 seconds Do the exercise twice	Hold for 20 seconds Do the exercise twice
Slow Neck Roll	83	Roll your head twice to your right and twice to your left Do the exercise twice	Roll your head 3 times to your right and 3 times to your left Do the exercise twice
Complete Breath	55	Hold your breath for 5 seconds	Hold your breath for 10 seconds

	Do the exercise five times	Do the exercise five times
Raja Yoga	228 —	—
	*	
	*	
	*	

SLEEP

Name of Exercise	Page Number	Advanced Count	Potential Count
Complete Breath	55	Hold your breath for 5 seconds Do the exercise five times	Hold your breath for 10 seconds Do the exercise five times
Four-Way Neck Stretch	116	Hold for 10 seconds Do the exercise twice	—
Wings	215	Hold for 10 seconds Do the exercise twice	Hold for 20 seconds Do the exercise twice
Alternate Nostril Breathing	223	Inhale for the count of 6, hold your breath for the count of 6, and exhale for the	Inhale for the count of 8, hold your breath for the count of 8, and exhale for the

			count of 6	count of 8
Ninety-Second Relaxer	161	There is no advanced count for this exercise; repeat the last count: take 30 seconds each to lower your body, hold the position, and raise your body Do the exercise once	Do the exercise six times	Do the exercise eight times —

*   *   *

TENSION

Name of Exercise	Page Number	Advanced Count	Potential Count
Cow	52	Hold for 10 seconds Do the exercise twice	Hold for 20 seconds Do the exercise twice
Slow Neck Roll	83	Roll your head twice to your right and twice to your left Do the exercise twice	Roll your head 3 times to your right and 3 times to your left Do the exercise twice
Lion	153	Hold for 10 seconds Do the exercise twice	Hold for 20 seconds Do the exercise twice
Cobra	120	Hold for 10 seconds Do the exercise twice	Hold for 20 seconds Do the exercise twice
Raja yoga	228	—	—

* * *

TENSION

Name of Exercise	Page Number	Advanced Count	Potential Count
Refreshing Breath	46	Hold for 5 seconds Do the exercise twice	Hold for 10 seconds Do the exercise twice
Chest Expansion	178	Hold for 5 seconds backward and 10 seconds forward Do the exercise twice	Hold for 5 seconds backward and 20 seconds forward Do the exercise twice
Wings	215	Hold for 10 seconds Do the exercise twice	Hold for 20 seconds Do the exercise twice

| Ninety-Second Relaxer | 161 | There is no advanced count for this exercise; repeat the last count: take 30 seconds each to lower your body, hold the position, and raise your body
Do the exercise once | — |
| | | * | * | * |

TENSION

Name of Exercise	Page Number	Advanced Count	Potential Count
Rock and Roll	210	Rock back and forth 5 times Do the exercise twice	—
Bow	184	Hold for 5 seconds Do the exercise twice	—
Cobra	120	Hold for 10 seconds Do the exercise twice	Hold for 20 seconds Do the exercise twice
Three-Way Neck Stretch	206	Hold for 10 seconds Do the exercise twice	—
Raja Yoga	228	—	—
	*	* *	

TENSION

Name of Exercise	Page Number	Advanced Count	Potential Count
Cleansing Breath	62	Do 5 breaths Do the exercise five times	Do 10 breaths Do the exercise five times
Wings	215	Hold for 10 seconds Do the exercise twice	Hold for 20 seconds Do the exercise twice
Four-Way Neck Stretch	116	Hold for 10 seconds Do the exercise twice	—
Curl	80	Hold for 10 seconds Do the exercise twice	Hold for 20 seconds Do the exercise twice
Complete Breath	55	Hold for 5 seconds	Hold for 10 seconds

Do the exercise five times   Do the exercise five times

* * *

TENSION

Name of Exercise	Page Number	Advanced Count	Potential Count
Cow	52	Hold for 10 seconds Do the exercise twice	Hold for 20 seconds Do the exercise twice
Wings	215	Hold for 10 seconds Do the exercise twice	Hold for 20 seconds Do the exercise twice
Slow Neck Roll	83	Roll your head twice to your right and twice to your left Do the exercise twice	Roll your head 3 times to your right and 3 times to your left Do the exercise twice

Name of Exercise	Page Number	Advanced Count	Potential Count
Cobra	120	Hold for 10 seconds Do the exercise twice	Hold for 20 seconds Do the exercise twice
Alternate Nostril Breathing	223	Inhale for the count of 6, hold your breath for the count of 6, and exhale for the count of 6 Do the exercise six times	Inhale for the count of 8, hold your breath for the count of 8, and exhale for the count of 8 Do the exercise eight times

*   *   *

TENSION

Name of Exercise	Page Number	Advanced Count	Potential Count
Refreshing Breath	46	Hold for 5 seconds Do the exercise twice	Hold for 10 seconds Do the exercise twice

Cow	52	Hold for 10 seconds Do the exercise twice	Hold for 20 seconds Do the exercise twice
Chest Expansion	178	Hold for 5 seconds backward and 10 seconds forward Do the exercise twice	Hold for 5 seconds backward and 20 seconds forward Do the exercise twice
Four-Way Neck Stretch	116	Hold for 10 seconds Do the exercise twice	—
Rock and Roll	210	Rock back and forth 5 times Do the exercise twice	—
Raja Yoga	228	—	—.
		* * *	*

APPENDIX A

EXERCISES THAT MAY BE DONE IN BED

Abdominal Lift
Alternate Leg Stretch
Alternate Nostril Breathing
Back of Leg Stretch
Cleansing Breath
Complete Breath
Eye Movements
Finger Clasp
Four-Way Neck Stretch
Half Lotus
Leg Stretches

Lion
Ninety-Second Relaxer
Preliminary Back and Leg Stretch
Raja Yoga
Rock-A-Bye-Baby
Shoulder Stretch
Slow Neck Roll
Spread Leg Stretch
Tailor
Three-Way Neck Stretch
Wings

APPENDIX B

EXERCISES THAT MAY BE DONE IN A CHAIR

Abdominal Lift
Alternate Nostril Breathing
Cleansing Breath
Complete Breath
Eye Movements
Finger Clasp
Four-Way Neck Stretch
Lion
Shoulder Stretch
Slow Neck Roll
Three-Way Neck Stretch
Twist in the Chair
Wings

APPENDIX C

AN ALPHABETICAL LIST OF ALL THE EXERCISES TOGETHER WITH THE BEGINNING, THE ADVANCED, AND THE POTENTIAL COUNTS

Name of Exercise	Beginning Count	Advanced Count	Potential Count
Abdominal Lift	Do 5 lifts Do the exercise twice	Do 5 lifts Do the exercise five times	Do 10 lifts Do the exercise five times
Alternate Leg Stretch	Hold for 5 seconds Do the exercise twice	Hold for 10 seconds Do the exercise twice	Hold for 20 seconds Do the exercise twice
Alternate Nostril Breathing	Inhale for the count of 4, hold your breath for the count of 4, and exhale for the count of 4 Do the exercise four times	Inhale for the count of 6, hold your breath for the count of 6, and exhale for the count of 6 Do the exercise six times	Inhale for the count of 8, hold your breath for the count of 8, and exhale for the count of 8 Do the exercise eight times

Arch	Hold for 5 seconds Do the exercise twice	Hold for 10 seconds Do the exercise twice	Hold for 20 seconds Do the exercise twice
Arm and Leg	Hold for 5 seconds Do the exercise twice	Hold for 10 seconds Do the exercise twice	Hold for 20 seconds Do the exercise twice
Back of Leg Stretch	Hold for 5 seconds Do the exercise twice	Hold for 10 seconds Do the exercise twice	Hold for 20 seconds Do the exercise twice
Backward Bend	Hold for 5 seconds Do the exercise twice	Hold for 10 seconds Do the exercise twice	Hold for 20 seconds Do the exercise twice
Bow	Hold for 3 seconds Do the exercise twice	Hold for 5 seconds Do the exercise twice	—
Cat	Hold for 5 seconds Do the exercise twice	Hold for 10 seconds Do the exercise twice	Hold for 20 seconds Do the exercise twice
Chest Expansion	Hold for 3 seconds backward and 5 seconds forward Do the exercise twice	Hold for 5 seconds backward and 10 seconds forward Do the exercise twice	Hold for 5 seconds backward and 20 seconds forward Do the exercise twice
Cleansing Breath	Do 5 breaths Do the exercise five times	Do 5 breaths Do the exercise twice	Do 10 breaths Do the exercise twice

Name of Exercise	Beginning Count	Advanced Count	Potential Count
Cobra	Hold for 5 seconds Do the exercise twice	Hold for 10 seconds Do the exercise twice	Hold for 20 seconds Do the exercise twice
Complete Breath	Hold your breath for 3 seconds Do the exercise twice	Hold your breath for 5 seconds Do the exercise five times	Hold your breath for 10 seconds Do the exercise five times
Cow	Hold for 5 seconds Do the exercise twice	Hold for 10 seconds Do the exercise twice	Hold for 20 seconds Do the exercise twice
Curl	Hold for 5 seconds Do the exercise twice	Hold for 10 seconds Do the exercise twice	Hold for 20 seconds Do the exercise twice
Eye Movements First Second Third Fourth Fifth Sixth	Do the exercise 3 times Do the exercise 3 times Do the exercise 3 times Do the exercise 3 times Do the exercise 3 times Do the exercise once	—	—
Finger Clasp	Hold for 5 seconds Do the exercise twice	Hold for 10 seconds Do the exercise twice	Hold for 20 seconds Do the exercise twice

Exercise			
Four-Way Neck Stretch	Hold for 5 seconds Do the exercise twice	Hold for 10 seconds Do the exercise twice	—
Half Lotus	Hold for 10 seconds Do the exercise twice	Hold for 30 seconds Do the exercise twice	Hold for 60 seconds Do the exercise twice
Knee and Thigh	Hold for 5 seconds Do the exercise twice	Hold for 10 seconds Do the exercise twice	Hold for 20 seconds Do the exercise twice
Leg Stretches	Hold for 5 seconds Do the exercise twice	Hold for 10 seconds Do the exercise twice	Hold for 20 seconds Do the exercise twice
Lion	Hold for 5 seconds Do the exercise twice	Hold for 10 seconds Do the exercise twice	Hold for 20 seconds Do the exercise twice
Locust	Hold for 3 seconds Do the exercise twice	Hold for 5 seconds Do the exercise twice	—
Neti	Do the exercise twice	Do the exercise three times	—
Ninety-Second Relaxer	Take 30 seconds each to lower your body, hold the position, and raise your body Do the exercise once	—	—

Plow	Hold for 5 seconds Do the exercise twice	Hold for 10 seconds Do the exercise twice	Hold for 20 seconds Do the exercise twice
Preliminary Back and Leg Stretch	Hold for 5 seconds Do the exercise twice	Hold for 10 seconds Do the exercise twice	Hold for 20 seconds Do the exercise twice
Raja Yoga	Do the exercise once	—	—
Refreshing Breath	Hold for 3 seconds Do the exercise twice	Hold for 5 seconds Do the exercise twice	Hold for 10 seconds Do the exercise twice
Rock-A-Bye-Baby	Rock your leg from side to side 5 times Do the exercise twice	Rock your leg from side to side 10 times Do the exercise twice	—
Rock and Roll	Rock back and forth 3 times Do the exercise twice	Rock back and forth 5 times Do the exercise twice	—
Shoulder Stand	Hold for 30 seconds Do the exercise once	Hold for 1 minute Do the exercise once	Hold for 2 minutes Do the exercise once
Shoulder Stretch	Hold for 5 seconds Do the exercise twice	Hold for 10 seconds Do the exercise twice	Hold for 20 seconds Do the exercise twice

Side Stretch	Hold for 5 seconds Do the exercise twice	Hold for 10 seconds Do the exercise twice	Hold for 20 seconds Do the exercise twice
Slow Hip Roll	Roll your hips once to your right and once to your left Do the exercise twice	Roll your hips twice to your right and twice to your left Do the exercise twice	Roll your hips 3 times to your right and 3 times to your left Do the exercise twice
Slow Neck Roll	Roll your head once to your right and once to your left Do the exercise twice	Roll your head twice to your right and twice to your left Do the exercise twice	Roll your head 3 times to your right and 3 times to your left Do the exercise twice
Spread Leg Stretch	Hold for 5 seconds Do the exercise twice	Hold for 10 seconds Do the exercise twice	Hold for 20 seconds Do the exercise twice
Squat	Hold for 10 seconds Do the exercise twice	Hold for 20 seconds Do the exercise twice	Hold for 30 seconds Do the exercise twice

Name of Exercise	Beginning Count	Advanced Count	Potential Count
Standing Breath and Chest Stretch	Roll your torso once to your right and once to your left Do the exercise twice	Roll your torso twice to your right and twice to your left Do the exercise twice	Roll your torso 3 to your right and 3 times to your left Do the exercise twice
Standing Twist	Hold for 5 seconds Do the exercise twice	Hold for 10 seconds Do the exercise twice	Hold for 20 seconds Do the exercise twice
Tailor	Hold for 10 seconds Do the exercise twice	Hold for 30 seconds Do the exercise twice	Hold for 60 seconds Do the exercise twice
Three-Way Neck Stretch	Hold for 5 seconds Do the exercise twice	Hold for 10 seconds Do the exercise twice	—
Tree	Hold for 5 seconds Do the exercise twice	Hold for 10 seconds Do the exercise twice	Hold for 20 seconds Do the exercise twice
Twist in the Chair	Hold for 5 seconds Do the exercise twice	Hold for 10 seconds Do the exercise twice	Hold for 20 seconds Do the exercise twice
Twist on the Floor	Hold for 5 seconds Do the exercise twice	Hold for 10 seconds Do the exercise twice	Hold for 20 seconds Do the exercise twice
Wings	Hold for 5 seconds Do the exercise twice	Hold for 10 seconds Do the exercise twice	Hold for 20 seconds Do the exercise twice

BELOVED EXILE
Bantam Trade edition/July 1984
second printing August 1984

Bantam paperback edition/June 1985

Library of Congress Cataloging in Publication Data
Godwin, Parke.
  Beloved exile.

  1. Arthurian romances. 2. Great Britain—History—
Anglo-Saxon period, 449-1066-Fiction. I. Title.
PS3557.0316B4   1984   813'.54   83-45995
              ISBN 0-553-24924-X

Published simultaneously in the United States and Canada

Bantam Books are published by Bantam Books, Inc. Its trademark, consisting of the words "Bantam Books" and the por-
trayal of a rooster, is Registered in the United States Patent and
Trademark Office and in other countries. Marca Registrada. Bantam Books, Inc., 666 Fifth Avenue, New York, New York 10103.

PRINTED IN THE UNITED STATES OF AMERICA

O   0 9 8 7 6 5 4 3 2 1

Again for Quackenabush, who wanted this and nothing else, no nonsense, get on with it.

And for Doris—a little on account.

Contents

I

"Lady, the King Is Dead"

See that day as I remember it. A day in June, River Severn rolling to the sea, diamonded with sunlight, gulls gliding over the quays on a mild breeze that lifted the Red Dragon standard over Camelot. A quiet enough day for the end of my world.

On Camelot's ramparts they recognized the rider from the north. A lank red-haired man in plain linen tunic and breeches, his ring mail and sword stowed behind the saddle. Bedivere ap Gryffyn, Arthur's standard-bearer.

Most of Arthur's cavalry, the *combrogi*, were still in the north with Gareth. Camelot was near-deserted. I waited in the small audience chamber where Yseult once bade farewell to Trystan, listening to Bedivere's long stride echo down the stone passageway. My heart had been light all day, glad for the good weather, the royal and personal reunion with Arthur, the future we could burnish till it shone. Then Bedivere strode into the room, hot and dusty, and dropped to one knee before the dais. My heart stopped when I saw what he carried.

Bedivere's movements were stiff. The edge of a soiled bandage showed at the open neck of his tunic. He held out to me the ultimate symbol of British power, the imperial sword.

"Lady, the King is dead."

Between blow and pain, there is that instant of numbness, an unreal moment when I saw my hands go

1

out to grasp the jeweled scabbard before my mind fumbled and grasped at reality.

". . . dead?"

No, Good Jesu. Arthur and I were the best. That summer I lay down the sword of rebellion, sent Lancelot home to his grim Eleyne for good and all. On the field where we might have commenced civil war, we made a summer fair instead. Arthur and I were radiant with futures, stealing away to swim in a brook and make love for the first time in an age, my body accepting and trusting his with a passion and hunger I hadn't felt since the death of our child, and we fell asleep under the same blanket, close and content as children. We ruled a land finally at peace from Cornwall to Solway. Next year, with the unified west behind us, we would bring the Saxons under British rule or drive them into the sea. Each of us had made the large mistakes and paid the exorbitant price of those with a talent for rule. Now there was time for peace and loving, and the winning would follow.

But Arthur was dead and the man who told me so was one I never liked or understood, who once put me in irons at Arthur's command. The numbness washed away, the pain began. I wanted to go mad or find strength in God or whatever the trusting claim to discover in adversity.

"Who killed him, Bedivere?"

"Modred, Lady."

That was cold vindication. From the day I first heard of Morgana and Modred, Arthur's Faerie wife and son, I knew they'd be his ruin.

"Is that little bastard dead?"

"Aye."

In bald words Bedivere told me of the fatal ambush, of being at Arthur's deathbed in the monastery. Men called Bedivere the right hand of Arthur, the only man my husband would trust to bring me the imperial sword and the letter that named me his choice to succeed as ruler of Britain. Not a year before that I publicly humiliated Bedivere and Gareth, called them dolts and dogs. Now I needed Arthur's two able commoners before all the high blood of Britain. That alone should have tweaked me with the first glimmerings of humility, but I was a queen. Think first, act, and then feel. It must be so. The naming

of a new ruler demanded the Council of Princes and a ritual choosing by the people. It could also mean civil war. I needed the combrogi behind me.

"Bedivere, can I count on you and Gareth mac Diurmuid?"

His blue Belgae eyes appraised me, visibly pained by the shoulder wound, Modred's last treachery. Their color was startling as sapphire against copper in his windburned face.

"May I be straight, Lady?"

"Were you ever else?"

"The combrogi were sworn to Artos alone. Only death could break that oath. Without him there's nothing to hold them together."

"There's me."

Bedivere was a man of few words, most profane and all blunt. "You're the Queen, but no Arthur."

"No Arthur? You saw me on the field. My shoulders are still raw from mail, but by God I wore it. If we don't move now, someone else will."

And that quickly as the news of Arthur's death spread south. I could count on young Lord Bors and his handful of cavalry who'd escorted me home, perhaps even Gareth, commander of the combrogi. But Bedivere was vital, known to all as Arthur's first minister. No one else, not even myself—and that truth always galled—was so privy to my husband's mind.

"Lord Bedivere, I need you. Swear to me."

"No, Lady."

Stubborn peasant; with so much hanging in the balance and so little time I wanted to leap at him and drag the oath from his mouth. "Swear to me!"

I tried to fathom the refusal in his eyes and stance. Not dislike, not even suspicion, merely that Bedivere was a right hand from whom the governing head was gone. From the age of five there'd been Arthur to follow. Not a man without a mind or will of his own, still Bedivere was numb with that death as myself.

"Artos was educated," he said. "I have to piece things out. I'm thinking if I swear to you by Holy Church, what is it I'm bound to? Artos could be Christly wrong sometimes, but he always stood for one country. You'd have raised the north against him as a separate power."

"When he left me no choice. I executed Morgana, but what man will say that was against the good of Britain? Was it her death or Arthur's reprisal that split the country?"

"True," Bedivere allowed. "Artos was wrong to trust them. I told him as much, but . . ."

"But what? You say I am no Arthur?" My mind already churned with the need to move and do. "If I'm not Britain now, who is? Who will be? Senile Mark of Cornwall? Old Maelgwyn? Constantine who'd rather fight than think? Some Dobunni without Kay's talent for administration? His own son is an incompetent. Conant or Vortipore who know as much of unity as they do of Greek? Who, Bedivere?"

Bedivere winced. His hand strayed to the bad shoulder, then dropped. He was too proud to show weakness before a woman. For such a woman, crowned or not, there's a time to demand of men and a time to whisper.

"You're tired and hurt. Come, Bedivere, sit by me."

He accepted rather stiffly, settling in the other chair on the dais. Over the years I wondered now and then if Bedivere ever looked at me as a woman. Not that he attracted me at all, one just wonders these things. This much of him I knew: he couldn't be roared down, not even by Arthur. But he might be persuaded.

"You were straight with me, Gryffyn. I'll be the same. There's never been any love lost between us. Put that behind and be my right hand as you were his. You know there's no prince in Britain saving myself fit to hold this sword. If I lose it, we're no longer Arthur's dream but a rabble of tribes. You know the nobles."

Bedivere settled wearily in the chair, a man stirring deep waters. "When I saw Kay dead at Badon, I wondered, where does it stop? Each time I went home to Myfanwy and the girl, I prayed there'd be an end to war and we could just sit and grow fat. Arthur always called me back. And I always came, looking back longer at home each time. I was his man from the first. We were of an age. Now he's gone and I could whisper to fifty, I'm that close to it. Aye—I know the nobles, and I think unless I go home now I'll be riding till I'm prayed over and buried. Swear to you and we start the whole thing over again from the beginning. And I'm bloody sick of it all."

"You think I'm not?" I told him. "You at least could see your child grow. You were there the day I lost the only one I'll ever have. So I grow flowers. I'm good at growing things. I could spend days on end just hoeing and watering. There's never enough time, that's what gives life its meaning. I could take off this embroidered kirtle and put on homespun and pick up my hoe, and that's where Constantine or someone else would dispose of me on his way to the crown—and to you, Bedivere. Don't delude yourself. Arthur's right hand is like Arthur's flag, highly visible. They'll give you less of a choice than I do. What is it you don't trust—my ability, my courage?"

"Na, na. You were always a queen. Almost before you were a woman." He gave me a hard smile. "That might've been your problem, Lady." Bedivere rose to face me. "I don't know. Kay's dead, Artos is gone. I don't have the handle of that yet. All I want is to see Myfanwy and the girl and get crying drunk. When I'm sober again I'll think of tomorrow."

"There's no time for that! When there is, I'll cry with you. We were all born a hundred years too late, but so be it. Are you with me?"

Bedivere moved to the casement, gazing out at the pear tree beyond. "Last year you called me a peasant dog."

"I apologize for that here and now. Before the court if you wish."

"No need, it's true. I am a peasant. Not even born free. Without Artos, I'd be a groom like my father or a centurion of horse at best. The same for Gareth. We saw both sides of Artos' dream: why it was good and why it had to work. And why it never will. The night Cerdic attacked Eburacum—how many years ago?—Artos put Gareth and me in the first line of attack because it was common sense. And Agrivaine balked. He wouldn't take second place to commoners."

"Agrivaine was good at balking all his life."

"How different was he from the rest, then? Artos saw something the rest of them never did. He could bind them all together, even make them laugh at their own foolishness. God, how many times did he come over me like my own da scolding: 'You're thick, Bedwyr!' That night in Eburacum, and Agrivaine wasting precious time

with his pride, Artos said, 'If we can't agree tonight, it won't matter tomorrow to Cerdic and the flies.' When he was wrong, he was the worst. But that wasn't often."

Bedivere slapped a callused hand on the casement sill, punctuating his thought. "I swore to Artos because I knew that much of his heart. He wanted you to rule after him. I'll stay until you're chosen."

"You'll take oath with me?"

"No," said Bedivere. "Swearing's done before God. I'll save that. You've my word until the choosing. What's to be done?"

A straitlaced man, the Gryffyn. An oath between lord and man carried the same legal weight as a Roman contract, and that he wouldn't give me. I consoled myself that Bedivere's word was better than most men's oaths over holy relics. It must content me.

"Come back tonight with Lord Bors. I don't know how many friends we've got, but as for time there's damned little. We've got to call in the post riders between Camelot and Badon. We need them here. But get you some food and rest now." I moved past Bedivere to the door, already organizing the work in my mind.

"Where will we find you, Lady?"

"In the scriptorium, getting things done. As I did with Arthur. And Bedivere—there will come that day when you swear to me as you did to him and for the same reason. Because I am the best."

As news of Arthur's death filtered through Camelot, silence deepened about the imperial palace as it must have lain like a pall across all Britain. In that hush see a hundred busy men scurrying south with the same tidings to lay at the feet of ambitious princes. Arthur is gone: there must be a choosing and who better than this man or that? Or me? Who's between us and the crown but Guenevere, and she is no Arthur.

What mantle did you wear, Arthur, that I never fit? My authority was as unquestioned, my common sense sharper, my sentiment certainly more restrained. When we played the game together, was I not wagered as deeply as you? Art is instinctive, but craft is learned. I mastered the discipline of rule when you were a mere centurion of horse. What magic did you cast over men?

Bedivere was as good a soldier, Gareth as shrewd a tactician, Lancelot as great a commander, even Gawain more stubbornly honorable a king. Yet all these followed and loved you while you were wrong as often as you were brilliant. They'll sing of you as the savior of Britain and patron of the Grail while I'll be remembered as a rebellious whore. No shock there; men are not tolerant of competent women. They give us respect in place of trust. It's safer.

Imogen, my dour Brigante mistress of chamberwomen, spoke one brogued word to the rest of them and they waited out of sight but within earshot while I hurried to the scriptorium. This small chamber was for Arthur and me the heart of Camelot. Often we ate and worked alone here, the clutter of state scattered about to be taken up again as soon as our lips were wiped. The chamber overlooked the south courtyard, well placed to catch most of the day's light. There were no luxuries here, only a firepit, a shelf for documents, a writing desk, a plain oak table and several hard chairs. They sufficed us. We learned early to be working rulers. Any other sort didn't last long.

Whether it was the sight of this chamber where we worked together at kingship for so long, or simply the feelings I suppressed with Bedivere now bursting forth, I don't know. But I faltered at the door, purpose lost, making false starts toward different points of the room. The chamber was full of Arthur, crammed with his life, aching with the fact of his death. I began to shake, whispering his name. It came out as a whimper, strangling on the love and loss of him. Suddenly the bleak weight of a future without Arthur crushed in on me. One woman with a handful of knights—Sweet God, protect me. I have never lived without fear, and so I have learned courage, but now I have no courage left. I am so frightened. Cold to my marrow. It's too much, I'll never manage it all. It was Arthur, after all, not me. I'll never—

I halted, rigid and furious at the waste of energy.

"Think, you fool!"

My hands shook violently. I gave them employment, spreading the maps on the table. The whole game lay before me for perhaps the thousandth time. And it was all new.

See my world.

Within my lifetime Rome has crumbled like a rotted house. The Western Empire doesn't exist. Clovis the Frank is master of Gaul, sacking churches when it profits him to be a barbarian, harrying the barbarians when expedient to remember his baptism and Christian wife. The Visigoths ramp over Hispania where Seneca and Martial were born, when to be anything but a Roman citizen was beneath contempt. Theodoric is master of Italy, fumbling at kingship, dispensing order and assassination from Ravenna while Rome decays on the Tiber. Light gutters in the west while, in Constantinople, the Eastern Empire bargains with barbarians and tries to rewrite a common code of justice from ancient Roman law.

Trade in the Middle Sea has slowed owing to the Vandals who exact tribute from every boat. Vandals, Allemanni, Suevi, Saxons, Franks—Germans all. Rome should never have allowed them west of the Rhine. Now the maps are puddled with them, even mine.

See my country. Draw a wavering line from the Isle of Wight northeast to the land of the Lindissi, once tributaries to my own father. To the east of that line is Saxon country now. If there was one policy Arthur and I agreed on from the start, it was the reclamation of our east. If there was one crippling impediment in the British soul, it was that never enough of them would support us until it was too late. Arthur broke the Saxons at Badon, but they're second and third generation folk now. This is their home, many of them half-Brit like Cerdic.

Dear, ambitious Cerdic, late King of the West Saxons. May he be in hell a hundred years before heaven knows he's dead. Arthur invited him to our coronation and later personally killed him at Badon. He should have done it years before, but Arthur was always too lenient toward men he admired. I would have crucified the bastard or hired biddable Saxons to cut his throat. That's the game: you accomplish what you can with statecraft. What you can't, you buy.

My country. My petty, jealous, anarchic, song-hearted people. For Arthur and myself existence was shaped by practical Roman writers and lucid Greeks to sound thinking and efficient administration. But we ruled dis-

parate tribes whose political thought hadn't changed in a thousand years. Land belongs to tribes, not men, and borders shift with every quarrel. Our ideals are lofty, our heroes preposterous, our very language more often sung than written. The priest who replaced the druid found our souls already addicted to the unattainable and dispensed it in Christ's miracles. The Church didn't seed our passion for God, it merely cultivated what grew in wild profusion. The sacred oak became the Cross, the mistletoe the crown of thorns, the magic cauldron of Cerridwen the mystic and holy Grail. We are a people enthralled by holy light while weeds grow about our feet, readier to fight the next village than join with them for common safety. Such a people need brigands, butchers or saints for kings. Arthur and I were all at one time or another, but we created what Vortigern dreamed and Ambrosius designed: the combrogi, the nucleus of cavalry bound to the crown before any tribal loyalty. Two hundred *comites*, petty lords and a few commoners like Bedivere and Gareth; and with this anomaly we patched Britain together. Our unity was always fragile, an unbalanced burden that Arthur and I juggled perilously with treaties, friendships and a few good spies. The patchwork garment was meager; shift it to one side and you felt a draft on the other. But it was a start. We would bring back the best of Rome. Next year.

The map blurred. I rubbed at my eyes, trying to grasp the game as it stood now.

To the south in Cornwall: old Prince Mark, sick and frail now. He once bid for the crown with an attempt on Arthur's life and would sell the whole country for protected trade with the Middle Sea ports. My advantage: Yseult, his consort and my loyal friend. My danger: Mark's nephew, Constantine, already straining at the dynastic bit. There was little Dyfneint, tributary crown to Mark, ruled by Eleyne of Astolat and—to the extent that flesh can work stone—influenced by Lancelot, her husband. He loved me once, perhaps still, but I sent him back to her. The odds for at least nominal loyalty were with me.

To the east: Prince Maelgwyn, Arthur's staunch friend and our buffer against the Saxons. He held Mount Badon, strongest fort in the south Midlands. Vigorous,

forthright, no man's fool, but aging now with sons whose loyalties and abilities were yet to be tested.

In the west: Aurelius Conant, Prince of the Silures and Demetae. Vortipore, Prince of the Ordovices. In their mountain strongholds they had no real respect for central power. We knew them only through our tax collectors who needed military escort to make their assessments. Once when Conant sent back the severed heads of our officers, Arthur moved against him with the speed and efficiency of Caesar. The combrogi dashed by night deep into Conant's territory. By the next sunset a thousand of his own cattle were feeding the flies. A frightened herdsman was sent to Conant with the heads of several lords who'd opposed royal justice. An extra stake was included with Conant's name notched in Ogham. He paid his taxes without further incident, but I wondered how Conant would swing now.

My real strength lay in the north, still in my hands though I had promised Arthur to give it up. Not yet; the game was changed. I might well need it. Eburacum was a walled Roman city. If pressed I'd be safer there than in Camelot. The first of many letters that day must go to my Parisi ministers.

Guenevere to her beloved Parisi and Brigantes . . .

Any way you looked at the map, I had few allies without the combrogi, but the country must know there was still a hand on the rein. I put the maps aside and began to write. Time meant nothing when work absorbed me; it was something of a start to look up and see Imogen squinting at me from the door.

"Will y'sup wi' the ladies tonight?"

"No, I'm busy. Just fetch me something here."

"Well, then, I'll be bringing your warm cloak and laying a fire at supper."

"Yes, good." I put a completed letter aside and began the next, forgetting Imogen, but she was a rock in the doorway.

"If I bring your supper, you'll not set it by to get cold?"

"What? No, no."

"The King, be his soul wi' Christ, was always after you to eat more."

True. Arthur's last letter contained not one word of dying, only reminders of work and my own irrelevant

health. It must have been sound as iron; since my still-born child I never took conscious care of it, a kind of contempt for the one part of me that so disgracefully failed. But even at the end Arthur found time to worry about it.

Tell Imogen I order her to be a nuisance until you finish everything on your plate at every meal. . . .

Suddenly I ducked my head away from Imogen. Maddening, passionate, caring Arthur. Always my love, not always my lover, somehow always the loving enemy. The price of being talented equals; yet in his last letter not one cry to me on the brink of the dark. He went with dignity and a joke, damn him. I don't think I'll die gracefully. While life still boils in my veins and there's a throw of the dice left, they'll carry me out kicking and screaming.

Imogen still hovered. "You'll be all right, then, Lady?"

"Yes, Imogen."

She grunted skeptically as if I'd be anything but, bobbed a habit-shallowed curtsy and withdrew. I went back to my letter.

Guenevere in the name of Artorius Imperator, to the Princes of Britain. God's peace be with you as it rests on our united realm.

There's optimism for you, scheming to hold a crown when I might shortly lack a head to wear it.

I wrote steadily through the waning light, conscious with every loop and stroke of other princes writing, planning, dusting off old ambitions, perhaps sharpening swords.

How quiet it was.

Listen to the sound of that tranquil, dangerous summer. Hear the whisper of sand through the glass, time running out.

The letters speed, answers return. The Parisi and Brigantes are squarely behind me, the north still in my hands. From the Midlands Maelgwyn pledges loyalty "providing" I honor Arthur's policies. Two sides of the game board are secure for the moment. Cold silence from Conant and Vortipore, too distant to care, but from the south a disquieting piece of intelligence un-

knowingly offered by my dear friend Yseult in a chatty letter.

Mark felt so much better this month that we planned a feast for Midsummer Eve. Would you not think the younger lords would vie to be there, but the table was all ancients like myself. Every bard of note in Cornwall but none of the younger blood. They were all at Constantine's hall. . . .

I pondered the Latin, written in the hand of one of Mark's court scribes. If Yseult's Gaelic mind sometimes skirted the fringes of meaning, the secretary always clarified. The young Cornish lords gathering to Constantine. At a feast he usually competed with his uncle for the best bards, but if they were all at Castle Dore, it might mean Constantine's assembly was not primarily a revel.

Your head against a turnip it wasn't. One day toward the end of June, a post rider dashed through Camelot's gate and ordered it barred behind him. Stationed south along Severn, he'd seen the three ships and waited, hoping it was Gareth. It was not.

"The blazons are all Cornish, Lady. Constantine and others. Nigh forty knights to the keel, horses and arms."

But from the ramparts Bedivere, Bors and I saw only one ship glide serenely into view, Constantine's banner over the mast.

"The rest will wait," Bedivere said cannily. "He wants to know how many we are."

Or how pitifully few. Less than twenty knights, a handful of men-at-arms, the rest women, children and servants. Just then I'd have pawned the imperial sword for half of Gareth's combrogi who were still at Solway preparing to sail home with Arthur's body.

Young Bors voiced my own question. "Does Constantine know where Gareth is?"

"Which is to ask are his observers as good as mine. I don't know."

Bedivere pointed as the ship turned in toward the quay. "I don't think so. Look there, Lady. He's not in mail. He's not going to risk an attack until he knows our strength."

"Then he shall see it."

From the day of Arthur's death, we knew this might happen. Now they were come, the first flies around the unguarded honey. Constantine would come in all the trappings of courtesy, unarmed, observing the Peace of Britain which enrounded Camelot like a defensive halo. But his eyes would be everywhere, and he must see our readiness, such as it was. For the rest I would smile, charm and lie like a mountebank.

"Bors, I'll need yourself and Regan—and Lord Ifan, I think. Bedivere, let's to work."

Prince Mark of Cornwall—Marcus Conomori as he styled himself—could boast as clear a Roman descent and certainly more royal blood than Arthur. He always considered us usurpers, even though Arthur was chosen by Ambrosius to succeed him, and might have been crowned had not Arthur been the people's hero. Throughout our reign we never turned our back on Mark for very long.

In childhood and youth, Mark knew close ties with Rome as a reality and the protected sea trade that swelled his father's treasury. Unlike Arthur, he couldn't change his views when that reality faded to myth but always looked to the sea and the continent more than internal affairs. His advisers could better tell you what was current in Brittany or Hispania than in the interior of his own country. A Cornish emperor would mean a Britain largely left to shift for itself or be a mere tributary to a maritime province, the dog wagged by the tail. Either way led to chaos.

Childless Mark had a number of nephews. Trystan was the favorite until his affair with Yseult drove him from Castle Dore with prudent speed. Mark turned then to little Constantine who grew up, as it were, in the prince's aging lap. The boy's sentiments were no broader than his uncle's. He rankled under our suspicion of his family and nursed that grievance to a cause. The house of Cornwall would rise again and vindicate itself before all detractors. He would subdue the Saxons in one vigorous campaign that wouldn't halt at Badon but would sweep to the eastern coast and occupy once more the lost lands of the Cantii, Belgae and Iceni. His logistics for all this were hazy, but they reduced to the fact that Constantine, once crowned, would simply *command* the allegiance of

the various tribes (who didn't give a political damn
about Cornwall) and food, money and troops would fall
like manna from the sky. Good fortune, say I.

He had certain advantages: he was a natural fire-
brand, a good warrior. I watched him bound down the
gangway to the quay, bare brown arms and legs swinging
from a short Roman tunic, long chestnut hair ruffled by
the river breeze. He had an energetic, lunging stride that
reminded me of Geraint, but the likeness ended there.
Geraint's energy had been totally innocent. Constantine's
was always a little abrasive with arrogance and purpose.
As a vessel of discontent, he was a rallying point for the
young while the mature held off. He harbored grudges,
an expensive habit for leaders, and jumped too quickly
at small gains while larger ones eluded him. He kept efficient military order for Mark, but conquest is only a
means to government, not an end, and government is an
art disciplined to a profession. Arthur and I were profes-
sionals. This young man striding up the sea path toward
my gate was an ambitious amateur.

For all that I still wouldn't underestimate Constantine.
We were ready for him as he neared the river gate with
his two companion lords flanked by Bors and Bedivere.
Constantine could hear the hoarse bellowing of men-at-
arms on the high ramparts, and saw the practice stones
flung westward from the onagers again and again. From
the east wall more men grinned down at him and at his
anchored keel so easily in sinking range. Inside our gate,
there was humming activity. Servants ran and fetched,
two Grail knights practiced with sword and shield in
that unique, agile style refined by Bedivere. Another led
a horse by the visitors with Gareth mac Diurmuid's
shield hooked to the saddle. The smithy smoked and
clanged with employment. On their way to the great
hall, the Cornish met a knight or two at every corner
they turned. I doubt if any of this was wasted on Constantine. If his spies reported Camelot helpless, that report lost credence with every step he took.

I let him discover me in the middle of some merry nonsense with Bors' pretty wife, Regan, and several other
ladies of the court. A sheaf of state documents lay on the
dais by my chair where Lord Ifan, a stiffish Grail knight,
stood at ceremonial attention, the imperial sword

crooked in one arm. When Bedivere announced him, Constantine and his companions approached. They might have knelt but only inclined their heads in respect.

"Long life to the Lady of Camelot." He did not refer to me as queen or empress; that would imply a right Constantine did not yet recognize. "Bless the soul of our departed King. May he be with Christ."

"Amen," Bedivere added pointedly.

"My Lord, if you come in peace . . ."

"Lady, I do."

"Then so we receive you. What a surprise. Dear Constantine, you were a handsome boy and now I declare you've grown into a devastating man. But there, I'm hot from foolery with these idle women. Lady Regan, bring us something cool to drink."

"Yes, my Queen." The lovely girl skipped off to obey.

"Lord Ifan," I noted, "whatever are you frowning at on a day as lovely as this?" Without waiting for his reply, I took my place on the dais and picked up the documents. "These warm days I try to mix a little pleasure with business. There is little enough pleasure in Camelot now."

Constantine rose to the occasion. "Lady, you have the sorrow of all Britain with you."

"And all its welfare."

"If you are chosen, Lady."

I didn't miss the minute difference in his courtly tone, and looked up from the page I was scanning. "What? Oh, I will be. Surely—where *is* that letter?—you have heard I have Arthur's own voice?"

"Indeed I had not, Lady. In any case—"

"It's true," Bedivere prompted at his shoulder. "The King said it to me more than once. I carried the letter to the Queen."

"Which you may read." I handed it to Constantine. As he grasped it, I glanced at the casement and rose. "There they are. Goodness, they do raise a lot of dust."

A furious cloud of it, framed in the casement, from behind a hill some half-mile to the north. A few riders trotted briskly back and forth along the crest observing the activity beyond. I turned to smile at Constantine's puzzlement. "The combrogi and Maelgwyn's Catuvellauni are at practice maneuvers. The day was too fine to waste."

Lady Regan bobbed back in again with a pitcher, followed by a serving woman with a tray of goblets.

"And with some half-thousand hungry knights, the supper board will be crowded tonight, but you are welcome. Some wine, my Lords?"

"He . . . is in Camelot?"

Yes, you're still an amateur. Not fast enough; your hesitation shows. I played it with impeccable carelessness. "Who, Lord Gareth? Of course. Oh—you meant Prince Maelgwyn. Yes, they're both here to escort me to the choosing. And I suspect you'll be there. You'd be foolish not to. There may come that day when you will make a worthy king, Constantine."

Off balance, he cleared his throat. "True, I will stand to be chosen."

The Cornishman on his right took a step forward. "My Lord will be the next king."

"I don't think so. Not this year, anyway."

Constantine's tone stiffened audibly. "Lady, Britain must look again to her best interests."

"That is true. At more leisure I'd hear your views on a workable policy with Picts and Demetae. Or for that matter on interior trade. Do you know who forges our best iron? Where our best wool comes from, the going price per bale and how much it's worth oversea? What is your policy toward the British Church, the orthodox dioceses and radical monasteries, and how would you favor the one without the other calling you heretic, since you may need both behind you? 'Best interest' is like subtle poetry, my Lord, easier to pronounce than to understand. Do have some cool wine."

Regan offered me a goblet and was pouring another for Constantine when the tense hospitality of the audience was suddenly shattered.

"No."

We turned to stare at Lord Ifan, who stepped down from the dais, moving toward us with a marked limp. No older than Constantine, he had the weathered look of the combrogi. "By your leave, Lady, no." It was not a request but a peremptory command. "Offer no cup to Cornwall in this place."

I gaped at his bad manners. "Ifan, what on earth—?"

Constantine braced himself. Bedivere and Bors moved

closer to him as if in protection. Regan and the other women withdrew a little in sibilant confusion as Ifan turned to me.

"Has the Queen forgotten how the Cornish sat warm at home while we froze at Badon with the King? But for Lancelot and Dyfneint, there wouldn't have been a Cornish shield on that hill."

"That's enough," Bors reminded him. "They are here unarmed and in good will."

"Good will?" Ifan stumped to the casement and pointed to the dust beyond. "If it weren't for a full cohort out there, how safe would the Queen be with this false creature—?"

"I said enough!" Bors moved to restrain him.

"Combrogus," Constantine answered with steely quiet, "don't presume on your honors or my good nature. You see how I've come: one ship and a few men—"

"Liar!"

Now it was my place to still him. "Ifan! Not another word."

"—to state my claim in the choosing," Constantine finished a little hotly. "Is this treachery?"

And then suddenly there were two more armed knights at the hall entrance. I paid them no heed.

"Aye, one ship," Ifan groaned. "And how many more in wait? Two? Three?"

And still another of my knights appeared at the nearer entrance. The three converged on us. Constantine's escort began to look a little uncertain.

"Ifan, leave us," I snapped. "And don't show yourself in my presence again until that temper is schooled."

Still he hung there by the casement, righteous and shamed in the same breath. "My Queen, I—"

"Boy." It was Bedivere, firm as iron but gentle. "You wear the Grail on your shield. That's an honor even I can't claim. Then wear it well. Leave us. Bors, go with him, help to cool that anger."

"And you ladies—Regan, all of you." I dismissed them. Bedivere, the three armed knights and I faced our slightly shaken guests. "Constantine, I commend you for an even temper."

He shrugged it off, not without some visible effort.

"That farmer's son? But I won't forget he called me a liar."

"His loyalty overtipped good manners. May you have as loyal around you someday. My Lords, Bedivere, you needn't hover so. In peace he came and in peace he'll go. Constantine is not so false he'd think treason in my own palace." I let my gaze wander to the casement. The riders on the crest still milled against the curtain of dust. "Nor so foolish as to attempt it in so careless a manner."

The last knight to enter moved a step toward me, hot and dusty from the saddle. "Lady, Maelgwyn and Gareth ask will you come view the field or shall they attend you here?"

"Here, I think. I was on a horse all last month. Bring them here. Now, Constantine." I took his arm and led him apart from the others some distance across the hall. The spot I chose for privacy was calculated. The flagstones at our feet still showed the faint but unmistakable stain of Morgana's blood. Every prince in Britain knew that stain that tore the country apart and who had ordered it done.

"All right, boy, let's speak plainly. I won't question your motives or count your ships, but don't think a grieving widow is helpless without Arthur. We were crowned young; I taught him much of kingship. In turn he attempted to teach me a certain charity toward rivals—with indifferent results, I admit. When that sword that Ifan carries is placed in the stones, and when the tribes of Britain have cried *ave* to your pulling it out—*then* I'll go back to Eburacum and leave Camelot to you. And God help the British. Until then I'm your Queen, and all the things you've heard about me are laudably and regrettably true. I'm not above the knife when I need it, and if I thought you came with treachery on your mind, you wouldn't leave. Any of you. Is that clear, sir?"

He studied me before answering. I had the chance to read his eyes. They didn't show much—he wasn't that green—but the respect was there, if only for an adversary.

"You're no coward, Guenevere."

"Damned right, not and live this long. Nor foolhardy nor cruel where it gains me nothing." Suddenly I put my arms around his neck and kissed his cheek. "Still, I never

could resist a handsome man. You'll have dazzling children someday. However—"

I steered him back toward my waiting men, raising my voice for them to hear. "It is true the combrogi and Maelgwyn have no love for the Cornish, wrong or right. I'd change that, but for the moment it's wiser if you leave. There might be incidents we couldn't check. We thank you for coming and your good wishes."

"The Queen's right." Bedivere nodded. "In your position, Artos himself would withdraw."

"My very dearest love to your uncle and aunt. Lord Bedivere will see you to your ship."

Constantine bowed to me; I acknowledged it. Our glances were a veiled classic. Smiling, I knew he had the daring to usurp the crown over my corpse. With the same courtesy he knew it wasn't going to be that easy.

"Until the choosing. For I mean to be king."

"As God wills. Speed the interval in health."

"But speed," Bedivere reminded him. "Maelgwyn will be here any minute."

I smiled them out of sight as Bedivere and one of the knights escorted them down the stairway, then instructed the others to send back Bors, Regan and Ifan.

"Nicely done, all of you, but now I need a post rider to track that ambitious young man until he meets his other ships—whether they turn south or wait."

Interest as well as instinct drew me to the scriptorium where, from the casement, I could observe Constantine in the courtyard below. He was alone with Bedivere, punctuating with rapid gestures what were evidently serious words. They paused near the gate, Bedivere still listening. Constantine spread his hands in a what-else-possible? attitude and smiled confidently at Bedivere. He rested his hand on the older man's shoulder before they passed through the gate. I could well imagine the assurances Constantine issued as I mused my way back to the hall: for Bedivere, honored as widely as Arthur, the future could be even brighter, more honorable.

I had his word but what I knew of his heart was pessimistic. Bedivere probably saw little difference between me or any other prince on the throne. For him, as he said, it was starting all over again. He wanted the humblest

and most expensive of gifts, home and peace. If Constantine offered that, what price Guenevere?

When Bors, Regan and Ifan entered the hall, all three of us breathed a deep sigh so simultaneous it was comic. I opened my arms to them.

"You dears! Come kiss me, you were *perfect*. Ifan, you might have been a player. Never have I seen such outrage struggling against propriety. I declare you were seething visibly when I dismissed you."

Bors wondered. "You think Constantine suspected?"

"Who cares? He took the bait. Now you and Regan pack for a pleasant journey. I need two ambassadors, and none so fit as my dearest children. And Ifan—go tell our ladies the enemy's fled and the field is theirs!"

Give us all some credit. We knew someone would probe at Camelot's strength in those weeks after Arthur's death, and where could I muster it? Maelgwyn's loyalty was conditional; I couldn't strip the Wall of my own Parisi in the face of Erca's Picts. To ask anywhere else was a blatant confession of our helplessness. We prayed Gareth would arrive in time, wisely assumed he wouldn't, and fell back on my father's tactic of constructive dishonesty.

When Constantine walked into my hall there were fewer than fifteen combrogi in Camelot, counting Bedivere, Bors and Ifan. We created a cohort of cavalry out of two dozen perilously mounted women dragging gorse bushes round and round a dusty field, and pure bluff.

Appearance was everything: the walls teeming with men at catapult practice, knights on display, distant riders observing unseen but furious activity that raised a great deal of dust. And just as Constantine was questioning the efficiency of his spies, a new diversion to push him further off balance—Ifan's outrage and expulsion from the hall, a few armed reinforcements at the correct moment, a reminder that the Cornish were not popular with my troops. Then my quiet show of candor and steely resolution in sight of Morgana's blood, my magnanimity in sending him home unscathed. To attack in the face of all that would have taken more confidence in his scouts, more men than he had or monumental stupidity. Constantine did the logical thing, exited gracefully. One doesn't gain a crown by dying young.

That evening I gave a private supper for my gallant and saddle-chafed combrogi wives, and at each place was a spiky leaf of the plant that saved Camelot. Some washed the leaves in gold and wore them with merry pride, my Ladies of the Gorse Bush. They all thought it rather fun except for Gareth's Rhian, whose appearance in her husband's breeches (too small) and cast-off mail hanging from her shoulders like wet laundry was the jest of the table. Rhian considered women in men's clothing a profanation and herself a martyr to necessity.

I enjoyed that supper. There wasn't much to laugh about those days, but we did our best. My ladies went to bed mellow enough, but Bedivere and I paced the high ramparts through the night while the watches came and went, waiting for a flare of light that would tell us Constantine was returning. Every available keel and hulk along our banks was packed with flammables, the east-facing catapults armed with pitch-missiles, to burn the Cornish ships before they reached the shore. It would be our last defense. But my post rider returned near morning to say Constantine had turned south. We'd won a bloodless victory.

"I wish we could win them all this way," Bedivere observed, rubbing sleepy eyes.

And yet as his tall figure moved away down the rampart, I wondered again what Constantine had spoken to him. He didn't take oath with me. We were bound by expedience, not love. It seemed he'd listened very carefully to the Cornishman. That's a difference between Arthur and me. He could and did wonder sometimes whether a close friend would betray him. My only pause would be the price. What would it take for Bedivere—or any of them—to put my head on a pike?

I sent Bors and Regan with gifts to Castle Dore and Astolat. Grail knights were welcome anywhere. They were to drop a word in those select quarters where silver bought me ears: watch Constantine.

In early July Lord Gareth sailed home to Camelot with my husband's body.

If Bedivere was Arthur's right hand, Gareth mac Diurmuid was the left. Lord-milite of Arthur's cavalry, he and Bedivere were day and night for contrast. Beside the

lank Gryffyn Gareth was short and disproportionate, a
huge breadth of chest and shoulders and a long torso on
short, bandied legs. Though the best horseman I've ever
seen, on foot he rolled like a round-bottomed curragh in
a heavy sea. Cheerfully positive against Gryffyn's laconic
gloom, his Leinster tongue needed no literacy to give it
lilt. In the sod hut of his birth there might be little to eat,
and that plain as they fed their few pigs, but always a
warm peat fire and stories to while away the wet Irish
night. Gareth could never letter out more than his name,
but the turn of his most casual speech could make a legend out of driving the cattle home.

"And why not," he said once. "After dark there was
naught to do but pass the *uisge* and a word."

I humiliated him once but Gareth was a forgiving
man. Prickly Rhian rankled more from that ill-consid-
ered outburst than he did. Sentiment aside, the little
Irishman had no ties of loyalty in Britain save Arthur,
who brought honor and advancement and meaning to
his life. Lady Rhian might have her own opinion of my
methods and morals, but her husband's loyalty was one
of the few things I could count on. Gareth did not disap-
point me.

His three ships slipped around Conant's southern coast
and up Severn to drop anchor at our quays. The combrogi crowded one deck—dear God, so few?—their
horses another. The third, shadowed by a black sail, carried my husband. Waiting on the sea-path I kept my eyes
away from the ebony-sailed vessel and searched the others in vain for Gareth. Beside me Lady Rhian pointed to
the funeral ship.

"There. Where would Gareth be but with his oath-
lord?"

Just forward of the mast stood a rough catafalque on
which rested a casket hewn from the heartwood of a sacred oak. It was draped in red and white, Arthur's colors.
I chose them myself when my Parisi women sewed his
first standard. Four men flanked the casket in full mail
despite the warm day, bare heads bowed, hands folded
on their sword pommels, rigid in formal mourning as if
they grew from the deck itself. Only their wind-tousled
hair stirred. Stillest of all was Gareth mac Diurmuid.

I saw Rhian glance sideways at me. Leinster-born like

Gareth, pig-poor before Arthur titled him lord-comite, she once had the conviction to stand against me openly when I had Morgana killed. She followed Gareth from Ireland when he was no more than a common soldier enlisting for pay in Ambrosius' new cavalry. Protruding from the tight cuff of her neat kirtle were hands still red and strong from years of a washtub and a hoe. She had no children; her life revolved around Gareth and the Church. Like him she was loyal and tough. Unlike him, her mentality was peasant-thick, pliant as stone. It was difficult to wedge a new idea into that mind, impossible to dislodge an old one. The quality was nature, not breeding. There but for the grace of birth went Lancelot's wife, Eleyne of Astolat.

"Use him well, Lady." Rhian's murmur was stiff with pride. "Remember, he need not have come at all."

Vindictive woman. I nodded, mumbled something and moved down the path to the quay to step aboard the funeral ship. As my foot touched the deck, Gareth and his guard went to their knees, foreheads bent to their sword hilts. I knelt, uttered the formal prayer, crossed myself and felt Gareth's hand under my arm as I rose.

"We thank you for your charge, Lord Gareth. You're a welcome sight." Then in a lower voice: "Why so few?"

The little lord-milite looked back at his waiting men. "Three and thirty, that's the sad number of them."

"So few to believe in me?"

His head wagged forlornly. "Am I not wearied out ranting and pleading with the rest? Their lord is dead, that's all they know. They went home."

Use them well? Good God, they were all in the world I had to use. Less than half a hundred in all. But they were combrogi. The term has bemused foreigners now and then. It means "companion" or "one of us."

They began as Roman cavalry, the Sixth Alae under my father, Cador. For centuries cavalry were an afterthought in the army; the main salient was always the foot legion. Alae were mere scouts, messengers and escorts, recruited from the fringes and dregs of the empire. Ambrosius changed that. He made it an honor to join, inviting the best blood in Britain. Two squadrons on the Wall of Hadrian were commanded by the Princes Gawain and Agrivaine, a third by my brother Peredur.

Trystan headed one, Bedivere another, Arthur the tutoring, guiding genius behind them all. His own brother Kay forged them longer swords than cavalry ever carried. From his battles with the Goths, Lancelot brought ring mail, the improved battle lance and the stirrup.

For a time they were Roman in name, never in spirit or practice. When Ambrosius did away with the last vestige of the legion and made Arthur Count of Britain, the only way to hold jealous, restless lords together was a personal oath of fealty that made each equal under Arthur's command. King-to-be like Gawain, royal nephew like Trystan, chief's son, younger son, bastard, commoners like Bedivere and Gareth, it made no difference. They put their swords in Arthur's hand and swore by Christ, Epona or Mithras to be his man. They took the blade back as plain lord-comite, as combrogus—one of us.

It was never easy to maintain that equality in the face of tribal heritage and stiff pride, but their performance was something else. No enemy in Britain was a match for them. Though most would yelp with injury and parade their pedigrees on the merest hint that they worked at a common trade, they were the first professional cavalry Britain or the Western Empire had ever seen, and the finest.

Look at these men, threadbare, dirty cloaks rolled over one shoulder, coaxing their horses down the gangway like spoiled children. Young or young-no-longer, they bear a common stamp. Flat-bellied men more at ease in the saddle than afoot, faces windburned to reddish leather and lined from constant riding in wind, sun and rain. Their finery is rarely displayed. Over the years they have discarded every unnecessary piece of gear or fancy that will slow or tire a horse. But they go into battle in the newest ring mail, wielding a longsword in one hand where most men would need two, each blade weighted and balanced to the owner's arm, forged from Damascan iron that has more strength and resiliency than any other.

The younger men grew up in Arthur's service. Some of them, like Bors, have had their swords blessed by the Abbot of Ynnis Witrin, their shields blazoned with a gold cup. They are Grail knights, present when Peredur found the holiest relic in Christendom, and now under the pro-

tection of the Church. Any man, even a king, who attacks them without cause or right risks not only his life but his soul.

"I, Gareth, son of Diurmuid, swear on my life that head and foot I am your man to obey your law and look to no other lord for increase. That I will hold faith with none but you, saving God and Holy Church. By which sign I swear in the name of Christ Jesu."

Gareth's nicked and darkened blade was heavy in my grasp. I held it with my right hand covering his on the consecrated pommel. "I, Guenevere, in the name of Arthur, swear by God and Holy Church to be your faithful lord and affirm you as my lord-milite as you were his, be his name blessed. Amen."

So Gareth and I bonded to each other as lord and vassal. One by one his men followed him to kneel before me. There was a small Roman incense altar provided for those who might hold with older ways. Only one knight chose it, and that after a moment's hesitation. He was one of my own people, a Brigante with a daub of Pict in him, if I know the look. But this oath bound him as tight as the others.

Britain as a whole likely accepted Gareth as lord-milite with less reservation than they did me. Despite Arthur's published will, I was not yet chosen. Anything could happen. A current of urgency ran swift under the pageant of royal and holy ritual, even to the choice of Arthur's tomb.

Where should I bury him? Maelgwyn, who owed his restored crown to Arthur, offered to found a chapel at Badon where they fought side by side. Arthur's crypt would lie beneath the altar with a perpetual endowment for masses. My Parisi, whom Arthur saved at Eburacum, would do the same, and so on through the numerous wide-flung abbeys whose good will Arthur and I nurtured over the years. His Dobunni relatives, especially old Flavia Marcella, sued for burial in the province of his birth.

In hindsight you might ask: Why not in Camelot itself? Because honor to my husband was not the only consideration. I simply couldn't afford to bestow that honor without some profit. That granted, whom did I need

most? The Parisi and Catuvellauni were safe in my pocket, the Dobunni divided and insignificant, Cornwall an opponent, the far west totally unreliable. No single tribe was that valuable alone. Only one institution transcended them all, the Church.

The clergy adored me, not without prudent effort on my part and misgiving on theirs. They were strong but not yet religious masters in Britain. Conversion filters down from the crown to the subject and not all that quickly, Church historians to the contrary. Like Arthur's family, mine gave hospitable room to Christ without evicting the older tenants. Royal women of the Parisi were always identified with the old goddesses of fertility and our beds were privileged—indeed, prescribed—as evidence of that joyous virtue. My grandmother, mother and I made a pleasure and a profit of a necessity—one learns more about men in bed than out—but how could our priests preach chastity to the many while condoning the few? To their credit they managed; in turn I was scrupulous in my observance of the remaining commandments.

I'd worked for that adoration and now I needed to lean on it. The Church must be behind me.

Because the Grail was found at Ynnis Witrin, Abbot Brochan's was the most prestigious monastery in Britain. He'd already requested the honor of interment in his precincts. Ynnis Witrin—I believe the Saxons now call it Glastonbury—was on the northern border of Dyfneint within the holding of Eleyne and Lancelot. They were tributary to Mark but loyal to me, so with one stroke I gained two more voices toward my permanent election. If that seems bald and calculated, remember I had few friends, forty-odd knights, a dead king to bury and no other choice but to relinquish the sword or be murdered by someone like Constantine. Which looks more viable to you?

The letter was written: *Guenevere in Arthur's name to her father in Christ, Brochan, Abbot of Ynnis Witrin. I ask your blessing . . .*

Yes, quite calculated. Less than twelve hours to Ynnis Witrin, all of it by water. As a margin of safety, Bors and Regan would not notify Mark until he barely had time to arrive, much less inform Constantine. The funeral pro-

cession would be my party and that of Astolat. If Mark
could not appear, our profuse apologies . . .

I rarely misjudged my enemies and made few mistakes
as queen. Burying Arthur at Witrin was a blunder. The
letter was sealed and with it the history of Britain.

We embarked before midnight. Only Brochan, Lancelot and Eleyne, Bors and Regan knew the exact time of
our arrival. Our three ships were captured Saxon keels,
swift shallow-drafted vessels both seaworthy and able to
navigate the silted, fen-choked rivers of our coast. Morning found us almost at Witrin, and I congratulated myself on shrewd common sense.

In the stern of the lead ship Imogen whiled the last
hour before Witrin brushing out my hair which must be
unbound for mourning. She worked over me with one
eye on Bedivere and Gareth standing forward of Arthur's
guarded casket, leaning over the prow gunwales. I would
have wagered Christ to fight with Mary quicker than a
tiff between those two ancient companions, but it happened at Camelot—and confirmed my chilly suspicions
about Constantine's solicitation of Bedivere. They were
drinking in the refectory and must have had too much,
not the usual way of either. Imogen was looking to my
supper in the scullery and eavesdropped, fascinated. One
of her few soft spots was for Gareth mac Diurmuid.

She drove the brush across my scalp, her voice low so
the steersman wouldn't hear. "Look at the two of them:
still bonny friends, though the Gryffyn's summ'at hard to
like. Arthur's oldest and closest, but you could say the
same of a wart. Give me Gareth any day."

Imogen's Brigante burr softened a little. "Many's the
time in the old days I looked after the mac Diurmuid
when he passed, and that lonely wi' my own husband
and bairn dead. A sunny man, a smiling man." She
jerked her narrow head toward the ship off our bow that
carried my men's wives. "God gi' me to understand
someday *why* he married that bog-running Rhian."

She scooped her fingers into the mass of my hair and
caught up a handful to worry at a snarl.

"Well, then: there's the two of them alone at the refectory table drinking to y'lord husband's memory. And
Gareth says—very civil—Why is't you'll not swear to the

Queen? And tart Bedivere answers he'll stay to see you chosen and the rest is his affair.

"Now, Gareth's nae a mean bone in his body, but a wee bit further in's cup than usual. Says he, You all want to go home as if the troubles were over. Then Bedivere says, Even combrogi grow old. I want to go home while I still know the way.

"Then they filled the cups again, Lord Gareth very thoughtful, saying, Do you know that's all I heard from the men, that sort of style? Arthur is dead, it's all up, my oath is broken and my home a long way and dear in my heart. And didn't I need all the wit of my tongue to keep the tenth of them with me, and those more out of loyalty to me than anything else? It's as if my lord never lived."

Imogen reached for the fine-toothed ivory comb in my lap, bending close to my ear. "Then how does it look to those few, Gareth says, when the oldest and closest will not swear to his lord's Queen? Won't they feel fools? And Bedivere comes back sharp: And what of *my* wife? Myfanwy's spent her life seeing the front of me come and the back of me go and what else but waiting in between?"

Imogen went back to the brush. "Mind, Lady, that's the laundered gist of the Gryffyn, leaving out the worst. I'll hazard his confessions, when he deigns to make them, are mainly to do with shameful speech. Ah, Jesus, he moans, I don't know the right of it. How much fight must a man have in him, Gareth? Even in the legions a man went home when his time was done. Twenty-five years, and what's left of it? Kay dead, Artos dead. I knew I was done with it at Badon. Done, Gareth.

"Well, Lord Gareth is on his third cup of uisge and beginning to feel it. Says he: Don't hold up Badon to me. Wasn't I there riding in the cold while you slept warm? Aye, says Bedivere back. There's Kay dying in the mud and you rode right over him!"

I winced to think of what that did to Gareth. Kay took his mortal wound from Cerdic, saving Arthur's life. He was already half dead when Gareth's men charged the Saxons, trampling Kay and nearly Arthur as well. They were all over muck; Gareth couldn't tell one from another, but he agonized months over that accident of war.

"Well!" Imogen punctuated her story with long strokes of the brush. "Gareth's a gentle, Christen man, but that

was a sore point. Says he and not so gently, I never thought to say this of an old friend, but you're a cruel bastard you are, opening a wound I prayed to close. I won't drink with such a man or one who won't swear service with me.

"*Listen*, says Bedivere, getting hot himself. You know Guenevere. All her love for us you could drop in that cup and never taste it. Don't I know that, says Gareth. You're thick, Bedwyr, as Arthur always said. It's the holy *principle* of the thing. Guenevere is Arthur's wife, bound by the Church. One flesh, one oath!

"Ah, go to hell, you're worse than a bloody priest! And Bedivere heaves up from the table all unsteady. And then Gareth rises, too—very slow, very deadly if I know the look—and says, But I'm right and ready to fight to prove it if that's what you want."

Imogen bent close to my ear, tense with her story. "I thought they'd at it then and there, and the two of them like crossed swords over the table. Then Bedivere says— soft, I could barely hear—Gareth-fach, what I want most is to cry. Guenevere asking on one side and Constantine promising on the other. For God's sake let up on me.

"And there's Gareth looking like something in him will break. On a sudden he smiles—well, like a smile but all crumpled about something inside. Jesus, says he, that's the truth of it. I have to bury the best King I ever knew, and I don't want to think on that sober.

"Nor I, says the Gryffyn, so let's drink to him. And the two of them sat down again weeping like mothers for a lost bairn. There now: you're combed out."

As Imogen set the gold coronet on my brow, I looked forward of the guarded casket to where Bedivere and Gareth stood together, intent on any movement from either shore, a vigilance they learned long ago on the Wall. Gareth sagged a little. Bedivere's arm slipped around his shoulder in a natural gesture of understanding. Two men I really didn't know yet. I and Britain might be a lost cause; if so, which of them was the more tragic, the believer or the realist who saw it all might come to nothing? There was an uneasy sense of things beyond my cleverness.

They loved Arthur, they obeyed me. The two are not the same. Deep love, like a tall tree, is a long time grow-

ing, and I didn't know very much about the emotion
then. Felt it sometimes, bought it, used it, understood it
not at all. To youth and even vital prime, age seems a
lessening and a narrowing toward death. It's not that at
all but a widening out to where love has so many more
targets, becomes so many different things with varied
faces, and the hasty scrawl of a hurrying life becomes
meaningful writ. So many loves: the river widens until
we know so much more than we can utter, that the sure
silence of it must be God's own hand on our shoulder. But
that takes a great deal of living. That summer day on
River Brue, I still used men more than I loved them. I
was forty-seven and thought myself wise, when I was
still a child learning at life's knee. I knew nothing, not
even that I'd left Camelot for the last time.

"Lady!"

Gareth pointed to the north shore where a small party
waited on the bank. I recognized Lancelot in his customary dun and black, Eleyne and Galahalt beside him. Not
too happily I noted Yseult in her favorite green and
Prince Mark like a tall, tired old willow beside her, and I
wondered how in God's name they were here so quickly.
They had earlier notice than was planned or good for me.
Then how close might Constantine be?

"*. . . and Constantine promising.*" It gave me no assurance to know my survival instincts were still infallible.

The royal houses of Cornwall and Dyfneint were cere-
monially grouped before the monks of Ynnis Witrin and
behind Abbot Brochan. The abbot was once a knight under Eleyne's father, Caradoc, and never lost the warrior
stamp. He moved as if armor still hung about his shoulders. His vital stride, the breadth of his shoulders and
corn-yellow hair could remind you of Arthur from certain angles until you noted the hard mouth and the ascetic conviction of the ice-blue eyes. Some abbeys
existed at ease with a pleasant measure of jocularity at
table. At Ynnis Witrin, under Brochan's iron order, they
labored in their own fields, missed no holy offices whatever the day, ate plain as Anchorites and eschewed as
much of the world as possible. I knelt to receive the Abbot's blessing, offering up my donative of silver denarii.

"In the name of Arthur, your patron."

"And so we receive it." Brochan signed me with the cross and had barely grasped the purse when his almoner bustled forward to relieve him of it. "Bless our daughter in Christ. Long life to our Queen."

While a detail toiled the heavy casket ashore and the combrogi saddled their horses, there was time for the muted greetings of a funeral party. Old Mark, feeble but with eyes shadowed and subtle under heavy black brows. Dear Yseult, still beautiful in a fleshy way, hugging me like a sister. Lancelot was gravely formal; but that all Britain knew it you'd never think he was my lover only months ago. Even in that short time his heavy, square frame had thickened, as if in leaving me he simply surrendered to girth and middle age. I tried to find something in his glance that remembered. It wasn't there. And yet no one knew better than I the deep passion, even the lyricism of Ancellius Falco whom men called Lancelot. Reaching for God, he found me. It was a lovely need, and I filled it more practically than heaven ever could.

Eleyne's hair was going the way of mine, fading to a colorless state that Imogen would one day realize was more gray than anything else. I envied Yseult her thick ebony mop that silvered so exquisitely in just the right places. But Yseult was my age and Eleyne barely forty. She went from youth to decline with no lingering, nothing, apparently, to linger for. In all the years I knew them, as often as I'd slept with Lancelot, I could never convincingly picture the two of them in bed. Eleyne was not homely but plain, lacking that vivacious lunacy that had flamed her brother Geraint, self-saddled with a leaden sense of God and duty derived through her descent from Joseph of Arimathea. An implacable woman; we would never have been close even if I'd never led Lancelot astray. For that matter she regarded him as having gone from her only briefly and returned to his rightful place like a stone falling back to earth.

Eleyne was personally loyal to Arthur, even more so when Lancelot married her. She doubtless considered me as much of a whore as Yseult and with better reasons. Her moral contempt for Yseult and Trystan she never bothered to conceal. Eleyne was not a sensitive

person but she was iron, and there's nothing better for
bolting a door. I always used her family with enormous
courtesy.

"Lady, the house of Astolat grieves with you." Eleyne
embraced me formally and without enthusiasm.
"Galahalt, attend the Queen. She will be uncovered. You
will bear her coronet."

I hadn't seen Lancelot's son since he was ten or so. At
fifteen Galahalt evidenced his father's broad build that
would ripen more to power than height, but the face was
Eleyne's, stolid and humorless. I removed the gold circlet
and placed it in Galahalt's hands. The boy lowered his
head and stepped back. *My God, he already looks like a
chapel mosaic.*

"We embarked as quickly as we had word," Mark told
me. "Hardly time to gather an escort."

No time at all. The official nuncio should not have delivered our message before last evening. Yet his dozen or
so knights, standing aloof from those of Dyfneint, bore
no stamp of haste in their appearance. They were
groomed; their gear and that of their mounts was spruce
and shined.

The formal greetings done, Gareth formed our combrogi escort, some ahead and some behind the funeral
wagon. All would be mounted except myself and Imogen, who wouldn't hear of riding with me afoot.
Gareth's men carried lances as well as swords and
quickly donned their mail. At the rear of the column, two
riders led an extra horse for me. This mount was not part
of custom. Gareth knew the situation and was taking no
chances. In the stir of mounting and forming, Lord Bors
and pretty Regan came forward to greet me.

Bors was no more than one and twenty, Regan seven-
teen. To anyone watching, these youngest of my courtiers
glowed and preened under my affection, but beneath
Bors' robust forthrightness and Regan's flighty innocence
were mature and capable observers—the term I preferred for trusted spies as opposed to those I merely
bought. Regan ducked her curtsy; as I hugged her to me,
she kissed my cheek like a daughter and whispered,
"Constantine sent messengers to Astolat."

"And?"

"Sounded them on the succession."

"My dears, it's so good to see you again. Regan, I believe you're getting plump . . . who's with me?"

"Astolat for sure," Bors murmured. "Lancelot wouldn't even hear the envoys and Eleyne sent them packing home with insults."

"Nay, *please* you, Lady!" Regan flustered convincingly. "I've not gained the tenth of a stone in weight, but I think I am breaking out here on the neck."

I leaned close to inspect the creamy, unflawed skin on her throat. "Mark didn't wait for messengers, but sent to his nephew straight on Arthur's death."

"Interesting. Was Mark's invitation delayed?"

"To the hour you wished."

"Then how in hell is he here?"

"We don't know," Bors confessed uneasily. "How or who, we can't fathom it."

"Darlings, we've been sold. And we can only smile and pretend we don't know it. Take your places."

Mark bowed again as I passed to take my place behind the funeral wagon. Nearly eighty he was then, and still I couldn't read those hooded eyes. He tried to kill Arthur before his choosing and came so close to succeeding that Arthur came bloody from the hill of the sword to our wedding. If Mark was jubilant at my husband's death, he'd declare a holiday over mine. If he planned treachery, this was a good day for it.

We should post picket riders. Even as I thought it, I saw Gareth speak quietly to two of his knights, who dropped inconspicuously to the rear. As we moved away from the river, they lagged even farther behind. My eyes must see no object but the casket, but Imogen glanced back from time to time.

"They've nipped out of sight, Lady. They'll be your eyes."

I trudged on through the summer morning, not feeling much safer.

In my tongue Ynnis Witrin means "isle of glass." The abbey tor and the lowlands skirting it were encircled by a wide marsh which must once have been a lake. The bog would still be impossible to cross without the raised causeways north and south. It has always been a sacred place. At the hill's summit where Joseph of Arimathea founded his wattle church, our druids once sacrificed

red-haired chosen to the sun. Holy Well itself, now the spiritual property of Jesus, once had its own protective deity.

The burial of a king can't be a total secret. At Holy Well near the foot of the hill, some hundred of Eleyne's free and unfree peasants were gathered and waiting. They uncovered and knelt as the wagon passed. The reverence was all for Arthur, I'm sure. They knew me only as a recent rebel, but Arthur was their immortal, raised even in his lifetime to the eminence of Apollo. They fell back as we gathered about the well. The other wives ranged themselves about me to hear Brochan and his monks sing that hour's office for the dead.

The psalms rose on the still air. My eye drifted to note the wives of my combrogi and subject lords. It seemed all I knew were present except Bedivere's wife, Myfanwy. Queer absence, considering her husband's position. Lady Myfanwy had known Arthur as a child and his generosity after she married his most trusted friend. Then again, perhaps not so strange. Did Bedivere sell me or did he just know the risks we took here? He was not sworn to me. He'd look after his own first.

Only months ago my brother Peredur found the Grail in this well, and it was that most holy relic the people came to see and wonder at as much as their dead king. Wise Brochan knew this, and though display of the Grail was no part of the office, he used it well. The genuine Grail was an ordinary bronze bowl, not even of high quality and far too plain for the exalted vessel expected of legend. Brochan had it set in silver. When he elevated it before the awed throng, the blaze of polished surface suffused his hands, as if Brochan held out to his flock the very light of God.

What he did then smacked more of the old religion than any Christian mass. He dipped a censer into the vessel which held water from the well and blessed the multitude with it, as druids once dipped the male symbol of the sky-knife into the female receptacle of earth. It was what the people knew and understood, and no British priest with any common sense would call it sacrilege. Where God has many names, you give men one they can read.

Built over Joseph's primitive church, the abbey was

not very impressive by city standards. The whole was enclosed in a wall of vitrified stone. Inside were a number of small beehive stone cells for the seclusion of each monk, a large refectory, a timber stable and the small oratory itself, its narrow interior showing the effects of Astolat's obsessive (and possessive) generosity. The walls were mosaicked with portraits of the Apostles, Peter and Paul, and the latter-day pillars, Germanus, Augustine and Ambrose. Pelagius, popular with most patrician families in my grandmother's day, was emphatically disavowed in Astolat. The altar was a simple sandstone slab cut with a *chi-rho* cross. Several large slates of the chancel floor had been taken up and excavated beneath to receive the body of my husband.

The small oratory barely contained our company. I knelt beside the casket as Brochan spread his arms to the Cross and began the mass for the dead. The deep-timbred Latin was richly stained with his Dumnoni dialect.

> *Requiem aeternam dona eis, Domine,*
> *et lux perpetua eis . . .*
> *Exaudi orationem meam;*
> *ad te omnis caro veniet*
> *Kyrie eleison, Christe eleison . . .*

The stone floor was cruel on my thin knees. I tried to keep my mind on the mass, but a sodden blanket of weariness descended on me. For weeks I'd thrust away the reality of this death, muffled it in hard work and preparation. The long walk to the abbey I spent in fear and the suspicion that corrodes the best of rulers. Now I was naked to the moment. This rough wood within my reach contained a man I loved, a body I exulted in. It was physical loss, an amputation. We were one flesh and half of me was going into the ground. No, wait. Not yet—

> *Sanctus Dominus Deus Sabaoth!*
> *Pleni sunt Coeli et terra gloria tua*
> *Hosanna in excelsis!*

No, merciful Christ, not this clear a truth: that I would never see him again until we stood before God for judg-

ment. Out of so many years, why did we have so little
time?

> That day shall be a day of wrath,
> of calamity and misery;
> that day shall be a mighty one;
> Grant them eternal rest, O Lord . . .

I'll need that mercy more than you. Darling, will you
hold my hand then, very tight? I think you'll have a better case than mine, and I want to go with you, wherever
it is.

> *In paradisum deducant angeli . . .*

Oh, Brochan, shut up, shut *up*. Leave me alone, let me
love my lover here and now, alive and stained with im-
perfect earth. Let me touch him once more—

> There may the choir of angels receive thee
> and with Lazarus, once a beggar,
> mayst thou have eternal rest.

"*Dominus vobiscum,*" Brochan intoned.
"*Et cum spiritu tuo,*" murmured his acolyte.
Brochan turned back to the altar. "*Requiescant in
pace.*"
"Amen."
It was finished. Eight monks took up the slack on their
ropes while four others removed the supporting timbers.
The casket began to sink beyond my reach, and then it
was all too real, the last of Arthur alive ramping through
my brain and body.
"No . . ."
Never, never until Judgment Day. All those years of loving and fighting, country-love and gut-love, my body and
will against his or clasped to his and containing it, so
interwound that one grew to the other. Never till Judgment, and it was that denial in the face of love, powered
by love itself in that last moment, that made me claw
once more at my love and enemy as he went into the
ground.
Damn you for leaving me.

Never to see you lope across the courtyard at Camelot, the imperial cloak for which lesser men would pawn their lesser souls, slung in a careless bundle over one shoulder, the whole meaning of purpose and energy in your stride. I remember that, Arthur.

I stretched a hand to touch the casket once more before it was gone. *Don't go. Don't leave me, damn you—*

Never again the loving that was a battle and the battles that were love frozen in the cold muck of duty. Damn you for that last falsely cheerful letter, cheating me of my grieving share in your death, so even that I must do alone. Even at the end I don't know if you thought of me or Morgana, cried to me or to her, and damn her too, the filthy bitch. I would have heard you down the length of Britain—but there was only your letter and silence, and I'll feed my own entrails to the fox while they bury Good King Arthur as a goddamned legend. Christ, Arthur, this isn't *us*, not you and me. Break out of that lie and hold me, fight me, make love to me. I can't think, only reach to hold you back, keep you yet where I can rend and kiss. You've left the worst of it, the dirt of it to me, and why wasn't there more time for love? Why didn't I come to you instead of Lancelot or say the things I felt, and why have you gone and left me with the bleeding mess of it all? I love you and hate you for this, and I *damn* you . . . love you . . . damn you, Arthur—

The casket thumped softly on deep earth. Silence for the space of a breath, then the clatter of hooves on the courtyard stones and the combrogus ran through the portal, elbowing his way to the chancel: Dai meqq Muir, my Brigante pagan, still buckling the sword about his ring mail. Brochan bristled at the lack of respect, but Dai had no time for niceties.

"Sorry, but he that's dead would do the same. Lord Gareth, there's Cornishmen moving between us and the ships. Threescore I counted."

In the general eddy of fear and consternation, the second picket rider pounded up to the entrance and ran inside, mail and sword dangling in his hands.

"Get the Queen mounted and gone. There's a hundred riders coming from the north."

Gareth didn't even blink. "Constantine."

"Aye, his flags."

"How far?"

"Three miles. Coming slow."

Which meant we had only minutes to clear the north causeway or be neatly trapped on this hill.

"Like we were already cooked and ready to carve," Bedivere ground through his teeth. "This was planned."

"Combrogi, mount," Gareth ordered. "See to the—"

"Not yet!" Bedivere's clear voice shrilled sudden and high as a banshee's. "There's a Judas here, and I want him first."

"No time for that," Lancelot urged. "Get the Queen to safety."

"You said it yourself, Lancelot, not three months gone. There's no place left for honor. I'm sick of being sold."

"Amen to that," Gareth said out of desperate disgust. "We've bled a long time. If I go, some bastard goes with me."

Even as my mind worked to control the moment, Eleyne pointed at Mark. "There he is! Who was it tried to murder our King before the crown was safe on his head? Who would have murdered my own brother into the bargain? Mark, I say."

The old prince played shocked surprise as if he'd invented it. "Not true, woman. Here in the Church and on my soul, you lie."

"Who profits most from the Queen's death?" Eleyne persisted as her own knights edged in about her. "Who will wear the crown, you or Constantine?"

"Woman, Mark is your own lord," Yseult reminded her venomously. "Don't perjure yourself. Guenevere, this is false. I have my husband's trust, and I wouldn't hear treachery in my own hall."

No, she wouldn't. Or much of anything else, either. Yseult was an innocent. "You're a loving woman, sweet," I answered sadly, "but Mark was always a traitor."

Bedivere turned on the old prince like a judgment. "So he was."

It happened very quickly. Before anyone could intervene, Bedivere and Gareth did the thing forever. Bedivere's motives I might question—and did—but not Gareth's. His love for Arthur, his lord's needless death just when there seemed an end to war and agony. Twenty-five years of Gareth's life went into the ground

with Arthur. Now, at the grave, this final betrayal. It was too much for even gentle Gareth. He yanked Mark forward and whipped him around, arms pinioned, as Bedivere's dagger went into the old man's breast. Whatever sound Mark made dying was drowned in Yseult's wail of horror and Gareth's command.

"Combrogi! Swords!"

Forty blades hissed from their sheaths against the Cornish knights, Lancelot's among them as he, Galahalt and Eleyne took their place beside Bedivere. Crouched over Mark's body, Yseult screamed: "Kill them!"

Bedivere leveled his sword at the Cornish knights, quivering with murder. Lancelot moved smoothly to cover his flank.

"Yseult," I said, "for all I love you, this was well done." And so it was. Whoever sold me, Mark, Bedivere himself, I had one enemy less. They were my men and few enough. I must stand behind them and take responsibility for their acts. "By my wish and on my head."

Brochan looked down at the body of Mark. "By my God, Guenevere, you and your men are unfit for holy chapel. A prince killed in God's own house and you call it well done? Leave this place."

Bedivere snorted in cold disgust. "Don't waste your sanctity, Father Abbot. This whole country's whored for a hundred years. God couldn't find it for the muck. Gareth, let's move."

"Right, then: two by two out the door. See to our women. Rhian, look lively now. Bors, take the Queen."

Bors hurried to me with frightened Regan's hand clamped in his. "Lady, if we must die today—"

"Sod that!" Bedivere cut him off with the sharp edge of his own tension. "No one's worth a damn dead, didn't Artos teach you that much? Get the Queen to horse."

"Guenevere!" Yseult rose over her husband's body, cold. "I always knew you could murder, but I looked away because you were my friend. Was it so easy with Morgana?"

"Oh, my dear, it was never easy; it was necessary. That's the difference between us. I was always a queen. You were never anything but a wife."

"Nor one to keen over any husband," Eleyne said with

an indecent relish. "You lay with his nephew before your wedding sheets wanted changing."

"Enough, Eleyne." Miserable bitch, I despised her thoroughly, ally or not. At least Yseult was a woman and always a friend till now. "I'm sorry, Yseult. Pray for me."

I hurried from the oratory with Imogen close behind and Yseult's high-keening curse for farewell.

"Pray? Whoever kills you, Guenevere, you and your whole filthy combrogi lot, it's them I'll pray for till my knees grow to the floor—"

This is how I leave you, Arthur. You came wounded to our wedding from Mark's first treachery, I run from your unfilled grave through his last. Bedivere's right, we've been whored for years, and still no one's worth anything dead. For all that, I'm all they've got . . . all they've got, and if I live through this day I'll trust none but myself. I'll rule as you wished, but for that I must live. For you and all of them.

II

Lie Down with Serpents

f you can tolerate Gildas' ungodly Latin and his lip-smacking condemnation of other men's sins, he gives a biased but clear picture of my country's downfall. Disappearance is the better word; surely it was that swift.

We didn't know it that day but our dash to the north causeway was to become a headlong flight across a Britain crumbling as we rode. When it ended, the illusion of unity was gone, the separate pieces Arthur and I joined with such care mere fragments once more.

Were you the cement after all, Arthur? That flashing, inconsistent mind of yours, common yet touched with genius, flawed by sentiment, rippled with laughter and impatient scorn of tradition? That slight a feather to turn the scales against anarchy for a little while? I think you made all the difference by being just who and what and when you were. The end would have come anyway, has come, but you were allowed to die in the brief light we kindled, while I've survived well beyond the dark into a very strange morning. That made for a profound education; indeed, I'm stuffed with the virtues of learning. I could write a better history of my times than Gildas, but when you're running for your life, you can't stop to ponder the view.

If Constantine trapped us this side of the marsh, the game was done. We sped across the causeway four

abreast, clearing it as the first Cornish came into view around a low hill. Northern Dyfneint is rolling moor and down; there was no cover or chance for flight. Gareth had to fight and protect an encumbrance of women at the same time. His blunt little face contorted as he studied the ground ahead, then conferred swiftly with Lancelot and Bedivere. If we women were frightened—a pallid estimate—we had no time to mill about. Lancelot wheeled on us.

"Form on the Queen."

Eleyne, Rhian and Regan hurried their nervous mounts in beside me, Imogen edging as close as possible, as the men sheathed us smoothly in a formidable wedge. Constantine outnumbered us, but we had the better position. He was still deploying his men in two lines of attack when Gareth's command sent the wedge of us like a loosed arrow at the raveled edge of his line. I am a competent rider but not when a hundred lances are seeking me out. Eleyne rode with a rein tight as the line of her mouth, Rhian cursing in Irish, Regan white and wide-eyed, searching for Bors in the confusion.

"Where is he? God, where *is* he?"

At full gallop our men's lances swept forward. The Cornish were barely under way when we ripped through their line like wet parchment, rolled over the fallen and sailed on. Arthur always said battle gave you a heightened awareness of absurdities. Boiling with terror and excitement, I remember even now clear flashes of total irrelevance: the dainty yellow flowers woven around the helmet of a Cornishman as he plunged past us, Eleyne riding close to me like a shield, a small dagger ready in her hand if he broke through; Regan hoarse with fright and something more as she twisted desperately about to find her husband. It seemed terribly important to her.

"Where is he? I haven't told him."

"Never mind, child; look to yourself now."

"But, mum, I haven't told him."

"What?" I bawled.

"I'm pregnant. I haven't told him!"

And in the middle of that, sight of the darkening sky, and thinking, *It's going to rain.* And Rhian breaking off her curses to screech almost comically at Regan: "Could it not in the name of Jesu wait a breath? There he is, fool!

Not a dog's bark away from you. And there's Galahalt! *A-
ho! Dia dhuit a Galahalt!*"

Eleyne's boy reined in at her side. "Father says we've
got a chance. Stay close together." And he was gone again
as our wedge reversed, closed around us and once more
carried us at the disordered Cornish, trampling the
wounded who tried hopelessly to crawl out of the way. I
remember hoping in jagged shards of prayer that none of
them were ours. The center of the wedge was the safest
place for me; neither I nor my women were ever exposed
to Constantine's advantage, but we ran against time. If
the troop by our boats had a chance to join the battle, we
were dead.

The combrogi fought as an efficient engine with well-
greased gears. Where the Cornish lords took eight or
nine seconds to form, Gareth's men needed only four or
five. Time and time again the stubbornly honorable Cornish flashed out alone or in twos, shrilling their challenge to single combat. The combrogi never broke
formation, never stopped moving, always one thought
ahead of Constantine, who fought with a ferocity blunted
by his lack of discipline. Our second attack completely
disorganized him. I saw him dash down his front, trying
to re-form some sort of line; in that moment Gareth and
Lancelot changed tactics. The wedge opened out like a
bird taking wing into two straight ranks, the first already at full charge as the second swerved into line behind Bedivere.

It was the same attack that broke Cerdic at Eburacum,
so precise it looked more a dance than a maneuver. The
first line hit and spread wide apart to let the second line
through. During the second assault, the first line
wheeled and re-formed. Not a movement for untrained
horses or undisciplined men. Constantine was forced on
the defensive from the beginning and never had a chance
to attack in force. Just when he anticipated the wedge
again, he got something else and lost more men, but the
shift left myself and the women vulnerable for a moment. For two reckless Cornish knights that was enough.
Where they'd expected quick victory, they were fighting
just to stay alive, and it lashed them to a red fury
through which they saw one clear fact: except for
Galahalt and his groom, I was undefended. They could

reach me now. They dropped lances and drew their swords, lashing into a gallop. No war cries, only that hurtling determination. Galahalt and his groom spurred to intercept, but they were awkwardly placed. They hit one of the knights from both sides. His horse coughed with the impact, stumbled and went down on its haunches. The other knight battered Imogen's mount aside and came on at me. I had a flash of Eleyne drawing in on my other side, the knife in her hand, the Cornishman's sword raised, Rhian stretching out, screaming in Irish as her sturdy wrist caught his and took the power from the blow. He ignored her, snapped straight in the stirrups and dove headlong, dragging me from my saddle.

We struck the ground together, both of us jarred by the shock as he groped for his dagger. Then there were three of us rolling on the trampled down as Eleyne was suddenly there. A vicious flurry of movement, his knife raising, mine slashing up, Eleyne's somehow between us. Mine went into his throat first. Eleyne hesitated only a tiny breath before she finished him efficiently. Then it was Galahalt dragging me to my feet, bruised and queasy. "Stay close, all of you. Regan, I mean you! You want that child to be born? God bless you, Eleyne. Rhian, are you hurt?"

Not hurt, only frustrated, rubbing her wrist. "What would I not give for a good club. A stone, a clod. Anything."

Poor Galahalt looked sick after Sawel finished the other knight. "It's well, Mother. Father's lost not a man. It looks like we have them."

True. So far we'd suffered no losses while Constantine had left a dozen on the field. Gareth was between us and the Cornish now. Again they were slow to act, and in those vacillating seconds our men formed in the protecting wedge around us. Lancelot pushed through to me.

"We're going through to the road this time. Don't stop for anything."

"Finish Constantine!" I panted at him. "Never mind the others, get *him*."

"Guenevere, there is no time. We're too few to be sure of it. Better you alive than him dead. Wife, we're making for the Sulis road."

"Aye, husband, and well done."

"We're going to live!" Rhian crowed with jubilant release. "Was't not my Gareth did it? We're going to live."

"Of course." Eleyne gave Rhian one heavy-lidded, disdainful glance. "Did you think else?"

Gareth's arm swept forward. I closed my eyes, winced as my bruised body protested further punishment, and dug heels into the mare's flanks. Constantine barely opposed us this time. His men were already beaten in their hearts, no longer that superior in numbers and hopelessly overmatched. As we flashed through them, I turned in the saddle to see Constantine glaring at me, stymied but still vibrant with purpose, and couldn't resist one parting sting with all the satisfaction of the quick bird eluding the cat.

"Not this year, boy. I told you: not *this* year!"

Not that day at any rate. You were an amateur to the end, Constantine, and made an amateur's unholy mess of it all. Whatever inspired you to think you'd fit a crown? And why is it always your mucked-up kind that needs one most? My God, history is depressing; for that reason I've decided to give up drinking *next* year, not this.

He didn't pursue us. We thought he might after his second squadron came up, and didn't slacken our speed until we reached the Roman road eight miles west. All through the day we expected them behind us, but our rear pickets saw nothing.

When Gareth called a needed rest at the junction with the sea road, we all breathed easier. This was Dobunni land where loyalty to Arthur was a matter of blood relation. None of our men had more than superficial wounds, no horses were lamed. The rain came while we grazed them, a steady downpour that promised a long, wet, hungry ride to Aquae Sulis. I huddled in my cloak, envying the mare her graze when a familiar pair of boots halted in the narrow vision of my hood.

"My Queen, may I have a word?"

"Of course, dear. And you needn't be so formal. We're alone."

Lancelot offered me his arm to rise. "You're not hurt?"

"Despite appearances, no. I must look as if I died yesterday."

Lancelot smiled tenderly. "You will never change. You

always slighted your beauty and always made sure no woman outshone you."

"Good policy. You've seen me in the mornings: frowsy as a mudlark before my women do me."

His smile broadened, less tentative. "Well . . . some mornings. You seemed always beautiful because you made me feel that way."

"That's the secret, darling. Yseult was a born dazzler, but I had to work at it. What did you want?"

"We ask leave to part here. It was Eleyne's decision," he hurried to assure me. "I would stay, of course, but Eleyne is the crown power, and she's right, Guenevere."

"Yes, of course."

"There's no danger for you now, but perhaps for Astolat and our own. We must be there."

Sound thinking; were I not so battered and soggy, I'd have urged it myself. By taking my part they were in actual revolt against their Cornish overlords. Constantine would come down on little Astolat like this damned rain. "Yes, it's best. Do go on."

Lancelot hesitated, obviously wanting to speak further. My gentle, tormented lover-that-was, never able to accept his own passion when it wasn't pointed at God, a bulky man with the face of a patient monk now going to jowls and the downward set of unresolved disappointments.

"I'm sorry, Guenevere. I couldn't believe it when your letter came, it—stunned me. I wanted to come to you. Comfort you if I could."

"Dear Lancelot, thank you."

"I once hated him because of you. And yet, Britain without Arthur? It's a contradiction."

"He had his flaws. He couldn't let love go when its time was past. You and I can be wiser than that."

He accepted that much. "I suppose we are. But it's hard to forget."

"Us? Impossible, my love, so let's not even try. Look at us as a national treasure. You can tell your randy grandchildren you were once loved to exhaustion by the wickedest bitch in Britain."

"Damn you, Guenevere, aren't you ever serious?"

"Always. I just won't go wet over it. Come." I took his arm. "Let me give thanks and farewell to Eleyne and

your people. *Oh*, this miserable rain. Just our luck it'll keep up all the way home."

When our farewells were said, Eleyne brought Galahalt forward to kneel in front of me, the boy still pale from the battle that must have been his first.

"High Queen." No one but Eleyne could make it sound so undeserved. "We want no thanks but this. Take my son to be with you at Camelot. Keep him safe, he and his groom, Sawel."

I put my hand on Galahalt's head. "He will be as my own in fosterage until Astolat calls him home."

He'd be that and one more cord to bind Astolat to me. Cheap enough where I needed every alliance I could find. The groom Sawel was a small, agile man with long arms dangling forward from stooped, muscular shoulders in the manner of an Afric ape. What note I ever took of him showed a totally blank expression, eyes bright but opaque, the shallow alertness of an animal. Devoted but not overkeen. He would look after his lord.

Eleyne took Galahalt's moon face in her hands. Her bleak rectitude, like a cold light, always warmed when she gazed on her son. I wondered often if the woman of her didn't gasp for air inside the armor of her duty. One of God's loons, a mouse-colored, iron-hard woman. Did she make him pay after I sent him back to her, or was she too lofty for that, too? I only know that light never showed for him; what spontaneity Eleyne felt in love was all for Galahalt now.

"Follow the Queen, serve her well. And let you remember, as God is watching, you are a royal son."

"I will, Mother. But I'd rather help at home."

"In time, my joy." Eleyne embraced him once more. "I do love you so. Be in God's hand."

So Astolat went seaward and we pushed on to Aquae Sulis.

Near nine that night, still summer twilight, we lurched through the gates of little Sulis and ordered them barred behind us. Never really a town, it had no magistrate, only a minor decurion to administer the baths which centered on the curative waters of a natural hot spring. Imperial architects whose like we have not seen in two hundred years designed them in the days of the long peace. Arthur and I came here often in our

youth. The great tepidarium was a lovers' delight—we sometimes reserved the vast expanse of it to ourselves— and if you've never made love in a warm bath, you've missed a major advantage of civilization. When age and winter wet ached my bones and his scars, the pleasures of Sulis were as beneficial if less intense. On this dreary night at the end of it all, I wanted only to be clean and to sleep. Thus we decline.

The place was nigh deserted; I'd guess no more than threescore citizens in the twenty walled acres. Only a few of them stirred at our arrival, peeping around corners before their priest ventured out to us. The place looked wretched as I felt. Uther Pendragon kept it up handsomely in his time, Kay somewhat less, but in late years Sulis had been badly neglected. Where the buildings once glittered white in the sun or ivory in moonlight, they were dingy now, the statues of Minerva overturned or broken, the portico of her pretty little temple strewn with garbage.

"Tell the keeper, if you can find him, we'll quarter in the bath," I told the apprehensive priest. "My people need food. Have someone bring it."

"And water and grain for the horses," Bedivere snapped. "Tell the men to treat them well; they're not cart animals."

The priest squinted up at me in the torchlight. He looked seedy as Sulis itself, sparse ginger hair not recently tonsured, grimy hands like bear paws, bunioned feet straining at the straps of his sandals. Longer a plowman than a priest, I'd hazard. "If there's a clean place in this sty, some of my people may want to hear mass. You will say it for them. And take confessions if they require it."

"Will the Queen want a confessor then?"

For what, overconfidence? I'll keep that to remember against the next time, thank you. "No. Just see to the food first."

Beds would have been a luxury, any sort, but we stayed together in case of alarm. We bedded down on the unswept, bird-limed upper gallery of the bath and eked a supper of leek and cabbage soup with occasional nuances of hare, none of it very fresh. We wolfed it down anyway and soothed our punished flesh in the great bath

with perfunctory modesty, men at one end, women at the other. I helped Regan into the water myself. Dear babe, she didn't even show yet, belly as flat as mine.

The bath stank now, rank as their soup. It hurt me to see lichen and green scum on the cracked tiles, feathers and dead insects floating on the water. Slumped against a column on the gallery, too tired to fall asleep easily, I looked down into the fouled bath where ghost-Arthur broke the surface, skin summer-brown and darker than his hair, diving again to come up beside the giggling girl-sprite of me, and we thrashed about panting for air as much as ecstasy. . . .

Oh, enough. Silly bitch, you never used to be sentimental. "Sentiment is a dangerous indulgence in a king." I told him that when he was bringing Morgana and beautiful, vicious Modred to Camelot. Not so long ago; why did it seem ages? Days, doors, walls. Things come between people. I couldn't bear for him to touch me after the baby died. Just for a little while, I thought. But the little became longer and longer in different chambers until being apart grew to habit; until, like exiles, we no longer knew the way home. Lovers have a language that can be lost—how to speak, how to touch, when to *try.* We forgot everything but the starved and stubborn love that wouldn't let go or bend in compromise. Such waste. Such fools. And we were so clever, too.

Of all the times for my cramps to begin. Most women are fortunate enough not to have them. Not I; twelve or thirteen times a year since I was scarce older than that there'd be something vital to do when I wanted only to double up and grit my teeth. The dead child made a mess of my loins, but that part went on, regular as taxes.

Nearby Gareth rested against the stained wall while Rhian worked hyssop ointment into his nicked shoulder. He looked discouraged and older than ever I remembered. *Get up and move, woman. You'll feel better, and the people need you.*

"How is it, Gareth?"

"Nothing, Lady." Not his usual cheer, but eloquent. The man was worn down to the bone.

"We'll feast in Camelot tomorrow night."

Down the long gallery then, stepping around men and women sprawled or curled into lumps of exhaustion, to

where Bors and Regan huddled together, her head on his chest. There's youth for you. They looked more worried than tired.

"Good cheer, children."

Regan's head moved a little on her husband's breast. Bors nodded at her supper bowl, still mostly full. "She was sick after mass. Of all the cursed times to be so blessed."

"Regan, you told him?"

"Yes, mum." I cherished the way she sometimes called me "mum" like "mother." At least she'd be free of that other curse for a few months.

"Try to eat, Regan. The sickness won't last. Tomorrow we'll be home and have such a time making linens for the babe. Rest you gentle."

I made a circuit of the gallery among my people, passing what I hoped was an encouraging word, read their drained faces in the torchlight and saw not mere fatigue but a cumulative despair, the mirror of Gareth's. They'd ridden so long with Arthur for a dream perhaps not understood but worth the striving. Now within months of his death, the dream was tearing at the seams. I lay down beside Imogen, knees pressed up tight against my suffering belly. Not much sleep for me this night.

"Lady?"

The tall shadow loomed over me, holding out something.

"Oh . . . Bedivere."

"The bath keeper makes his own uisge. Here."

I drank from the small amphora, hoping the keeper's uisge was cleaner than his bath. The liquor tasted vile and raw and blessed. "How much do these people know?"

"Well, then. The priest's worried and the bath keeper's drunk. For the rest of them, they know there might be war over the choosing, but they've got nothing here worth a battle except us."

"Meaning me. What did the priest say?"

"Not a great deal, Lady. My confession froze the wee man's blood."

"Mark? Let that be on my soul."

"It needed doing for years," Bedivere agreed. "But I wonder, was it him sold us?"

Bedivere's face was shadowed; I couldn't read his eyes, but the question sat queerly with me. Constantine wouldn't cavil much over his uncle's death. Why should he? It gave him the Cornish crown in one guiltless stroke and might even be part of the plan. "If not Mark, what other man, Bedivere?"

"Na, you want the truth of it?"

"You always ask that as if the truth would send me up in flames."

"The riddle's not who, then, but who next."

"Very perceptive."

"You've got a dagger?"

"You mean, fall on it and save someone the trouble?" Bedivere laughed again. "That would save nothing."

"It saved me today. You still think I'm no Arthur?"

"Well, this much of one: whoever takes the sword needs your voice or your death. I'd keep that dagger close."

"I do, Bedivere."

He took another sip from the amphora and set it on the floor by me. "Rest well, Lady."

The uisge dulled me enough to doze snuggled against the warmth of Imogen. My thoughts broke up as they circled warily closer to sleep, reluctant to surrender vigilance. All these tired, sleeping people, all their fear and hope centered in me. One could wish for an end. *Parousia*, the Greeks call it, the end of all things. An end to my troubles and especially these infernal cramps. I should have heard mass and confessed; one shouldn't go to God unshriven. *Ave, Deus in Coeli:* the end comes when you please, but I'll still plan for tomorrow because the stupid thing usually comes.

In my shallow sleep the bath below me was warm and clean at first. Arthur swam toward me, and I reached down to take him in my arms and wrapped myself around him with a sob, and he burned in me as we sank into the red-clouded water already turning filthy and cold lady lady wake please lady—

"Lady, wake!"

Someone shaking me. My eyes opened, saw the figure over me. Animal fear moved my hand with the dagger—

"Hold, it's me. Imogen."

". . . Imogen?"

"There's folk at the gates crying to get in."

I sat up, rubbing hard at my eyes. "Oh, Jesus. Cornish?"

"From Camelot, Lady. They said it's *taken*."

"Taken? By whom?"

"God knows. I came back straight hearing that. There's few of them and sorry as the lot of us."

"Quick, fetch a taper."

With Imogen lighting my way, I stumbled along the gallery past people already belting on swords or still squirming up out of sleep, down the stairs and out to the portico where Bedivere, Gareth and Rhian faced the small, torchlit knot of Camelot's survivors. Mostly servants, a few men-at-arms, all on foot and muddied from the long journey, much of it through rain. In the flickering light their faces sagged with fatigue and shock. The attack must have been sudden. We didn't leave any force in Camelot; from these pathetic few we could guess how many never had a chance. This lot scarce had time to reach the boats, snatching up a few oddments as they ran, things absurdly important at the moment, as if saving these denied real loss.

"When did it happen, Bedivere?"

"Last night, they said."

"Last *night*?"

"Aye, last night," Gareth spat out of terminal disgust. "And ourselves no farther down Severn than a stone could swim. They knew the moment we left. Is there no end to the treachery?"

I went down to the huddled leavings of Camelot, seeing one of my own Parisi chamberwomen. Poor Morag: no younger than myself and less inclined to exercise, ready to drop where she stood. Her hands twisted and crumpled nervously at a piece of material.

"Who were they, Morag?"

She pushed the dull yellow hair gone frizzy with wet and lack of combing, out of her eyes. "Conant, Lady. Silures . . ."

"Archers," one man spoke up. "Hundreds of them."

Morag nodded, dazed. "Hundreds . . ."

"And Cornish," someone croaked from the rear. "Cornish too, right enough. They that wrap their filthy helms in flowers."

"There was everything but mercy," Morag whispered. "From the boats we saw their torches going through the palace. We heard women screaming."

Conant had ransacked the palace, obviously searching for the imperial sword, as if I'd be fool enough to leave it behind. As clear was the shape of the trap closing on me. Such a snare needed an intricate web of treacheries. Only a few knew where I was going or when, and the first to know from my own mouth was Bedivere. Then Bors and Regan.

Clear thought was impossible at the moment with the sight of these people and the crushing loss of Camelot. Not a fort but a dream. Iceni hands built it, but the dream was Arthur's and mine. We raised the Dragon over Severn Valley to stand for all Britain. That sanctuary of reason and enlightened rule had been violated only twice. Trystan's drunken murder cost him his honor and his place. Mine cost me my crown, a dungeon and almost a war with Arthur. But Camelot, like a child, was a thing we made together. We weren't always worthy of it but, in joy and sorrow, half our lives were lived there.

Morag held out the scrap of material to me. "I saved this."

The fine-carded wool of the little shirt, once white, was limp and colorless with age. Uneven stitches, the whole thing lopsided, knitted when I sat in council meetings pregnant as Regan and less concerned over it, while Arthur stalked among his princes like a worried stallion, proposing, coaxing, demanding, seeing further than any of them ever could—and thinking in my contented heart, *He makes me beautiful. He makes it all worthwhile.* And I let go and I loved and committed to him with a need as fierce as Morgana's ever could be, and the sum of our beauty came out of me dead. Yet I could never bring myself to discard this bedraggled remnant of almost-motherhood. In bad times when I could bear to be nothing but a woman, keening in my woman's heart where my queen's mouth must be silent, I'd take out the little shirt and muffle my crying in it.

"Oh, Morag . . . of all things."

The wool was stained, saturated with my tears. My tears, my life were in Camelot; my justice went out from its walls with Arthur's, the flower gardens planted and

nursed from scrub weed to blossom by my hands. And those Silures and Cornish tracked their filthy boots over stones purified with so much striving, so much hope? They walked on my very heart.

"Thank you, Morag."

The pattern of my life: brief moments of warmth embedded in the cold suet of duty. I gave Morag a little squeeze of thanks as the circle of anxious people closed about me, frightened, looking for answers where I had none.

"What now?" Rhian pressed her husband. "Camelot gone, what can we do?"

"That's for the Queen to say."

"Say what?" Bedivere put it flatly. "They've got us on two sides. We can bloody well run for it, that's all."

Combrogi were already hurrying for the stable and far from rested horses. The knot of people gathered closer about me as the only point of safety, Gareth and Ifan trying to push them back.

"Gareth, we'll make for Glevum. Tell them to hurry. Imogen, give Morag my purse." I pulled Morag close to me. "There's silver. I'm sorry, but we can't carry you people. The horses can barely get the lot of us to Glevum. I'll send for you if I can."

"But, Lady, if the Silures come—"

"They won't come here, it's me they want. If you can't stay here, there's an old legion brothel on the Badon road—oh, don't look righteous, Morag, they haven't done any trade for years, but maybe the roof's whole. God with you."

A young woman of the village began to sob harshly, jittering up to that hysterical note that could infect a mob. No older than Regan, holding a newborn child to her naked breast; in a moment she'd bolt and start a panic. Bedivere caught her firmly in his arms.

"No fear, lass. It's all right. It's all right now."

Turning from Morag, my mind churning over a hundred facts and necessities, I collided with a hurrying peasant as he plunged past, his elbow digging into my stomach. My cramps screamed at me. "You damned clumsy—"

"Lady?" Bedivere had one arm around the terrified young woman. She kept patting rapidly at the child's

dirty swaddling. I glared back at Bedivere; he could be responsible for all of this.

"What, then?"

"This woman and the others. They want to know if they should stay in Sulis or leave."

"Leave?" My voice sounded strained and ugly. "Why? Who in hell would lay siege to a ruined temple and a rotting bathhouse? It's their sty, let 'em wallow in it. Out of my way, woman."

I pushed past her, pushed too hard. Trying to hold onto the baby she lost her balance and sprawled in the mud. The baby started to wail. Bedivere bent on me one look of acid disgust and lifted the woman to her feet.

"Well, now, isn't this the dear old days come back again."

I seethed: "And well you know who brought them."

"What . . . ?"

"The map is burning under us. I've no time to be subtle, so don't come the startled innocent. Who knew before anyone else just where and when I'd bury Arthur? And who would leave his own wife at home—the only one not at Witrin—but the man who knew what was to happen? Oh, I saw you and Constantine in the courtyard. What did he offer you for my head, Bedivere?" We faced each other, me boiling and ready to put him in irons. "What am I worth? I'd give worlds to know."

"Oh, Christ." Bedivere whirled and disappeared beyond the torchlight in long strides.

"Bedivere, damn you—"

"Lady!" Imogen hailed me, mounted and leading my own horse. I swung up, still raging, and signaled Ifan to me as the combrogi formed near the gates. "This is an order, Ifan. You and two others: don't let Bedivere out of your sight. If he tries to leave our march, stop him in any manner short of death, clear?"

He blinked at me in surprise. "Lord Bedivere?"

"Is that *clear*, sir? Pick your men. Give me the sword."

The peasant girl still mooned up at me as if dazzled by the nimbus of a demented god. Glaring at her I felt a twinge of shame for my lack of control. She was only frightened like myself, wondering what would happen to her and the child.

"Woman, listen to me—"

And make her understand what? That I needed to be iron for now, safe in Eburacum where I could breathe, praying for no more treachery before I regained my grip on the throne and could strike *back*, once and for all, to ensure that the peace in which she'd conceived that child would last till it grew up? Then Gareth bawled from the gate—"Company formed!"—and there was no time. There never was. Patterns, I said. I thrust the imperial sword high overhead for all of them to see.

"Combrogi! My people, hear me! Camelot may be taken, but what was Camelot but a place of brick and mortar? This and no other is the sign of the *imperium*. Until the choosing, we are Britain, and to us will come the loyal tribes and Holy Church. If any of you doubts this, let him find what sanctuary he can. To Glevum!"

Gareth dropped back to my knee as we rode through the west gate, looking for Bedivere, who usually rode on point with him. "Is he to the rear, then?"

The question occupied all of us shortly. The cry went up for Bedivere to move forward, Ifan and his watchdogs ferreted in vain through the column and behind in the town. No one had seen Bedivere since mounting, nor had he lagged in Sulis.

Bedivere was gone. We'd a gutful of each other, true, but under my vengeful fury rankled a sense of loss over this man who was never a friend. That was a large difference between Arthur and me. He'd puzzle and mourn over such a desertion. I half expected it, was not surprised when it came, wrote Bedivere's name on the curse-tablet of my heart and went on without him.

We made slow progress through the night on mounts that had to be walked as much as ridden. The sun was high when we topped the last rise and saw the Roman square of Glevum beyond. Even at that distance, I made out furious movement in the streets.

"A good many riders, Gareth."

"But they're Dobunni," he decided after a long inspection. "It's untaken."

Untaken but not uninformed. Everywhere, on the walls, within them, men were preparing for a siege, shopkeepers hurrying their wares to storage. The praefect and decurions came running to us, bowing, ply-

ing us with questions. They heard Camelot was
breached, the combrogi disbanded, heard this and that.
This very sunrise Silure tribesmen rode to the gates and
threw up to the sentinels the badly spelled notice of my
own capture and death by Constantine. Their own Prince
Emrys was preparing to move into the city. Glevum
trembled with fear of a civil war for which they weren't
prepared after so long a peace. As they crowded around
my spent horse, I took the sword from Ifan, speared Conant's proclamation on the blade and held it high.

"Citizens, look at us! We've had the amusement of
reading our own obituary before. None were any more
accurate than this, though perhaps more literate. We will
not oblige them." I tossed the vellum to the ground.
"Britain is ruled. While Guenevere lives, so does Arthur."

We lingered in the city only to water the horses quickly
and bolt the soup and barley bread bucketed out to us,
then staggered the last mile or so west to Pendragon.

Until his death at Badon, Caius Pendragon was an able
prince of the Dobunni. In-laws are usually tolerated de-
fects in a spouse, but I dearly loved Arthur's half-brother,
Kay. His blood was Celt, his education Roman, his mind
pure Euclid. Were Arthur born legitimate and Kay the
bastard crowned by luck and destiny, he would have
made a prudent, methodical Claudius of an emperor, but
Kay remained a provincial, dark and squat as the tribesmen he ruled. His forges were Arthur's armory, his
downs the breeding ground for combrogi remounts, his
mind better equipped than ours, at first, to deal with the
prosaic minutiae of royal finance. In the first summer of
our reign, he took in hand the inconsistent mess of tribal
taxation and put it on a workable basis. There he sits at a
low table in my memory, digging in his nose, scratching
at his beard, worrying at the root of a problem: a muttering, contented little brown bear of a man—suddenly
brandishing a wax tablet at us as he solved it all. "There's
the deficit, I've found it. It's him, that Coritani bastard.
Juggled his expenses so he never shows much of a sur-
plus. Hasn't paid his corn tax in rutting years. Ho-ho,
we've got him."

A man you wanted to hug. I loved him.

Not so his widow, Blodwen, the "blessed white flower
of Cair Gloiu." Thus her father inaccurately presented

her to Kay whose vision went fuzzy when it came to women. In the Dobunni manner he had several wives, all rather casual, but he sent them packing when the white flower opened her petals for him. I never liked Blodwen, but never underestimated her either. There was mettle under that nervous, distracted exterior and a formidable singularity of purpose.

You were never comfortable around Blodwen. You sensed some part of her mind was doing the secret sums of her own ambition. She was polite and respectful, but you felt like an interruption of her own straight line between points perceived by Blodwen alone. She never relaxed in company, never voiced her deep feelings on anything, but spoke what she imagined you wanted to hear, those nervous hands wringing each other throughout. A chieftain's daughter from a minor holding, she still had the shrewdness to make herself Kay's first Christian wife and, as the religion increased among his people, so did the security of Blodwen's position. She knew she was adored, her son Emrys his father's only legitimate heir, and bugger the rest of them. Thus she was deferential to Arthur and myself, doggedly possessive of Kay, an irritant to Emrys, who inherited Kay's love of horses and smithing but not his royal instincts, and stoic under the pettish tyranny of Kay's mother, Flavia Marcella.

Ambrosius Aurelianus was incorrectly called "last of the Romans" while Flavia lived. She must have been seventy that year, and at least that often she'd reminded Blodwen: "Don't play the patrician with me, woman. My great-grandfather was born within sight of Tiber, and why he came to this misbegotten backwater I will never perceive."

They endured each other like dogs guarding their own territory, grudgingly acknowledging the other's. Blodwen ruled the villa and her son, Flavia reigned as matriarch. To Blodwen the city below was Cair Gloiu. To Flavia it would always be Glevum, built by legion veterans. If you dined with Blodwen you sat at table. With Flavia you reclined in the old way and ate with the right hand only. Blodwen's family once hurrahed in the streets for that ecclesiastical ratcatcher, Germanus. Flavia's father supported Pelagius in the days when education and

the British Church had some perspective and tolerance to them. Arthur and I grew up in the last of that benevolent light. To Blodwen it was largely unknown and suspect. She worshiped Christ in her own chapel; while Flavia was at least polite to him in her own chambers, the chi-rho shared space with her household deities. How real they were to Flavia I can't say, but they were her established order of things, and her loyalty to them waxed the more stubborn as she aged and they faded, like Rome, from reality. When Christian apologists inflate a roadside sermon into a "conversion of thousands," you may be sure Flavia, widow of Uther Pendragon, remained at home, aloof, acerbic and spoiled, and never more than a little drunk.

"Oh, you're the Empress, girl, you *have* to be something officially. But it's all so vulgar, a religion for plebes. The minute someone like Pelagius tried to civilize it, they howled him down. That's what happens when the plebes get their paws on anything: ignorance is deified, culture is a sin. You aren't virtuous unless you live in unwashed ecstasy and unpleasant clothes. Oh, some of the older bishops are tolerable—Anscopius, that sort—but I do not like this new lot. I don't appreciate being told by a peasant priest with breath as decayed as his Latin, that I'm a goat to be culled from lambs when the world ends on Saturday week. Nonsense! Pour me some more wine, Guenevere. Oh, I do love the way you keep your figure. If one has to wear those tight kirtles, you have the line for it. Artorius is so lucky. Would I could say the same for Kay. Isn't Blodwen depressing? Why *her*, I ask you?"

"I know he treasures her. Perhaps she's good in bed."

"Let us hope. Where was I? No, child, the world has gone its tedious way for ages and will go plodding on, and it damned well won't stop for holy louts who can't even agree on the will of their alleged savior or how to attain his elusive salvation. There, that's enough, it's dull as Blodwen. We need to be part of Rome again. At least we were organized."

The villa bustled with preparation even from a distance, servants hurrying to load chests and sacks into several unyoked carts outside the stables. We gave them a bad moment. They probably thought us Silures at first.

"It is the Queen! It *is* the Queen, no less than she. The Silures lied!"

I half fell out of the saddle and snapped at the groom when he knelt to me. "Where's the Prince, man?"

"Somewhere in Gloiu, Lady."

"And Lady Blodwen?"

"Ah, she's about. They move tomorrow."

"See Lord Gareth about the horses, and mind them well. They're spent as ourselves."

I tended to stagger a little entering the villa gate, but Blodwen and Flavia were waiting on the portico. Blodwen came dutifully down the walk to meet me. We embraced with the enthusiasm of fish. "A thousand welcomes, blessed Queen. We heard you were killed."

From her careful manner, I couldn't tell if she was glad or disappointed, but you never could with Blodwen. "So did I. It's all rather unsettling. I see you're ready to go."

Blodwen gazed about with that familiar preoccupation. "At the coming of the sun."

"Yes, that's wise. We'll only strain your hospitality a few hours. We ride for Eburacum at first light."

"And leave the south?"

I caught the faint tinge of disapproval. "It can't be helped. Camelot's gone, they've got me south and west. I can only rally in the north." I swayed a little with the exhaustion of too little sleep and too much fear. "God's Eyes, just quarter my folk. I've got to rest."

I tottered past her to melt into Flavia's open arms.

"Guenevere! Come kiss me. They told us—oh, you're positively disheveled. Where have you been?"

"Mother. Wonderful to see you. Tell them to brew me some celery tea, a bucketful."

"That again," Flavia clucked. "I never saw a woman have such trouble being female. You shall have it," she promised with a dry little peck on my cheek. "And a bath, you grubby girl. Will you dine with me?"

"I can't, much as I'd love to. I must dine with Blodwen and Emrys."

"State business?"

"What else?"

"Bother. Blodwen! I suppose you'll sit the Queen to trough tonight as usual. See it's not too dreary, there's a

good girl. And have your women send in some celery
tea."

Flavia occupied the villa's best room, directly over a
stokehole fed with coal and warmed for her most of the
year. After a hurried but welcome trip to the bathhouse, I
stripped down again in Flavia's chamber while Imogen
oiled and strigiled me and I gulped the painkilling celery
tea. Flavia shook her head over me.

"You've gone to gristle, child."

"Eating's an afterthought these days. That's enough,
Imogen. Help me dress."

"I want to talk in private," Flavia said when Imogen
had laced the kirtle up my back. "Send your slave away."

Imogen bristled. "I'm nae a slave. I'm freeborn."

"I have no slaves, Mother. We couldn't condemn the
trade and keep them."

"Not even prisoners?"

"More trouble than they're worth. The Picts are too
crude and the Saxons tend to suicide."

"But I would speak to you alone."

"Imogen, please bring me more tea."

"Cheeky sort," Flavia grumbled when Imogen withdrew.

"Oh, she's been with me for ages. We've grown old together."

"Old? Nonsense; you're not yet fifty."

"Don't count, Mother. I do that myself."

"Be serious. You are in trouble. You've lost the south."

"I'll get it back."

"Yes. Meanwhile, there are realities." Flavia ferreted in
a small boxwood chest and extracted a glass vial. "If
they take you, it's the sword or worse. You'd be a valuable prize to show. They could walk you in chains by
Constantine's horse through every city he takes. Uther
did it himself in Cornwall. It's not pretty. I would not see
that happen to you."

I understood the mercy she offered. "How quickly does
this work?"

"In water or wine, a few minutes."

"Good. If there's someone in need of a swift journey, I'll
speed them."

"Don't be flip, my girl."

"No, darling, but it's not my style. You don't win by

preparing to lose, and I'm going to win." I drained the last of the tea. "If I can get rid of these rutting cramps."

Flavia winced in distaste. "Don't be vulgar, it's so British."

"So am I. I think in your language, but I feel in my own. They almost got me yesterday, Mother. I hate blood, it turns my stomach. But if I go I'll go cutting, not draped over my couch like Lucrece in a tragic mural. Oh, where *is* Imogen? I need more tea—Jesus, Mother."

Hunched on the edge of the bed I wrapped my arms around the old bones of her, buried my face in her shrunken breast. "It's all on me now, mum. I'm not beaten. I want to turn and *fight* those sons of bitches, and all I can do is run. Look at the few I've got left. Even Bedivere's betrayed me."

"Old Gryffyn's boy? Why, I virtually raised him with Kay and Artorius. He wouldn't."

"He would and he has. Deserted us at Sulis. Sold me out to Constantine."

"Not little Bedwyr."

"Mother, it's now, not then. It's grab what you can. It had to be him."

"My Kay would not hear you say that," Flavia insisted. "You must find the strongest men in the country and align them with you."

For Flavia the problem was that simple. How to answer such a mind. Imogen did it for me, standing in the door.

"The Queen *is* the strongest man in this country. Tea, Lady?"

Dinner was ample but plain since everything was packed to move. Blodwen's servants carted out trestle tables for my company who dined in the courtyard while Galahalt and I shared the triclinium with the family. Flavia declined to join us; sitting in a chair at table seemed too far a fall from graciousness. We sat down without waiting for Emrys. Sawel hovered among the serving people, ready to his lord's wish. Imogen poured wine for me with a sharp eye to the manner of serving. My father for some time employed a taster as a precaution against poison, but none was needed this day. We all ate out of two or three common dishes, the wine mixed with water in our presence and poured from one amphora. I would

have preferred to dine with Flavia and bask in the brittle iridescence of her wit, but dinner that night was business. I had to gauge Emrys' loyalty—meaning Blodwen's—and be sure of their support.

Emrys had been crowned less than a year. His mother hovered over him and therefore over her people. Her conversation was carefully hooded. I could sense Blodwen measuring her words carefully, never really relaxed, fingers wringing in her lap. How strong is she? I wondered. What does she want?

As a dinner companion, Galahalt was a dutiful cipher. He spoke only when spoken to, those few words polite as his table manners were colorfully atrocious. His civilized father must have found him and his mother a bit much at times.

We'd barely started on the fish course, Blodwen and I circling each other delicately, when Emrys clumped in direct from the saddle, unwashed and fragrant. Nineteen that year, he was still filling out his first beard—tentative, more at home in the breeding pens and forges than with matters of state. He ducked a bow to me and allowed his mother a sweaty kiss which Blodwen parried with a frown of distaste—"Don't, boy, you're all sweat"—and plumped down at table while a servant presented a ewer. Emrys splashed water over his brown neck, greeted Galahalt casually though they'd never met.

"Will you be staying, Aunt Guenevere? Why weren't we told of Uncle Arthur's funeral?"

Blodwen pushed the ewer back at Emrys. "You shouldn't dip into a dish with the Queen and your hands still black. Ah . . . but it is true: why was it only Astolat was invited?" Her glance slid to Galahalt. "And family left aside to wonder at it all?"

Galahalt spat an inedible bit onto his plate. "The Queen was in danger. Secrecy was important."

"Such secrecy as we managed," I said. "We were ambushed and almost done for."

"Oh, no!"

"Quite, Nephew. Which means Glevum could be next. Can you hold it?"

He hesitated, and while he did, Blodwen stepped in. "We will hold the city."

Damned woman, she picked at his manners, bullied

him like a petty tyrant, even did his thinking for him. I needed to put her off balance. "I was betrayed by a Dobunni."

I dropped it quietly and fell silent, toying with my food. Give them time to mull it, wonder if I'd come to punish or what. At that moment Galahalt's bald truth didn't hurt at all.

"Bedwyr ap Gryffyn," he blurted. "He ran from our side the moment he heard Camelot was taken."

To his small credit, Emrys leaned across to Galahalt and corrected him. "Prince, you're speaking of my friend. He has been Uncle Arthur's man since he could walk."

"But obviously not mine, Nephew."

"The Queen has said he's a traitor," Blodwen observed with deceptive ease. "That should be enough."

"Has he come here?"

"No, Aunt."

"If he does, I want him arrested. Or seek him at home, that's a crown order. Send him to me alive. In chains, Emrys. Tell him they're the same ones he put on me. For the rest, his lands are yours. Everything he owns."

"His holding was bestowed by Arthur," Blodwen said. "The Dobunni have no power over him."

"Blodwen, Arthur is dead. I am the crown. Emrys has the power. Will you deliver him?"

He dropped his eyes and nodded reluctantly. "Yes, Aunt."

"In chains."

"It will be done."

"The rest is yours."

"I'll go myself. He taught me horse and sword, Bedivere did."

"Admirable. Just send him. It's not a harshness, Emrys, just common sense. While I rule I want my enemies where I can reach them."

"Amen," Galahalt spluttered through a mouthful. "My mother would have his head on a pole."

"The Queen has said 'while she rules.' I would speak of that." Blodwen leaned forward, clasped hands writhing together on the board. Where survival is concerned, I've acquired the premonitory instincts of a rat on a sinking ship. *Ah, here it comes. And what's your price, woman?*

"You wait on the choosing of the people, but you have Arthur's voice to succeed. In writing. And you travel with the heir to Astolat."

"Galahalt is my ward, not my heir. Astolat is unsafe now because his parents are loyal to me."

"Just so," Galahalt said. "I want no honor but that of God, Lady. Like my father."

Blodwen's fingers stopped twitching. "But for yourself, Guenevere, the crown power has always come from the south and in particular from Severn. Vortigern, Ambrosius, Arthur himself who was my son's blood uncle."

I might have expected it. "Your son to succeed me?"

"With letters published. It must be remembered that the crown strained our loyalty in the matter of Pwyll who was my kinsman and murdered by Trystan. You gave Trystan exile when even Kay called for his execution."

"That was policy, not favor."

"Even so, only through our loyalty did the Dobunni stay with you, and not all of them at that."

"Blodwen, we were ready to execute him. But we needed certain efforts from Cornwall. We bought them through Yseult—need I enlarge?—and Tryst's life was the price. Cheap enough."

"And still," Blodwen said, "there were those who said friendship swayed Arthur."

"Trystan was a dear friend, yes. He wasted his life on a hopeless dream and very likely his death on a meaningless gesture. That was his nature, but not ours. Policy came first."

"Then is this less than good policy?" Blodwen asserted. "A successor should be named, and who with more right than Arthur's own blood?"

"And Arthur's experience? His particular genius? Even your husband's wisdom? Tell me, Emrys, do you think you would make a good king?"

I caught the telltale glance he slid to Blodwen. "Do you think so, Aunt Guenevere?"

Was he merely unsure or disingenuous as Blodwen? I signaled Imogen for the ewer and dabbled my fingers, cleaning them slowly before answering. "We think— when I consider who's to have my place, I'm always *we*, Nephew—we think that if you work hard and learn to

trust your own judgment, you may be a fine prince-magistrate like your father. You must be that first. As for the succession—well, I could die tomorrow."

"God forbid that," Blodwen protested.

"Thank you, dear. I might, but don't wager on it. Meanwhile you've advanced an interesting suggestion. I'll think on it."

Damned right, and to this extent: while I considered they might not sell me, and if Bedivere were within Blodwen's reach, she'd serve him to me on a plate. The mother would, not the son. And if the son was my successor, Blodwen would be the uncrowned ruler. Not likely. Meanwhile, this one needful night, I could sleep like a human.

Before retiring I made a round of my folk and the villa itself and arranged for my guard. Gareth suggested three.

"Three's best, Queen of Sorrows. Briefer watch, more rest for the men. And what time shall we ride?"

"Early. I'd say four at the latest."

Gareth tilted his head to study the placid evening sky. "You'll have light at three and a fine day by the look of it. We could be on the Cair Legis road by four."

"As you think best. How are the mounts?"

Gareth winced. "Isn't that a sad tale? Stretched out in the stalls and ready for last rites. Pray God we don't have to push them, and to all the angels we don't have to fight. They're done. And if a man who knows horses better than women may be permitted, you need rest too, Lady."

We were walking along the wall toward the servants' quarters. I stopped and leaned against the cool plaster of the wall. "I do that. Send my guard along straight."

He read the wariness that seeped through my fatigue. "You mislike this place for safety?"

"Nothing's safe until Eburacum. And Blodwen wants Emrys to succeed me."

He swore softly. "Were they on about that and yourself so worn out?"

"They—that is, she—let me know politely I'll have to buy them. The world never changes, does it? Wasn't it so when Arthur was crowned?"

Gareth smiled with sad reminiscence. "We were youn-

ger then. We had more endurance and luck than anything else. We couldn't imagine living this long."

"And you've known Bedivere all that time?"

"Have I not? Since we were centurions on the Wall."

"Why would he sell me?"

Gareth took his reflective time answering; obviously he'd pondered it too. "I don't think he did, Lady."

"Oh, for God's mercy, man, what would you call it?"

"He left. Leaving is not selling." The firmness surprised me. Arthur's last letter urged me to trust Gareth's opinion, and by God I got it then.

"You're Arthur's Queen. You have my oath, and if you'd be knowing why, it's because you're all that's left of him, and the best as he was. You must be that or we're done. If Bedivere's broke his word, is that all there is to the Gryffyn? That was a man who stood by Trystan at his trial—and himself guilty as hell—because Trystan was a friend; who hunted Cerdic alone on the field at Badon when he thought the Saxons had brought me down. Because *I* was a friend." Gareth jabbed his arm toward the servants' quarters. "And of those few good men I brought home, the first word out of them was, Will Bedivere be there? Left he did and gone he is, but I put it to you, High Queen. Is such a man to be named in the same breath with selling?"

Under his respect I sensed a rage and bewilderment acid as my own. "He was puzzled in his mind," Gareth concluded. "He wanted to know the right of things."

"He'll have his chance to speak. Believe me, I want his reasons more than his death. The Dobunni will deliver him to me."

"Bedwyr's own people?"

"Alive and unharmed. That's my price for considering Blodwen's princeling as a successor. Don't look pained, Gareth. You hardly objected when Bedivere put chains on me. In fact you approved."

"You were wrong, my Queen."

"Possibly in the manner, not the motive. Half the country cheered when I escaped. I put it to you in turn, Lord-Milite: Are we a power in the land or merely fugitives from a revolution? How can we show strength if we can't uphold the law? For that reason, I want Bedivere."

And for the deeper thing that rested neither with

wrong nor right. Like myself and Gareth, Bedivere represented the last of Arthur. *Why* did that rock-stubborn last desert me when we stood for the same thing? My soul needed to know, groping for the right as he did.

"Then I'll ask—" Gareth snapped straight out of his fatigue. "No, by holy Padraic, as Lord-Milite, I will demand to stand by him when the trial comes. And won't there be a line of combrogi behind me?"

"Of course." I touched his shoulder. "The loyalty does you honor. He'll be fairly tried, I promise you. Good night, Lord Gareth. Set my guard and wake me at three. Rest you gentle."

The summer evening was still quite light when I retired. Blodwen had prepared for me my usual chamber next to Flavia's, a well-appointed room where Arthur and Kay had slept as boys. The door had no lock; Flavia used to look in at night out of habit especially if one of them was croupy or down with a fever. The first guard posted himself and one of Blodwen's women brought a cup of chamomile tea to help me sleep. Imogen sniffed it and subjected a few drops to the inspection of her tongue. The Coritani once tried to kill Ambrosius with this kindness, and my own family had been known to use a cup where a cohort failed.

Imogen proffered it to me. "Chamomile it is and very good."

We propped a stout chair against the door as an extra safety, then Imogen readied my bed and helped me out of the travel-grimed kirtle, clucking sadly over it. "Ah, this one's seen its last state evening, more's the pity, and it one of your best. I always fancied it."

I held up the muddied hem. "Not really worn at all. You take it once we're home. It's good linen. The fullers can bleach and dye it for you."

"Oh, that's dear, Lady. I just think I might." Tongue stuck out in concentration, Imogen draped the kirtle to her own wiry figure. "I do believe we're of a size."

"Not a quarter-stone apart. Just two stringy wenches off the moors, we are."

We blew out the lamps and got into bed. Just before dropping off, Imogen murmured, "Lady?"

"Uh?"

"Will we get t'home, you think?"

"Of course, silly woman. Things will be put right then."

I've never slept deeply or for more than two hours at a time, the habit of a mind reluctant to let go of problems. It was pitch-dark when I snapped wide-awake, far too dark for a summer night. Oh, she'd done it again, closed the shutters after I fell asleep. Imogen had intractable views on the harmfulness of night air. I slipped out of bed, groping for the casement, and heard the guard speak outside our door.

"Who's there? Name yourself."

Someone answered, muffled through the door.

"Oh, it's you. What do you want at this hour?"

Not me, please. It'll be half an hour before I can fall asleep again. I waited for the guard's voice. Nothing: good enough. But as I turned to open the shutters, the skin prickled and the hair rose on the back of my neck. I didn't argue with instinct, but snaked the dagger from under the pillow and crept close to the door, mouth already framing a call to the guard. That same instinct smothered it: *don't.*

The latch clicked. The door pushed against the chair, then again, harder. I flattened myself against the wall as the door crashed in with tremendous force, splintering the chair. Imogen came up as if she were shot from a catapult.

"Who is it? Who's there? Lady!"

Only darkness saved us. The male figure dimly outlined against the twilight of the portico could barely see the beds with the shutters closed. As he moved toward them, I dove at his back—"Guard! Combrogi!"—dropping the knife in my stiff-fingered fright but clinging to the broad back. Imogen bounded out of bed, adding her terror-shrilled voice to mine.

"Combrogi to the Queen! Help!"

For this dark lump of murder, I could only say he was strong. The muscles of his back flexed as he twisted under me. Then the white-hot sting across my cheek as his arm came up, then I was hurled away. In the same instant the clawing fury of Imogen was on him. Something clattered to the floor and slid, then Imogen's *oh*! as a blow took the wind out of her. The intruder slipped out

the door like a shadow. I tried to follow but felt strangely
dizzy. Poor Imogen was still trying to wheeze her alarm
to the guards as more feet pounded along the portico.

"Ah, the dirty *sothach*. Hit me in the stomach. H-help!"

"Guard, hurry, damn it!"

A torch thrust into the room, then a long arm and Dai
meqq Muir's homely but very welcome face. I fumbled
for the lamp and lit it from the torch. "Dai, where was
my guard? We were almost—"

"Lady!" Imogen gaped at me, moon-eyed with horror. I
felt the warm wetness along my cheek and temple and
trickling into my left eye. In the growing light it came off
black on my fingers.

"Dai . . . ?"

He took my arm and led me out to the portico. My
guard lay in that awkward position that means only one
thing. "I was just out the gate on my way to watch," Dai
said. "I heard only your cry."

I swallowed hard against a wave of nausea. "Nothing
else?"

"No." Dai bent over the body. "It's Gwenlys. Would not
think him so easily taken."

"He wasn't surprised. I think he knew who it was."

Lights flickered and grew in other parts of the villa
now as more of my men hurried to us across the courtyard. Gareth and Bors and Ifan headed them. One look
was all they needed: dead Gwenlys and the blood-
masked, shaking apparition of me.

Gareth's tone was dangerous. "Orders, Lady?"

"I want everyone in the triclinium. Everyone: family,
servants, the lot. Drag them if you have to, and their
filthy princeling and his busy mother. By God, I want
those two on their knees. Oh, leave *off*, woman." I shoved
Imogen away from trying to staunch the blood still pouring down my face and soaking into the neck of my night-
dress. "Leave it. I want them to see what they've
bungled."

With Ifan helping me, I took a chair in the triclinium
and sat motionless, fighting to control the rage that
called for quick slaughter. The chamber began to fill
with cooks, servants and stablers, prodded or pushed in
by my knights. Galahalt hurried in with Sawel loping

behind. Flavia was escorted by Imogen. The grisly sight of me brought the old woman hurrying to my side.

"Child, what's happened?"

"What you see. And they failed."

Emrys and Blodwen were shoved into the room by Gareth and Dai. They were in bed robes and bewildered as the rest.

"I said on their knees, Gareth."

Gareth complied ungently. I let the murmuring room grow quiet, let Blodwen and Emrys look their fill of me before speaking. The effort not to execute them summarily took the last of my will. What had there been for days but blood, betrayal and desertion, nothing safe in Britain, no one to be trusted with a closed eye or turned back. The people who'd struggled this far with me felt the same fury. Looking at Dai and Gareth, I knew one word, one lifted finger would be the death of Emrys and Blodwen.

"Woman, the first thing you and your princeling should learn about regicide is, don't muck it up."

"Regicide?" Emrys' eyes bulged as Dai's sword pressed hard against his back. "Aunt Guenevere, what . . . what charge is this? We did nothing, we—"

"Be still, boy."

"Is this how you measure our loyalty?" Blodwen demanded. "Drag us from bed, accuse us of trying to slaughter you? Whatever's happened, we had no hand in it. Emrys is Arthur's own blood. We are your fam—"

"I said be *still*."

"No!" she flared. "We are innocent. Jesu deny me salvation if we ever plotted against you."

"Blodwen, you were plotting the moment I got down at your gate. You made very clear the price of your loyalty, but you damned well couldn't wait, could you?"

"One good man is dead," Gareth broke in, that lilting voice turned hard and flat. "On the Queen's word I'll have your heads myself."

"It was someone Gwenlys knew by sight," Dai said. "No one else could get close enough."

"Then couldn't it be one of your own?" Emrys quavered. "We're telling the truth, Aunt. Mother and I—"

"Mother and you. You're a matched set."

"Guenevere, a moment." Flavia spoke with quiet authority. "I believe the boy. He hasn't got murder in him."

"Affection's a poor witness, Mother."

"Not affection but experience. Pity my grandson, he's a sorry prince but no more capable of murder than his father."

"Not alone, no." I looked from Emrys to quivering Blodwen.

"We didn't." She shook her head vigorously. "Are you mad, Guenevere? Here in our house where every eye would come first to us? God's truth, woman, think what you're saying!"

"Think what?" Regan thrust forward from Bors' side, her pretty mouth twisted with fear and hate. "I'm with child, and I've barely lived this week out through all the treachery. Take their heads, Lady, before they kill us all."

"But who are *they*, young woman?" Flavia drew the robe close about her throat against the barely cool night air. "Guenevere, I'll grant you Blodwen's an ambitious thing out of a thatched hut with a mud floor. But I'll say this much for my lamentable daughter-in-law. I think she's far too prudent for something clumsy as this."

A glance from Blodwen, classic in its complexity: this jealous, selfish, wine-sodden old woman still ruled a house in which Blodwen should be unquestioned mistress, always arrogant, always taking the best as her undisputed right, adding a sting even to her defense. "There, you hear? She has no love for me, never had, and even she won't accuse me of this."

"Of course not, Blodwen. You're a boor, not a brute. Guenevere, a word with you." Flavia approached and bent to whisper in my ear. I smelled the wine sour on her breath; she'd drunk far into the night as usual, her only pleasure now.

"My girl, cool that temper before you do something you'll regret. The boy hasn't the steel, she hasn't the stupidity. Don't lose the Dobunni altogether. Guilty or not, she's given you an advantage. Use it. Uther would."

I gripped the chair arms to still the violent shaking while my mind ran riot with crimson possibilities. Flavia spoke good Roman sense. So did flaccid Emrys for that matter. It could have been one of my own for all I knew. What did Gwenlys say?

Oh, it's you. What do you want at this hour?

That could be anyone. He'd know our own people better in the dark than Blodwen's. No—galling as it was, guilt was not that evident. To kill me here *would* be stupid, a failing I never charged to Blodwen. So I sat there in the mess of my own blood, a target needing to take advantage of the arrows, but the pause restored some sense. Kill them both and what Dobunni would defend Glevum against princes no more tyrant to them than Guenevere? Not death, then, but a hostage. Blodwen? Her son wasn't that competent to command nor perhaps so loving of his mother that she'd be good pawn for his loyalty. But the reverse was a different matter. Tuck Emrys away in Eburacum and Blodwen would walk through fire to keep him alive. My hand no longer shook when I pointed to the young prince.

"Emrys Pendragon, for the crime of high treason, I sentence you to death."

"No!" Blodwen writhed in Gareth's grip. "Guenevere, please, he did nothing. He's my dear son, he's *innocent*."

"Don't worry, he's not going to die. He's my hostage and there's a sword over his head. Whether it falls depends on you, Blodwen. You will hold Glevum for me and you will send me Bedivere speedily. If you don't, you'll have Emrys' head in a bag. It is that simple."

Trying to rise I just went limp in the chair, the starch squeezed out of me. I'd lost a deal of blood and could barely croak my orders to Gareth in a reedy voice. "It's gone three by the light. Prepare us to ride. And you, Emrys—look at me, damn you! Take a good look at your royal aunt and what you aspire to. I've been nigh killed twice in two days. This wound needs a day of rest. I've got to get out of this chair and ride for three. Because I'm the crown and I believe in something, if none of my princes share that belief. I don't know if you've the stomach for it or how vividly you imagine yourself a king, boy, but you're going to serve your apprenticeship at my own knee."

"Very good." Flavia nodded. "My boy, you'll learn more than you ever dreamed."

"Lord Dai, take this puppy and pack him up. Blodwen, you have a city to defend. Call your chiefs and be about it."

And that was my visit with loving family. With Flavia and Imogen I shakily made ready to leave in my own chamber. Imogen found the weapon the assassin dropped, a wicked-edged shaving razor, so sharp it opened up my face before I even felt it. Had it been inches lower, had it been my throat . . . Jesus.

"Imogen, I need some uisge."

"Not that slop," Flavia growled. "You'll bring it right up again."

"I'll do that anyway. Might as well enjoy it."

"Here." Flavia poured me some herbed wine of the sort she drank as a digestive. "To settle your stomach. You were wise tonight. You made the right choice."

"No, you did. They don't know how close they came to it."

"But I do." Flavia gave me a grave smile. "I know something of fighters. Blodwen's not weak; devious, perhaps, but she hasn't half your killer instinct, my dear. You would have regretted it. You're all Brit when you're that hot, and there's nothing worse for self-destruction."

We sat together on the low couch. "Bless you, mum. I really need you tonight."

"There, it's over now. And you will take good care of poor Emrys? Between the two of us, we could make something of that boy."

"I'm more worried about you. Come to Eburacum with me."

Flavia looked mildly surprised at the suggestion. "This is my home, child. No one will touch the widow of Uther Pendragon."

I wished that were as sure as she sounded. "And if Conant comes?"

"If it comes to that—well, you blithely compared yourself to Lucrece tonight, but I've always admired the woman. She took her own way out when the game was no longer worth the playing. So will I."

Flavia gazed sourly beyond the casement at the calm morning sky. "Caesar should never have crossed that wretched channel. Ye gods, how have I lived seventy years in such a place? It is not a joyful accomplishment. Imogen!" Flavia flourished her goblet. "Fetch us another

drink. And one for yourself, I should say. You're white as your mistress."

Why not? Poor Imogen could have shared my fate, and she knew as I did that the assassin could still be with us, waiting for next time. *Not who, Lady, but who next?* Someone close to me, someone I trusted, someone I loved. One of my own . . .

III

The Hand that Holds the Lightning

've learned and unlearned all my life; it's helped me to survive. There are no constants, nothing is immutable, only random circumstance from which our experience builds a coherent arc of life. And for that arc you have to be truly done with one thing before moving to another. There's an art in letting go. Lucullus attained what philosophers call virtue when he became bored with what the virtuous call vice. Moral souls may find this a shaky underpinning for existence, but I've thrived on it. It's kept the edge on my appetite for life. That's why I pray to live past a hundred. I'd hate to think today is as wise as I'll ever be, and something fascinating may happen tomorrow.

Tomorrow belongs to those who can learn. For those who can't, there's only yesterday. The Saxons came as pirates who had to travel light. Most of their cultural follies were left at home or dropped over the side on the way from colony to nation. When it's survive or die, you don't make the same mistake twice, unless you're British, in which case you repeat it thrice for consistency. As it is, the Saxons clung to the bare edge of existence in my country for sixty years, disorganized and never secure. Now they're moving west again, and while Britain tears at its own throat, they're turning it into England because they can learn and change.

I was a spent she-wolf limping back to her last lair, going forty-eight and my tether running out when I slipped from the saddle in the marketplace of Eburacum to wash my face at the well. Fitting that it should be such a full circle: there in the city of my birth where I first learned to bear the weight of a crown.

My father's palace was the old forum of Eburacum built when the city was organized as a veterans' colony. There'd been a legion on the Wall since the earliest days and gradually the city and northern tribes merged in identity and purpose. For the last hundred years and more my own family had been the tribal crown and Roman magistracy combined, building wings to the simple forum to sprawl it out into its present form.

The audience chamber and the entrance hall still bore the marks of Cerdic's last raid. Chipped statuary, an arm missing from Jupiter, Goddess Epona seated on a three-legged horse, deep charring here and there that could be scraped or scrubbed clean but still showed where fire had consumed the wood or cracked the marble.

With Gareth and Imogen I stood in the entrance to the audience hall, the original forum. Behind us the palace staff waited in small groups, not sure of their orders or my mood, and beyond the doors the growing hubbub as the people of Eburacum gathered gratefully to welcome home their princess.

"Hasn't been cleaned since we left." Imogen sniffed about distastefully. "Since spring, I'll be bound."

"See to that, Imogen. Take charge of my women as usual. Please send a messenger to Prince Maelgwyn: did Morag and that lot reach Verulamium. Also, I want him for council as soon as he can arrive. Prince Galahalt may have my old chambers, Lord Gareth and Lady Rhian my mother's old rooms. You'll find them quite suitable, Gareth. Let me know if Rhian needs anything. Imogen, I'll take Cador's rooms just off this hall. See they're cleaned and fitted out like the scriptorium at Camelot. I want to be close to the center of business at all times. From now on, this palace is Britain."

They waited for my rapid orders to continue, but a soft weight bore in on me. The forum resounded with echoes only I could hear. The tramp of Roman boots, the plucked music of riddling bards, the measured cadence

of Latin and half a dozen tribal dialects. There were still two chairs of state on the small dais where I first set eyes on Arthur the day my father commissioned the cavalry squadrons. Arthur, Bedivere, Gawain, Agrivaine, Trystan, Peredur. Not ordinary men at all; fated, every one for good or ill.

To Peredur, my dear son, the third numbered squadron.

My frail brother with his scholar's mind, who killed himself to find the Grail for a half-savage like Eleyne and perhaps the glory of God as Peredur alone perceived it.

Centurion Artorius Pendragon. Bedwyr ap Gryffyn. To these two officers for engagement of Saxon raiders against the heaviest numerical odds . . . the gold laurel of valor.

Lord, were they more than twenty then? Not a day of it, but they were the only regular army officers in the line of young nobles standing before my father. Blond Arthur, red-haired Bedivere, the horsehair crests still new and stiff on their helmets, scarlet cloaks fresh-brushed. And Arthur looked to me again and again. I was flattered rather than smitten. He was a well-made man, but not yet irresistible.

I sagged down on the edge of the unswept dais. Yes, it was just here we sat on the day he returned from Morgana, the palace in a panic and uproar and Cerdic poised to attack.

May I have some of your wine, Arthur?

From the same cup?

Why not? We're in the same war.

"Lady?"

It was Gareth who interrupted us then, too, all those years ago. None of us had the right to live so long or see so much. I first set eyes on Gareth one day at Peredur's side, watching his squadron on the drill field. This bandy-legged little man broke away from an argument with Rhian conducted in violent gestures and Irish maledictions, stumped to his horse and suddenly became a centaur, taking the mount effortlessly over one high hurdle after another. I was impressed.

Peredur, what lord is that?

No lord at all. An Irish mercenary from Leinster. My second in command.

A commoner in command of lords?

I know, sister. It's embarrassing. I have only one other

lord who knows as much of horse as this commoner, and he's not even British. Ancellius, a Gaul. The men call him Lancelot. Have you noted him?

Lancelot? No, I think not. I repeated the name and then forgot it in the press of more interesting matters. . . .

Gareth called me again. "Lady? The decurions are waiting. Shall we go out to them?"

"In a moment." I rose from the dais feeling stiff, wretched and plain old. There were, as usual, more orders to be given before rest.

"I want a double guard on my chambers at all times. All messengers are to be brought to me immediately but none passed through until they're disarmed, is that clear? Any dereliction will be punished by death. I'm sorry, Gareth, but you know it must be that way. I'm no use to Britain dead. Now let's be courteous but brief about this welcoming. We'll none of us be worth a damn without a few hours' sleep."

We went out to the palace steps, combrogi, princes and ladies ranked behind me, to receive the decurions and the shouts of my still hopeful Parisi.

Gwenhwyfar ferch Cador a Epona! Ave!

Hail Guenevere from the loins of Epona.

Gwladys! Gwenhwyfar, Gwladys! Long life!

We stood straight, arms raised in greeting, hoping our weariness and discouragement didn't show.

See my body. Strip off the muddy kirtle and ruined shift, pass them to Imogen and share the image my unkind mirror presented that fall. Skinny buttocks and belly, small breasts already sagging. The auburn of the hair gone to brownish streaks in the dull gray mop, artfully combed forward to hide the long scar. Eyes too hard for their intelligence and humor, ironic mouth puckered with middle age. The unadorned lump of flesh that tried to rule Britain alone. To think I even heard bards like Trystan sing my wit and beauty. No—Tryst wouldn't lie, and yet I wonder if Arthur went through a phase like this: yesterdays crowding in like old retainers eager to be pensioned on my heart. I *am* getting sentimental. It must be age. The young are far too busy.

See my life. I was born almost precisely at sundown on the last day of the kalends of October. For Celts this is the

beginning of the new year, the festival of Samhain, the time when the worlds of light and dark, of living and dead, are open to one another. Born thus on the edge of things, I was a quandary to the augurs who were to cast my future. A cautious lot and mindful of their livelihood, they played the fox, talked a great deal of obfuscation about the difficulty of reading cusps, and predicted for me a future of great distinction but few specifics. Later astrologers resolved these vagaries. Any *fool*, they said, could have foreseen greatness in my birth, even accounting for errors in the Julian calendar. It was all a matter of competent interpretation.

If you can't laugh at this, you need not tarry any longer with me or my life. I could never abide a lack of humor. It's dangerous. The worst people, kings and commons, are always devoid of it, and this depressing majority is still waiting and will always wait with mouths agape for some other solemn clown to read the stars for them instead of reaching for their own as Arthur and I did.

Peredur asked once, "What does God do more, laugh or cry?"

At the risk of heresy, I have my suspicions.

We knew early on that Peredur was more for Church than secular rule. But for Ambrosius' war he would have gone for holy orders the year Arthur came north. Even before that, Peredur's physical frailty and reclusive bent made Cador look to me as his successor. I was fourteen when my mother died; at an age when most Parisi women bore their first child, I began to learn government. I sat months in council, learning not to squirm with boredom, before I could follow the simplest threads in tribal policy; why this logical course could not be pursued, why that palpable insanity must be perpetuated for a greater good. Why we kept up the trappings of a Roman magistracy on one hand and a tribal principate on the other. Besides Latin and my native Cumbric, I learned, virtually from the cradle, half a dozen other British dialects and how to read and write Greek. The facility stood me in good stead, for I learned English very rapidly where most Britons find it unfathomable.

There were mathematics and rhetoric and history as well, but the emphasis was always on language. How to think in a different language, how to listen to men until

their *way* of thinking was clear and tucked away for recall. Until I could dine between a Cornish ambassador
and a Catuvellaun chief, catch their subtlest meaning
and the droppings of the loose-tongued Gaulish merchant several couches away but within earshot.

The little girl has finished her sums, lisped
through a passage of the *Germania* without too
many mistakes, and heard Bishop Anscopius say
the mass. Freed by her tutor at last, she skips down
the hall, making a game out of avoiding cracks in
the flagstones. She dodges through a forest of male
legs, brushes past the draped togas. Nurse will take
her riding, but Father must kiss her first because
she's his favorite. Gwenhwyfar ferch-Cador. Skinny
little thing doesn't give a damn who she interrupts.
The men move aside for her without question. She's
already used to that and will be all her life.

She hops up onto her father's lap. The chiefs of
the north prudently mask their impatience. Perhaps their own sons will bed this privileged brat
when the time comes. She is hugged and praised by
Cador, then slips down to run back through the leg-
forest to find Nurse.

Educated or illiterate, in our hearts we were still Celts.
Jupiter, Mars or Minerva might inhabit our temples, but
we remembered older altars and the giant figures cut on
the chalk downs. Our own early kings were less important than our druids. There's even now that part of me
that thrills uncritically to the mysteries of religion and
superstition while playing political chess with the
Church. Sophistication has eroded some of the awe, but
the deep soil remains, like the hard reddish earth under
our peat bogs. There are certain hills crowned by stone
circles where, on certain nights, I would not go even now.
The great stones were set in place by people who came
before us, at the command of gods older than our own.
Dark, stunted, evil people. The Church didn't have to
condemn them as minions of Satan; we knew the Faerie
to be the enthralled spirits of the dead. This knowledge
was another music always audible under the *Alleluia* or
Gloria.

The child is warned away from dangers like open
flame and yearns to poke slivers into it to see them
burn. The peasant nurse mutters of Faerie rades
and dances under the moon. Gwenhwyfar bursts to
see one though the thought terrifies even as it com-
pels. Later, when the moon starts her flow of blood
toward womanhood, there is a secret fantasy. She's
not ferch-Cador at all but one of the children of
Mabh, placed in a queen's cradle. She wants to
dance on the hilltop, leap through fire, even fly as
they say the Faerie can, couple with men and tear
them and lick their blood, consuming them even as
they take her, like a beautiful queen bee.

But this day there is sunlight. The fire is safe to
play with. She coaxes Nurse and the guard to let
her play within the ring of stones. With themselves
close by, the child takes out the gold *aureus* filched
from her mother. She lays it before the biggest
stone, hoping it will please the old gods enough so
they won't ask for her new golden torc. It's only a
message anyway: Gwenhwyfar gives this as token
of the Faerie gold hoard she seeks. Point her where
it is.

The child turns as the nurse-shadow flows across
her own.

It is not Nurse. Gwenhwyfar's legs turn to water.

The girl-thing is not much larger than herself but
grown-up. Mostly naked, she has a woman's full
breasts with big brown nipples like a woman who's
borne child and given suck. Gwenhwyfar stops
breathing. The Faerie girl has come out of nowhere,
as they always can, to crouch beside the stone, gray
eyes stabbing through the fear-numbed child. Under the loose black hair her cheeks are scarred with
dark blue marks where Satan marked her for his
own.

The child tries to cry out but her throat is
blocked. She can only mew weakly as the Faerie
girl glides closer. The wolf-hide wrap around her
thin middle is buzzing with flies and her feet are
caked with dirt. From the language of childhood
that holds all the true words for night and fear,
Gwenhwyfar knows those eyes bent on her. They

have peered over the foot of her bed a moment before she woke from the bad dream. Wolf is in that face, wolf in the alien way the girl opens a brown fist in a peculiar motion to scatter the white pebbles before she lunges and snatches up the gold coin.

"Nurse!"

Finding her voice and her legs, she breaks and flees across the sinister circle where the stones on the edge of terrified vision are waking, changing to their true, malignant shapes, an ambush of Faerie ready to pounce, to steal her away under the hill where Nurse or Epona will never find her. And now the guard is up and roaring as much from fright as anger. He should have been watching. He could be beaten for this, but the filthy things are silent as the dead they come from.

"Goddamned Pict bitch. Go! Get out!"

He won't heave a good pylum at her but he flings the first rock to hand. When Gwenhwyfar dares to peek out from Nurse's skirts, the circle is empty.

"Filthy pigs," the guard rumbles. "Kill them all someday."

"Na, na, be still. There, the bairn's took fright. Nae fear, sweeting, nae fear. It's gone."

The child remembers in the dark. The eyes return when the lamps are blown out. She translates literally from the infallible grown-ups. *It* is gone. *He* and *she* are people, but *it* is a thing, less than human. Faerie are *it*.

She scattered the white stones as her own offering before stealing mine. Arthur said the stones reflect moonlight, and the moon is the eye of Earth Mother as the sun is the eye of Lugh. Man-sun, woman-moon. And the moon, in her time, drew my blood from me and I became a woman.

Paul's notion of women and marriage never sat well with Britons, but then Paul was Hebrew. His church was seeded in one patriarchal society and nurtured in another at Rome. The farther north you go, the more and more powerful goddesses you'll find among the gods. Paul's apology for celibacy as a virtue has its adherents

(chiefly among men and, I suppose, those women glad to be done with it all), but could never be called a fervent tide, though it has eroded the sovereignty of women and nudged them down toward that second rank which Paul and his ilk regard as their natural place. Such declensions are gradual; in my own interminable lifetime, one of the clearest signs is the lapse of the custom of identifying tribal queens with the protective goddess.

My mother was named for Epona, the goddess-protectrix of the Parisi. Like her predecessors since we came from Gaul, Mother represented the fortune and fertility of the tribe. Many practices had modified since the coming of Rome. We no longer impaled beautiful sacrifices on stone altars, since Caesar objected and Jesus made it redundant, but the notion of the queen-goddess was too popular for the priests to denounce with any effect and far too useful politically for my family to abandon. We were an affectionate clan who made intelligent compromises. Mother knew and exhausted an astonishing number of men before she died. As a result of her favors, there wasn't an important man in the north whose mind was not an open book to our need.

At sixteen I knew the machinery of government; how much sovereignty Ambrosius would give us in return for holding his back door against the Picts; in whose bosom we must place a trust and in whose a knife; when to bargain, when to submit; when truth could be served whole and when it must be adulterated. And God knows, inheriting Epona's tastes as well as her privileges, I knew men. A round score ramped through my bed before Arthur came. I took them for reasons of state and pleasure, learned their minds, their expertise or lack of it, where they fumbled or failed, how vulnerable failure made them. They say every woman remembers her first lover. That is true enough, statistically. My first was a fool too full of himself to be of much interest to a woman. My last time with Arthur was ten times the fun. And there are other memories as poignant and painful, like Owain.

Gwenhwyfar slips into bed. Owain shyly turns his back as he undresses with movements all the more awkward for trying to appear casual. She watches, excited but with a tenderness beyond her

years. She might have taken off her nightrobe, but he'll want to do that. He slides in beside her, covered to the neck though it's a warm night. Tentatively he reaches for her, and she comes to him, nuzzling his smooth cheek.

He doesn't know exactly what to do first, interested and confused and a little frightened all at once. Between two fires, as the Picts say. His exploration of her is more spastic than passionate. He's been told you do this and then that and no doubt absorbed a great deal of self-inflating nonsense from men no more virile than himself, but none of it makes sense in the reality of now. Gwenhwyfar can sense his conflict and pops up on an elbow to smile at him.

"Whatever's the matter? Don't you like me?"

He struggles with it. "I can't. I mean I can't—now."

She strokes his body under the covers. No, he's not ready yet and never will be if he worries so over it. "Of course you can. We've all night."

Most of him wants her naturally, but the rest is still protesting something.

"You won't tell about this?"

"Tell what? Will they hang you for not being able this minute?"

A long silence. "I will be a chief when Llawdwen dies. A chief in his place."

"Well, so will I. And I picked you for tonight. I have very good taste."

"My father—"

"What of him? I shan't tell."

"I mean, I want to—"

"So do I, and for a start it's too hot for all these covers."

She slithers out of the light robe and sits crosslegged facing Owain in the dim light. The sight of her rouses him, she can see that much. And even this early she knows what he's struggling against. The expectation against the reality, his father's leering boasts and the fictional satyr he is impossibly expected to be. These pathetic lies have paralyzed him out of the man he is.

"You are very beautiful."

"So are you. Come snuggle." She beckons to him. "Talk to me, Owain."

"Talk?"

No, Da never said he had to talk to them.

"Tell me about yourself."

She cuddles herself in his arms until Owain relaxes, until his hands and lips forget the father's wishful fictions and know her with their own appetite, and the youth and health of the two of them are more than enough for the time. When that happens, when he's inside her, the boy is passionate and tender, his own man at last. The lamp burns down, the moon wanes. Resting, they talk like friends, laugh like delighted children, gossip like cronies. He won't come boasting from her chamber as Mark did from Yseult's, riving Trystan from his side forever, but Owain will be proud. For his own reasons.

So I learned men early: not a foreign country, not even enemies. We are more alike than different. Under the male urge to dominate women is a need for their approval. Oh, there were always those who strutted about my chamber expecting me to adore and submit as if they were the first. From such as these I divined the frailty behind the muscled chests that sought in dominance a kind of safe distance. I proved by my own axiom the irreducible equality of sexes and learned why fine rulers are so few: not for want of ability but for that peculiar detachment that makes true kings walk ever alone, chained to a power they can almost never unleash for themselves.

But I always regretted Owain. The self he found with me was soon buried under the father's brutal image. A year after he loved me, I had to condemn him to death. Not my father. Me.

She knows the law, she knows her royal craft, but the dispassionate ordering of death is new to her. For all that, the example must be made today.

Cador and Peredur are gone to crush a rebellion among the Brigantes. Insignificant as uprisings go,

not planned out, doomed from the start. Cador has sent these five prisoners home for his daughter's judgment. There are his advisers in the hall to counsel her, but Guenevere is the Parisi crown in Cador's absence. The judgment is hers alone to pronounce. Light enough; Cador has no taste for indiscriminate vengeance. Most of the rebels have been paroled, but an example must be made of these five leaders, ineffectual as they were.

Except that Owain is one of them.

She regards Owain's father. Damn you, Llawdwen, you're the miserable cause of this. You never saw the day you had the brains to lead a circle dance. You brought him here.

Llawdwen has no real grievance against Cador, none of them do beyond a hazy notion of Brigantia for the Brigantes—and precious little they accomplished when they had it. She curses the father virulently and his need of revolt for its own sake, for the gesture of daring, pulling the beard of Parisi authority with no thought of the aftermath, only that Owain must be a like swaggerer for bards to sing of in the home trevs.

And yet Owain followed him and was pricked on the list by Cador. And the example must be made. She feels the chair of state hard on her skinny bottom, but she must not wriggle in search of comfort. She writhed enough before they were dragged into the hall. She besought the stern counselors: must they die? Are they so important, dead or alive? Can't we mitigate . . . banish?

"You are the crown," they tell her. From what they don't say, she knows what she must do anyway. She is the crown and mercy here will be cruelty later. Other small men like Llawdwen will call it weakness. If this absurdity goes unpunished, the next will be larger and more dangerous.

She lets her eyes go over the five, one by one. "Which of you will speak?"

Owain steps forward. She tries to see the boy she knew, the potential. He touched her once, but he's all Llawdwen now, all swagger, even proud of the chains rattling on his arms and feet. In his eye is all

his knowledge of her, gone insolent and mocking. She's only a woman after all, and he had her like any sow. His father is watching. The lunacy must be played out to the end.

"Only that great Cador has sent us for judgment, we who most justly defied him." Owain mouths it with exaggerated respect for added insult. "What will his daughter do to Brigantes for being their own men?"

Behind Owain the other captives wait, flanked by soldiers. Their sardonic grins are frozen, clenched. She wants to talk to the Owain she knew once, but a cold settles on her, borne in on her by the weight of what she must be. Only for a moment she chokes on it. She's seen his parody of strength. He'll see hers for the real thing.

"Crucify them."

She can't look at him as he's herded out. She's that human. There will be enough of looking. She must be there when they put him up outside the city walls where he'll hang for a full day or more before dying.

For a long time after the audience chamber empties, Guenevere sits alone on the dais, awed by the first realization of complete power and its weight. As if she held consuming lightning in fists that must ever be balled tight, opened only on the tight rein of wisdom. The thought is only briefly drunken before it's sober again. She will look at Owain hanging on the cross with sadness but no remorse, none at all. It had to be done. Whatever ghosts haunt her will walk a narrow corridor in a locked wing of her mind. The crown is no longer too heavy nor the chair too hard.

She is a ruler now.

Women want to be loved, men to be assured. Men take each other at face value; from the supine position women more easily note the small depreciations. Some were all ardor, some smug with reputation the present failed to affirm. Some were brittle in their sickly need to dominate, or its obverse, the need to be dominated, even defiled, by women. Most were just men and no longer a

mystery to me. They came as I chose them, crude or sensitive, devious or honorable, but I learned to ration my heart. Arthur was the first to whom I went myself, telling my pride he needed me. That lapse of independence was the first thorn in our crowns. I never forgave Arthur my need of him.

Damn him.

Most people never know who they are, only what they're expected to be. But Arthur knew. When he came back from Morgana, the mark was on him deeper than those cut in his face. Cador's lords were always jealous of him, this upstart bastard in dirty leather, with mud on his boots and gorse burrs in his cloak, who prayed as infrequently as he bathed and cared nothing for rank. But men as different as Gawain, Trystan and Bedivere followed him and none could ever clearly say why, except that Arthur saw what was to be done and set about it, never looking back to see who followed. Which can be exalting but very hard on the faithful.

Was that it, darling, the element I lacked? I wonder.

After he left Morgana, you could sense—how can I put it?—a stillness in his soul. Out of this serenity came an acceptance that could live with imperfection, a laughter born of some vast, cosmic joke Arthur could never share. Winning or losing was just that to him and no more. No loss was insupportable. His laughter or his tears could flow for whatever touched him, and what touched him must have been, simply, a part of God. He was a paradox—readable as a page and fathomless, ambitious as myself yet striding easier under its goad, never so embattled. He treated men as equals, looked into their eyes to feel the essence of them, and in return they courted the honor of kneeling to him. Accessible to all and apart from them.

Did she give him all that? Something did. Somewhere between the scrubbed young centurion and the man who came back from the Faerie, Arthur became human and fascinating. I would have bled to bed him and straightly did just that. When it comes to bed, let an old woman tell you. Find a man with a capacity for joy and the loving will take care of itself. Love for us could be fierce need or merely affectionate, rarely perfunctory. Outside of Lancelot, I've never slept with a man more open to love or

ultimately harder to reach. Perhaps my taste runs to the enigmatic.

We were barely used to sharing a bed before it was sanctified and made royal: Emperor and Empress at twenty-three—Arthur always thought me younger; I never disabused him. The crown and all its cares came to bed with us now. How we worked and what a heaven-matched pair we were! We worked in bed, over breakfast, through the day and into the night, and saw by the light of our late-burning lamps the shape of a new country built on hard Roman common sense and planed from British oak. Arthur could be single-minded. He worked me, he drained me of every drop of experience that could add one more brick to the emergent state. That was the current gold in our crown and the worm in our marriage. Work became a habit hard to lay aside. At such times love could be a dutiful afterthought. Not often, but now and then, when a major problem absorbed Arthur, I could almost hear him thinking afterward: *There, that'll hold her a while. Back to work*—as he reached for the sheaf of documents always piled by our bed.

Well, I thought it too, love, and prayed more than once you'd leave Camelot for a few days or fall into some other diverting bed and leave *me* to get some work done or just putter in my gardens. Evidently the prayer was national. When I escaped from prison, the dust was barely settled behind me when a gaggle of hopeful and hard-breathing daughters was packed off to Camelot. Arthur availed himself of a few, one of whom had the temerity to hint of it in a letter I received just before the news of his death. Sexual egotism is not your sole prerogative, my lords, merely a wider opportunity to indulge it. I squelched the simpering slut with a brief frost in return—

. . . if memory serves, you and your father were at a Yule banquet some years ago. I remember him as an interminable speaker entrenched in the belief that digression is good for the soul, and yourself most vividly since you blew your nose in a ewer. I was polite with an effort; so, evidently, was my husband. If you were as inept on that occasion as you were on the other, I doubt further invitations to either function—G.

Someone told me—oh, years later, I don't know who—that she'd died of plague. God is good. Sometimes he's an absolute dear.

Like any peasant and his wife, loving became something to enjoy when we weren't too busy or tired. It is difficult after a day of ambiguity or outright dishonesty to relax into the role of lovers, or after another day of men far readier to praise your charms than admit your superior skill as a leader, not to regard your husband with the same bitter frustration. So he turns to his side of the bed, you to yours. The small healing words, the small touches that could join you again, are deferred and the unpaid debt of loving mounts.

Then I was pregnant. When I told Arthur, he placed both of his hands on my stomach. It seemed a dear gesture of affection; not for years did I learn it was a Faerie sign of reverence to Earth Mother and the getting-mysteries of women. That reverence done, Arthur was not viscerally involved. He had his own dreams for our child, more concerned with the grown result than the day-to-day quickening in my flesh. If he was spared the inconvenience, he missed the wonder. My body was changing, sending the most incredible messages to my heart. Briefly I woke ill in the morning; when that passed, my never-frail health became downright phenomenal. I developed an absolute craving for pears and honey and the color blue, waddled into council meetings with a sparkle and a burst of exuberant good will that must have aroused even deeper suspicions in princes like Mark who politely detested me. My moods went up and down over a hurdle course. Something was happening for me that needed no control or planning, and a *new* voice, my own, said: *you're a woman and this is your gift.* And God's Blood, how I'd needed it. I felt so complete now.

Clever little Gwenhwyfar: father's pet, adept student, shrewd princess, brilliant queen. Not once, till this miracle grew and moved in my womb, had I ever for one day lived for myself alone. Yanked from childhood straight to duty, witty before I knew true laughter, smiling before I tasted joy—I must have been very much as Trystan once described young Arthur, a well-functioning engine of administration. But now how *real* I was.

And how tired. In the last months when I needed more

rest, there was only more work, especially with the north and Cador where my relation and knowledge were more intimate. The child became a burden on my skinny frame, dragged from council to state function to scriptorium to bed. The daily score of letters became an ordeal as I wriggled awkwardly on the bench, trying to rest my back and think policy at the same time. The child began as part of me. I ended as an appendage to it until its time came.

Years later when Morgana was journeying south to Camelot, Arthur showed me the only letter she ever sent, dictated to a bewildered monk who labored to translate her primitive pride and woman's pain.

He racked me being born, but I bit on the cloth and thought on the hills at Bel-tein and you, my lord of summer. . . .

So she bore beautiful, vicious Modred, and the reality of us both circled about Arthur-Belrix, two dancers in an ecstasy of jealous commitment, a dark crannog for her, a soft bed for me, but I twisted in the same pain only to deliver his daughter dead. Then weeks of stillness, the guilt breathing softly against my breast where the child should be. I lost it. *I* lost it. It would not have happened if I were strong enough. Weak thing, too weak to be a real woman—until I sickened of the guilt and threw it at God who could live with it. He did this to me. So I lay still, listening to the prayers of the priest while something pagan stumbled on God's track to strike him in the face for my own loss. Man-god, man-priest, man-husband. Always men, and what in hell did they know of this tearing loss? Oh, Arthur was sorry and Arthur cried—in Bedivere's arms, not mine—and they went off to man-things again, and of course I had to be up and working again, hiding the hurt. Oh, and smiling! Even Arthur could be fooled with a smile. I learned to paint the rictus with one, facile stroke.

Yes, yes, then there was Lancelot. I did love him, and he was my salvation as I was his for a time, but that's another story for another night's fire.

So many years, so many people to care for, judge, buy and sell. When I killed Morgana, I believed it was for

sound reasons of state, not jealousy, and most of my
country agreed. Looking back, it was as much one as the
other. Any contrition I felt for Arthur's sake was never
without a nagging sense of right. The bitch and her
whelp were dangerous as Cerdic. Oh, yes, she was. He
was.

*I begged you not to bring them. I remember that night we
fought over it. I let you see my hurt, laid it out on the bed
between us. Do you know how hard that was for me? I
begged, goddamn you. And still you brought them . . . and I
had to watch.*

In the great hall with the lords and ladies of Camelot
whispering in disapproval, I remained in my chair of
state while Arthur made a fool of himself in a ring of
dwarfish clowns. They were ludicrous; most of their
clothes and bangles were stolen and much too large.
Morgana's cloak dragged the flooring stones. She and the
men scampered about Arthur with no more dignity than
children. Only the son stood apart, haughty and watchful. Arthur couldn't see the resemblance, but it was there
for me, the map of him in the clean set of the dark head,
the shape of the hands, the reserved energy of that com-
pact body. I let my heart go to hell and painted over that
image another of my own: a head taller, fair as his father,
a soldier-scholar like him, heir to north and south alike
someday. I might call him Phoebus . . . yes, bringer of
sunlight.

Then Morgana spoke to him and he turned on me.
Phoebus vanished; this was goatish Herne, something
from the woods that smelled of manure. Those eyes knew
their otherness, no part of any flesh or experience but
their own. Dead, trapped spirits coming at me across the
hall, across the stone circle, toward a terrified young
woman shivering on the edge of her bed and knowing her
own death only seconds away.

The battle began in darkness and confusion, the
Saxons and Picts scaling Eburacum's walls before
Arthur's men could counter. The Picts are in the palace now, running and shouting through the halls
below her. Gwenhwyfar hears them and knows her
family must be dead and the city lost. She'll die
too, and yet the terror will not harden to resigna-

tion. She can't pray. She wants to live and punish these inhuman creatures dirtying her home, killing the future.

Then one of them crouches in the doorway, grinning at her. He tosses his torch into the hall and advances on her. Grabs her wrist, pulls her up close to him, his face against hers.

The thin blade goes into him much easier than he would have penetrated her. His face, the loose-mouthed desire, goes comic with shock. She coils to strike again but there's no need. He staggers from her room to die in the hall. She sinks down on her bed, still smelling him. He actually touched her.

Then the shouting below is British. Lancelot and his men are back in the palace.

She looks at the greasy mark on her wrist where the Pict held her. She rubs hard at it, rubs it raw. She is still frozen there with the dagger in her hand and the blood drying on her fingers when Arthur finds her—

—and Modred stepped up onto the dais and laid his hands on my stomach. He said something in that ancient dialect of his. I caught only one word of it. So did my people. It was enough.

Adaltrach. Adultress.

Arthur did mean to hurt me with this, no other reason could obtain. Not only to flaunt his Faerie wife in my face, and the son she gave him where I failed; to this he added one more cut, told them of Lancelot and made *me* the whore, as if it weren't an open secret already. Arthur and I never spoke of it because—I foolishly thought—some part of us still touched above it all. Wrong again, lost again. Now he walked on me, and I had to strike him back where it would hurt the most. I left the hall, seething, collected my guard of Parisi knights and rode out of Camelot to a small chapel on the banks of Severn. The ride cooled the murder in me only enough to give it shape. There in the chapel, beneath sorrowing Jesus on the Cross, I gave the order.

"Brocan, you know what a danger she is."

"Aye, Lady."

"You know the house where they'll sleep?"

"It is known to us."

"Don't let them wake. Do it and make for Eburacum. There'll be bounty in this. Yes. There will be bounty."

Even Brocan saw the tumult in me and tried to urge caution, at least a subtler plan. "Perhaps if the Queen waited—"

"*Do it!*"

Without another word, he and his knights left to carry out my order, leaving me with Christ's carven reproach.

"Don't you look down on me," I glowered back. "You think you're the only one who ever bled?"

A hurt child with a royal arsenal of state reasons and public opinion, I butchered Morgana for all the pristine motives of a queen guarding the good of her people. Only Arthur wasn't fooled. He dragged me to her body and pushed my face in her blood.

Was she the stone that broke us, Arthur? Because my love was all yours, yours always shared with her? Because a part of us could bend and reach and another couldn't? Because—I'll howl it at you in hell—I was your equal? You never knew a woman who matched you as I did, in bed or on the throne, and we never accepted that until it was too late. Remember that day on the plain when we made peace? Agrivaine might have charged when you were on foot, but I planted myself between you. He'd damn well have to ride over me first, and the men wouldn't do that. We finally knew then how much of a love worked through us. I'd fight you any day for my rights in Britain and as cheerfully die for you. We would have been lovers anywhere, you and I. We should have been born peasants in a wattle hut, with ten Modreds of our own to raise, where we could love and rail and bully each other with the same passion but in a smaller war where it didn't matter . . . Lord, I can get so tired of living. Almost.

The country was breaking up and so was I. Inconvenient nature chose that autumn to stop my maternal clock and announce redundantly that there would be no more children.

"Well," I growled to Imogen, "that's fresh news, isn't it?"

My menses flowed and stopped, flowed again and stopped. A week of it once a month might be a minor bother. Six or seven unremittant weeks were depleting hell. My nerves wore even thinner until I wanted to scream at Imogen for her softest word and leap down the throat of anyone who opposed me. Like the country itself, my skin erupted in a nervous, itching rash that no slaves or salutary diet would help. Nothing was comfortable against my skin, especially nothing tight. I gave Imogen the blue kirtle she coveted, had several loose undershifts made from the last of my Egyptian cotton and went about in loose gray homespun, looking for all the world like a nun of some order of poverty.

Meanwhile the post riders from Glevum plied north via Cair Legis and kept me in some touch with Blodwen. Her dispatches were brief and artless, their lack of reproach reproachful in every dutiful line.

Guenevere, Queen—
Our southern roads are taken. The Cornish and Silures are moving against us. I thank God after all that Emrys will be spared if we should be taken. High Queen, look to my son.

> **Blodwen at Cair Gloiu**

And a short time later—

Blodwen to Guenevere, Queen—
Conant's forces attacked Cair Gloiu this morning. We are besieged, though the first attack was repelled. Bedwyr ap Gryffyn has been taken and will be sent straight, as you ordered. Thus you may judge my loyalty. I pray each hour that God soften your heart and that my son may be free and safe.

I couldn't expect Glevum to hold forever without the help no one could send. Constantine's strategy seemed to Gareth and myself a mixture of brilliance and ineptitude. Where we thought he'd descend on Astolat and wipe it out, he merely occupied the small but well-placed fort of Neth Dun More and several other vantage points, pocketing Lancelot's cavalry where they could do

nothing but sit out the revolution or waste themselves in useless sorties. Even Gareth was impressed.

"Very neat," he allowed. "Keeps Lancelot off his flank and rear with hardly the loss of a man. Tidy. He'll move against Badon next."

But advantages gained by Constantine were squandered elsewhere. He readied his forces against Maelgwyn's Catuvellauni on Badon, and then inexplicably paused while I puzzled his reasons, waving the map at Gareth.

"What's he waiting for, a star in the East?"

Not so far off the mark. Constantine had his own troubles with Aurelius Conant over his share of Camelot's treasury. In reply to peremptory demands for an accounting, Conant testily replied that there was not that much money or gold plate on hand. There wasn't, but I'd never tell. While they wrangled and burdened the south with maintenance of their armies, Badon prepared and I published my own appeal to all Britain.

Guenevere to all her people and her spiritual fathers, the bishops of Britain. In sorrow for her embattled country.

Is this the legacy of Arthur, this contention against the order he established? We do not covet the sword, but will pass it only to the lawful custom and choosing of the lords, people at large, and the Church of Britain. We will not surrender it to Constantine, nor to Aurelius Conant, nor to any usurper who brushes the law aside like a common thief. We call the tribes of Britain to attest our right by proclaiming these rebels as such, their acts unlawful, their edicts of no force. God will judge the right.

Thus I showed myself within the law and Constantine beyond the pale. Not that it would bother that idiosyncratic young man. My outburst to Gareth was more accurate than we guessed at the time. In a shambles of victory, Constantine was tripping over his own feet, now daring, now too cautious. And, for what they were worth, in the east or elsewhere, his stars were not in the mood. It seems his astrologer foresaw disaster in any large endeavor undertaken in haste. Thus Constantine vacillated this way and that while I used every minute, riding here,

striding there, scratching my rash, Galahalt and Emrys the bewildered tail to my comet. My chiefs were gathering shortly to firm our war plans. There were a thousand details daily. Despite our worries from the south, we couldn't neglect the Wall without finding ourselves throat-deep in Venicone or Votadini Picts. In case of siege, how much food and fodder could we count on? Should we move south? Where should we make our stand, Legis or Eburacum? And on and on with my benumbed princelings in tow and Imogen nagging at me to use the salves and not to scratch, and sending bowls of barley soup and other nourishing snacks to clutter my scriptorium table. Arthur and I ate this way for years. State dinners were business; alone we ate with one hand and worked with the other. It's often amused me to think that Church historians pawing through the blizzard of that year's correspondence might hold up a stained page and whisper, "Saintly and burdened Queen: mark where her very tears dropped upon the page." More likely it was soup or sauce, but I'll stand by the image if they will.

Hostage and ward, my princelings pattered after me and wondered at the pace of it all. Galahalt was too stolid to learn. He did not see the preservation of Astolat as a quirk of war but the intervention of God. The rebels *dare* not move against his father or his mother, the holiest woman in Britain. Courageous he was, like his uncle Geraint, but a dolt. If I'd told him to charge a cohort with a fruit knife, off he'd go, and no doubt Britain needed such, but there his attributes ended. He knew no Latin beyond the mass, read not at all and cared even less to learn. His attitude toward rule was no more flexible than Eleyne's. God made the law, his chosen nobles enforced it. Anyone in dispute of this was clearly unnatural and deserved the worst that could be meted out. The notion, even in my hard-pressed example, that rulers might have to bargain or cajole, could not penetrate the boy's complacency. He was born and raised to unquestioned power. One wave of his hand brought silent Sawel to his slightest wish, another sent him away. That was government to Galahalt. Set in his ways at fifteen, he rose at a certain hour, took a certain time over meals, heard three masses a day and could not adjust to

any break in routine. At such times he simply ceased to function.

Emrys was of a different stamp. He flourished in disorder. If dinner was a cup and a capon leg gulped on the move, he couldn't care less. I ran the baby fat off Blodwen's boy, but he kept up with me and even began to evince some glimmer of ability. Logistics, the how of things, interested him. In manner and dress he was careless as his father or Arthur. Whatever came to hand was the day's apparel. He thinned out from worry over his mother, hurried meals and the pace I set. A stone lighter, he looked more Arthur than Kay, a rangy, loping stride and the same habit of unfastening his cloak as he entered the palace and tossing it over one shoulder.

But he still lacked confidence in himself and the ability to make swift, firm decisions. This showed in his nervous habit of repeating the first phrase of a sentence before going on, or retreating from a point the moment someone challenged it. Of course, Galahalt had no such problem.

"How would you respond to chiefs who vacillated over sending you levies?"

The serene heir to Astolat responded, "I would kill the lords and take their lands."

"Suppose you needed them later. You probably would."

"Oh . . ."

"Emrys, what would you do?"

"First I would—I would find what they might want."

"Very good. Why?"

"Well, I heard my father say they always want something, especially when their taxes are due."

"And?"

"Well, then. I might—"

"Might, boy?"

"I would offer them a deferment of taxes, or part of them, until the next year in exchange for the levy of troops."

Granite Galahalt couldn't see the logic. "But they must pay their taxes."

"And I would have not only the troops but a better bargaining position next year. When they'd probably need favors from me."

Shrewd enough. I was pleased, but then Emrys invalidated it all with a self-deprecating shrug. "At least that's what Kay would do."

"And how long would you take to decide this?"

"As long as it needed."

"If you had less than half a day?"

"Impossible."

"Perhaps. That's why it's sometimes taken Arthur and myself as much as an hour. Think, decide and *do*, boy. If you don't, someone else will. That sound behind you is always sand running down the glass."

The last message from Blodwen was passed to Lord Bors who was sweeping the Legis-Eburacum road for signs of Conant. I was with Regan when my guards passed Bors into my chambers, taking a few pleasant minutes to cut linen for her baby. Little thing, she was swelling mountainously. Everyone thought it would be a boy. Bors looked grim when he knelt and handed me the message.

"From Glevum, Lady."

"Bors, come," Regan bubbled. "See the shirts we're making. I'm going to embroider them with samite thread."

"Aye, they're bonny." He kissed her with male absent-mindedness. "How is't?"

She touched his cheek, not put off. "Say how is't with you? Your lips are chapped. Why *won't* you use that salve when you ride?"

"Yes, yes. I will."

Regan knew her husband too well. "Is the news so bad?"

"Glevum's fallen," I told her.

Blodwen's bald note said it all.

Guenevere—
We were breached this morning. Though my people give only a street at a time, there is little hope. I hope this reaches you. I have done your bidding and held as long as I could. I entreat your mercy and parole for my son who betrayed you no more than I. May God forgive you this. I cannot.

                              Blodwen of Cair Gloiu

So that was it. The city, Pendragon, Blodwen and my dear Flavia—we had to assume it was all up and that they were dead or captive. "So it's done."

"Done," said Bors. "Legis could be next."

"It should be Badon. Have the guards send Emrys to me."

"Poor mum." Regan's eyes narrowed in sympathy. "You'll have to tell him."

"Yes."

"Do you still think it was them tried to murder you?"

"I don't know, Regan. Probably not. Go along now. It's time for your nap anyway."

By my order, Emrys was still guarded. He slouched into the chamber, careless in an old leather tunic and loose trousers, dropping the cloak on a couch.

"Lady."

"Sit down, boy. Some wine?"

"No, thank you. Does that silly guard have to follow me even to the latrine? I won't try to escape."

I handed him the letter. "This just came."

He must have read Blodwen's letter three or four times, letting each word burn into him. Finally Emrys placed it on the table and poured himself a cup of wine.

"I'm sorry, boy."

"Guenevere," he said deliberately, "my name is Emrys. I may not be a prince to your cut or fit to go unguarded, but I am no boy." He finished the wine in one draft, swaying a little, his voice tight. "There's little honor left me, but you could remember my name."

"As you wish, Emrys."

"There's something else I've got to say to you, Guenevere, and you can do what you will about it."

"Go on. Perhaps I deserve it."

"We had less will to murder you then than I do now."

"I couldn't be sure of that."

Emrys threw the cup across the chamber. "Sure? Sure? Aren't you the one that's always at me to be sure, damn you? You've killed my mother because *you* couldn't be sure!"

"How many times do I have to tell you? Decide and do. The country was falling apart under me."

"Not us. We were loyal."

"I was almost murdered, bleeding like a butchered hog. I don't always like what I have to do."

"She never betrayed you, never! And you—you put us down on our knees and—God, I hate you for this, Guenevere. I want you to know that. My God, that—that was *my* city."

"She sold it dear."

"Mother would."

"A house at a time."

"Aye, she would that. She. *She*, and where was I?" Emrys broke with it, sobbing out his shame. "Where in useless hell was I?"

My rash was on fire; I desperately needed to sink into a soothing bath, denying with an effort the savage need to scratch myself raw. I went to the weeping boy. "The two of you dead would have served no better. At least the Dobunni have a prince to call home."

"A prince?" he choked. "What kind of prince? Do you think I could face them now? You've ended that, you and my own uselessness." He shrugged away from the hand I stretched to him. "No. Leave me alone. You always sneered at Mother and me. Because we're country folk with country ways, eat at table instead of lolling on a damn Roman couch. You laughed at her, didn't you, you and Grandmother? You don't know how she had to fight for everything."

"You think I didn't, Arthur didn't?"

"I don't know. I don't know you at all. Do you—do you honestly care about anyone?"

There are times you must pity the young. All they know is truth. "I've had my better days, but none since spring." I fetched the map of Britain from the table and thrust it into his hands. "Here. You've had your cry and a go at my character, well and good. In a few hours I'll meet with Gareth and my chiefs. Bring this map to the council with you and be prepared to tell me what all of us need to know. Where will Constantine strike next. Badon? Legis? Or both?"

Emrys stared at the map, seeing only his mother. "How would I know?"

"Someone had better. We're guessing blind."

"You thought me unfit to guard my own city."

"You were. Blodwen did you no favor in that. When you

came in here you demanded not to be called boy. Very well, I'll accord your title, but you'll earn it. You may go now, Prince."

Emrys wiped his eyes. They were cold when he turned to me, inclining his head. "Till then, Lady."

Samhain was past. That day the autumn wind blew through the streets of Eburacum already astir with preparations for war. Parisi horsemen came and went, Gareth's cavalry clattered in and out of the gates. The tribal chiefs came in a swirl of tartan color; against their garish hues old Maelgwyn was somber in black cloak and worn ring mail and the new weight of sudden tragedy. Long a widower, now he was totally alone. His sons were dead, murdered by Constantine. To match the death of Mark, this was perpetrated in the same chapel at Witrin. Livid Brochan must be pronouncing anathema on all Britain by now; but this was too much, a surfeit of atrocity.

"Dear Maelgwyn, I can't believe it."

"Constantine's a rebel," the old man husked, "but I thought him at least a man. My sons were on pilgrimage, look you, and that—that creature cut them down in the chapel itself, at the very tomb of Arthur. Then he hacked my boys apart like—why, Lady? They weren't even armed. They had his safe conduct."

But one of them would have succeeded soon to Maelgwyn's crown; fresh blood to lead the Catuvellauni and perhaps the country itself if he proved strong enough. Constantine was pruning rivals as well as enemies, and Camelot was worth a year of penances. Emrys should count his blessings.

"Poor old man." I winced to Imogen as Maelgwyn lumbered away down the hall in his threadbare cloak. "They've cut the heart out of him."

"And put him square on your side if he wasn't all there before," she observed cannily. "Ah, mum, how oft must I say't?"

"Oh, it's this tight kirtle. I can't wear homespun for the council, and it's torture."

"Y'will naever get rid of it do you scratch!"

Despite Gareth's need for a decision, the council started sluggishly. Maelgwyn was listless with his grief,

Emrys subdued for much the same reasons, but attentive. He'd dressed in his best tunic with Kay's old senatorial toga thrown over it. Galahalt, included only by courtesy, nodded in a corner after a heavy meal. My chiefs were divided in their opinions on Constantine's options, duty vying with self-interest, and not offering much of value. Even Ifan, standing beside my chair with the imperial sword, began to droop with boredom.

Then a suggestion from Lord Penrwd, one of my eastern Parisi chiefs, brought the torpid discussion to life. With all our forces, he said, we were still much less than the combine of Constantine and Conant, and mostly cavalry at that. Since most of our fighting would be defensive—

Enter Galahalt, waking up: "Defend? We will *not* defend. High Queen, we will attack, won't we?"

"After Lord Penrwd is finished," I reminded him.

"We need plenty of foot inside the walls," Penrwd argued. "Good ones, and such are available to us. I have an offer from Prince Icel of two thousand mercenaries."

Icel? Icel? The unfamiliar name whispered through the audience chamber.

"I know of no Icel. Who is he?"

"Of the Iclingas, Lady. The Saxons south of Humber."

Ifan spluttered: "Jesus God!"

Most of them were speechless with the heresy, but not Maelgwyn. "What! Arthur and I broke them not a year gone. You want to invite them back and *pay* them as well?"

Penrwd said simply, "They're the finest foot soldiers since the old legions."

"I know," said Maelgwyn with audible acid. "I've known their language and their ways all my life. Put them on Badon, my own men will walk away flat."

"Put them in Eburacum," I added, "they'll walk away with everything but the walls. No, Penrwd."

"No," said Gareth.

"No again," Dai meqq Muir voiced in his slurred Brigante. "Remember what happened when Vortigern brought them in. We could never trust them behind us."

"I think—" Emrys began and then smothered it as the older men turned, annoyed at his stripling presumption.

I prompted him. "Yes, Prince?"

"Your Parisi lord is right. My father said—"

"Your father is dead. What's he got to do with it?" Maelgwyn was not a brutal man, but his pain spoke for him today.

"Aye, sir. He died at Badon with you and Uncle Arthur. But you were sometime his guest before I was born."

The subtlety was gentle as it was deft. Kay had extended the hospitality of Pendragon to Maelgwyn when the Saxons ran him and most of his tribe out of the Midlands. Arthur had to win it back and Maelgwyn's lifetime loyalty in the bargain. Emrys glanced about as if in apology for being alive. "I think Lord Penrwd is right. Father said the same thing. The Saxons are fine troops. We could use a few of them, perhaps not two thousand—"

"Did your father mention they're ambitious and shrewd as hell?" Maelgwyn glared at him. "Not just Icel, the buggering lot. Every one of them has a chance to be a thegn if he can grab enough."

An inconsistency bothered me. "Lord Penrwd, how can this Icel maintain nigh half a legion without at least our hearing of them?"

"Well . . . they're not exactly troops."

"What exactly are they?"

Penrwd scratched his thick-maned head. "There's a thing—I forget the word—a kind of irregular levy."

"The *fyrd*," Maelgwyn corrected. "They're conscripted, you could call it that. So many men from a district called a 'hundred.' They just drop their hoes, pick up their spears and march."

"At whose order?" I wanted to know.

"The thegns. Like Gunnar Eanboldson."

"What's he? Lord of what holding?"

Penrwd struggled with the unfamiliar. "Well, then, he's not exactly a lord."

"He is or he isn't. You just said he was a . . . thegn?"

"Well, some thegns are nobles. Some are not."

"Penrwd, your explanation is irritating me almost as much as this lamentable rash of mine."

Maelgwyn, who spoke the language, stepped in to aid the floundering Penrwd. "Thegn can be hereditary or just a man with a certain amount of land."

"I see." I didn't see at all. "Then what exactly are men like this Eanboldson?"

"Farmers," Penrwd said, giving it up.

"Farmers?" Galahalt's mirthless, horsy laugh brayed through the chamber. "We should pay farmers to fight?"

It was funny. We all laughed with the eloquent exception of Maelgwyn and the combrogi who'd fought those stubborn farmers. Vaguely I remembered Trystan describing the totally alien mind of these people—

If their princes don't lead them, they'll come by themselves.

But all I could see then, hear then, were those Saxons hooting with the Picts through these very halls and this chamber twenty-five years past—tearing, grabbing, smashing my home on the day I could have died.

"No, Penrwd. And no more talk of it. How effective will we be against our enemies when we need keep one eye on our allies? Enough. Let's to realities. Badon or Legis? Where will we be hit?"

The men were even more divided on this question for strategic and personal reasons. The western Brigantes wanted protection for Legis. Maelgwyn and some of the Parisi were sure the attack would come at Badon. Cerdic attacked it in dead winter, didn't he? A victory at Badon would put the whole south in Constantine's hands. Aye, true, but Legis would give him the entire west, an easier victory against a smaller force. Nay, look at the map, just look at it, sir! No. Yes. And on and on.

Gareth plainly didn't know. Our intelligence from the south was not that good just now; he couldn't say for sure, though he leaned toward Badon. The proponents for Badon began to sway the others. It was the strongest hill fort in Britain; the rebels *had* to take it. Then Emrys cleared his throat and rose.

"My Lords, if I may—"

"Oh, sit down."

"Sit down, boy."

Without another word Emrys would have retired from the debate, but I jumped in. "Prince Emrys, have you studied the maps I gave you?"

"Uh—yes, I have."

"Then I think we're ready for a fresh opinion. Come forward."

Emrys mounted the dais where he faced the older lords with the map in his hands, plainly uncertain of

himself. "How can—how can Constantine go against Badon when we know he can't?"

"Why can't he?" Maelgwyn snapped. "Cerdic did."

"With ten thousand. For a start, the numbers are wrong. That is, I think they are."

"You *think*," one grizzled chief roared at him. "Is this a time for guessing?"

"Bless you, sir," Gareth purred with a slight twinkle. "We've been doing that for the last hour. Go on, Prince."

"Prince Maelgwyn has a thousand men on Badon, and the best equipment," Emrys stated carefully. "The axiom for attack superiority is three to one."

"Constantine has the men," Gareth reminded him. "We're sure of that much."

"But I've studied his dispositions. So many are committed to Camelot, Dyfneint and Glevum. The men on Badon are recent veterans, conditioned fighters. Cair Legis hasn't fought a war since before Cador's time. Constantine knows this as well as we do."

Galahalt chose this juncture to bray again: "Do you think lack of numbers will keep him from Badon? He is no coward."

"No, no," Emrys conceded genially, "but in all—in all this strategy, I think we're overlooking the man. And the man is inconsistent. Like a chess player with a brilliant opening and no middle game, just flashes of inspiration."

I pricked up my ears at the unaccustomed sound of incisive thought. "That's true."

Emrys relaxed a little, unrolling the map. "He's not so committed to logic he won't pause to listen to his astrologer. We all consult them now and then. Blodwen's foretold I'd be a girl and should be called Julia for the month of my birth."

"Not half," Maelgwyn muttered.

Emrys ignored the insult and the snickers that greeted it. "We know this worthy has warned Constantine away from a large commitment at present. Now . . . with this news and his scattered forces, he'll think twice about Badon, where Arthur and Maelgwyn held off ten times their number."

The lords stirred and whispered to each other, but no one cried him down on the point, nor was there any more

sarcasm. Emrys had taken the maps from my chambers along with his grief and made sober use of them.

"Our Queen has remarked on allies who have to be watched more closely than enemies. We know the love Cornish and Silures bear each other, and Constantine already suspects Conant of withholding treasure—with cause, I should say. Now, if I—if I were such a man, knowing Legis the surer victory, I'd be there to make sure my own flag flew over the forum along with Conant's."

"All well and good," said Penrwd. "But we know he has to take Badon."

"Why?" Emrys answered calmly. "Why must he go for Badon when the sword is here? While he camps on Maelgwyn's doorstep with everything committed and no reserves, he knows we'll be merrily repossessing Camelot, Glevum and everything he's won so far."

"Damned right," I said. "Do you completely discard Badon as a target then?"

"No. No, I—I think he will move on it sometime but only when Maelgwyn is isolated. The sword is here. You are here, Lady."

Gareth rose and came forward to frown over the map. "Lad, you think neat as a horse thief. In my land, that's an honor. But riddle me this: Why Legis at all, then? Why not here?"

"Well." Still hesitant, Emrys looked again at the map. "The distances. An hundred miles against an hundred and seventy. Two days in subdued country against five across country full of Catuvellauns who'll rise against him."

Gareth shook his head at the map. "But will he think in that manner?"

"Remember his astrologer, Lord-Milite. He's already stretched his chances, and the days grow shorter and colder." Emrys took a deep breath, let it out, looked around at the other lords, and committed himself. "I say it will be Legis."

It made sharp, discomforting sense from beginning to end. There was really no more time to debate. "Are there any other views not yet heard? If not, we agree with Prince Emrys. We will commit to Legis."

A barely perceptible nod from Gareth, an audible sigh of relief from my western chiefs, disgruntlement from

Maelgwyn and those who held for Badon. The guessing carried us so far, then a decision must be made. Rolling up the map, Emrys whispered, "Lord, Aunt, what if I'm wrong?"

"Then it's our lot, isn't it? Don't worry. You made better sense than anyone here. My Lords! We'll recess for an hour and then consider disposition."

With something to charge at, even Galahalt became interested in Gareth's plan to intercept the enemy south of Legis, ripping at his flanks and rear so he could never throw his full weight against the small city. Gareth was a master of this wolfpack style of war. Last year at Badon, far in Cerdic's rear, he had destroyed his supply wagons, starving the fight out of his men. Flanked now by Bors and Dai meqq Muir, he issued crisp orders.

"Bors, I'll need scouts south of Legis as far as Viroconium on the west road, the same east. What's bog, what's firm, the forests, condition of the roads, the whole of it. Dai, now: let's rattle the chest and see what horse we can scrape up."

It was quickly decided the Parisi horse and such foot as they had would defend Eburacum. The Brigantes would man Cair Legis and supply it. Their few horse would be attached to Gareth under their own chiefs.

"And light, for Holy Christ's sake, light!" Gareth shook a stubby finger at them. "Not a hair more than they need. For food, a bag of oats, an apple or two. No more."

"That's for the horse," one Brigante observed. "What do we eat?"

"That," Gareth said. "In the matter of combrogi, now: have you ever seen a fat man or a slow horse? Light, my Lords."

The meeting was dismissed. Each man hurried off to his assigned tasks. Emrys waited for his guard whom I'd sent on an errand. I took the imperial sword from Ifan. "Ifan-fach, after today I'll appoint a new bearer. Gareth will need you."

The young knight glowed at the prospect. "Thank you, Lady. I was going to ask. It's been an honor, but . . ."

"Nonsense, Gareth needs you. And those Brigs will need every good example they can lay eye to. Go along."

Emrys' guard returned with a longsword and scabbard drawn from the armory. I dismissed him as well. "Re-

turn to your duties with Lord Gareth. Prince Emrys will no longer require a guard."

Emrys stared at the sword in his hand, testing the balance and edge. "This is from our forges, right enough."

"Put it on. No point in being a hostage now. You're my ally, Prince. You've earned that much."

"Have I?"

"You've uncommon good sense when someone kicks you into using it."

"It's from Kay, then. He was the proper horse thief. Do you think Gareth would let me ride with the combrogi?"

"I was hoping you'd stay here with me. You might come, against all odds, to like me a little. Don't leave me naked to the conversational mercies of Galahalt. Besides, Gareth needs trained men."

Emrys buckled on the sword. "My father bred Gareth's horse, and I've broken them since I was twelve."

Yet he'd never been in battle before. Despite my better instincts, I was feeling illogically maternal. It must be the damned change of life. No, I wouldn't hold him back now, owing him that much. "It'll be hard out there."

"To hell with that." Emrys gave the sword a final tug at his hip. "We're fighting back, Aunt. Us, by God! I'd be a water carrier just to *be* there."

The whole country was marching toward Armageddon that November and already feeling the ruinous pinch as both sides dipped into reserves of food, grain and other resources. Constantine didn't scruple to take what he wanted; with more reluctance I taxed my northern tribes only with service and the minimum of food and provender necessary for Eburacum to withstand siege. That fall the country consumed its own fat and the firm flesh beneath. If there was no resolution by spring, all Britain would suffer as crops went unplanted or were confiscated by chiefs who must answer in turn to demanding overlords. There were many small, internecine raids to fill these quotas. It was the shape of the future.

Arthur was six months dead, but the Church quite sensibly didn't call for a choosing with no point to it. Constantine and myself were the only realities now. A strong catalyst could tip the balance. The Saxons might have done it if they hadn't been so discouraged after their

drubbing at Badon. Years later I learned Constantine had tried to buy them. They refused out of a respect for combrogi that amounted to superstitious awe. *No* horses or men, they vowed, could move so fast without the witch power of flight, and was not Arthur himself half-Faerie? They gave Constantine no odds at all, but Icel would have hired out to me in exchange for land patents north of Humber. In Parisi land? Not likely, sir.

Yes, yes, I should have hired him, but the fear and prejudice ran too deep in me. Hindsight is always cheap and never wrong.

Gareth mounted three hundred cavalry to defend Legis, mostly Brigante with a nucleus of combrogi. Galahalt ravened for a place among them, his right as a son of Lancelot. Gareth parried with charming circumspection that a son of Lancelot and one of Galahalt's aggressive courage could hardly be spared from the Queen's personal defense. To that Gaelic tact I added my own entreaty.

"Galahalt, my dear, your parents would be wroth with you for leaving me, and with me for letting you go. Men of your quality are needed here in my own horse. I must command you in all love, stay with me."

He acquiesced in an adolescent huff, green with envy while Emrys rode off as Gareth's messenger-aide. For Lancelot's sake, Galahalt was on a short leash. He would charge a dragon without second thought—and why not? He was in full communion with God and Holy Church. The instant he died, by his theology, he would pass but briefly through purgatory, thence to heaven like his fabled ancestor, Joseph of Arimathea. There were not enough sins on his unused soul to fill a thimble. Thus Galahalt's cosmos, which is to say he was suicidal as Geraint.

All planned, all committed—done. We could do nothing now but wait. I snapped at the heels of my Parisi chiefs as Eburacum braced itself for war, mothered Regan, bequeathed a half-dozen more kirtles to Imogen, scratched my rash when she wasn't looking, suffered and cursed with the inventive obscenity of a drunken bard as my menses vacillated—and waited.

Dobunni refugees at Cair Legis report large numbers of horse and foot mustering in Glevum/Bors.

Mustering, yes, but to swing west or north? Badon was as close as Cair Legis. Which way, damn it? I pored over the maps of the west, trying to see the vital roads with Bors' own scouts. There are two roads north from Glevum to Cair Legis, each a journey of two or three days. *Aye, but Badon's closer . . . oh, stop, silly bitch. You're committed. Act like it.* The west road is more direct but runs over mountains most of the way. The east road crosses lower ground, part of it a sizable valley with more forage for troops. Gareth was barely rested at Legis, his Brigante lords still numb from the impossible combrogi marching pace, when the wax tablets began to arrive, borne by swift relays of post riders across the hundred-mile road to Eburacum, never more than twelve hours old. Usually written in the saddle with a worn stylus, the cursive script was jerky and angular, but I wish they'd survived. As history, they're a thousand times more relevant than any moralizing Church scribe. The men who wrote them, Bors and Emrys, were there.

14th noon. West road clear as far south as Virconium/ Bors.
14th vespers. East road clear one day south of Legis/ Emrys for Gareth.

"Of course they're clear," Galahalt yawned. "Everyone knows they will move on Badon. Sawel, fetch me an apple."

15th prime. West road clear half a day south of Viro/ Bors.
16th noon. No change in situation. Legis is manned and prepared. Many Dobunni refugees incl. Bedivere and his guard. Mother and Flavia not among them/ Emrys for Gareth.

My poor Flavia. Well, they had Bedivere at least, and he was mine. But where was Constantine? Were we wrong after all?

17th prime. No change. West road clear one day south of Legis/B.

"Well, we've done everything but pray," I lamented to Imogen. "Would that help, you think?"

"Aye, mum. Do you go to mass. God misses you."

Father in heaven, I'm not the one to be asking favors, not of your too-patient Grace, but at least let me know if I'm right or wrong. Have I wasted the time?

17th noon. Cornish cavalry moving north on east road toward junction ten miles east of Bancor. Number and disposition follow/Emrys for Gareth.

Thank God and my nephew. He was right.

17th mid-afternoon. Cornish and Silure horse and foot, siege equipment, company of stone slingers. Estimate 900 horse, heavily armed, strung out in poor order. Estimate 1,500 foot, mixed Silure, Cornish, some impressed Coritani, complement of Demetae archers, about 200. Much straggling due to camp followers—mountebanks, musicians and about threescore ladies of negotiable virtue and very sore feet/Emrys for Gareth.

The comment was my nephew's but the thoroughness that counted even the whores was Gareth's. But nine hundred cavalry! Constantine had his margin and more. Even looking at the sky that day, I could see only the map and that eastern road to Legis.

17th vespers. Con. main force camped with cook fires at road junction east of Bancor/Bors.

At midnight of the eighteenth, after hearing mass, I returned to my chambers where another rider was waiting with Emrys' latest message. Not a dispatch this time but a personal letter on a scrap of papyrus backed with a fragment of the Old Testament.

Dear Aunt, I hope you can read this. My hands are cold and a bit stiff, but we daren't light fires. Short of tablets so I stole this from our priest. It's only Leviticus; not too

relevant to men who'd die for a piece of pork as a change
from oats soaked in water or cow's blood, when we can
find an unattended cow.

We've hit them, Aunt Guenevere. Their foot is such a
slovenly lot, Gareth couldn't resist a raid to demoralize
them. They didn't put up stakes or even a bank and
ditch, just settled down with the women and the eating—and here come ourselves out of the dark and
through them like butter, scattering dead Silures and
Demetae all over the landscape and the rest running too
fast to leave footprints. Killed quite a few and roiled the
rest into a lovely stew, and not a one of us lost.

Must give this to the post rider now and get some
sleep. Gareth wants to do something about those 900
horse in the morning.

But I do feel better about everything now, even you./
Emrys.

I vented a snort of satisfaction to think Constantine
would leave his foot exposed with a hawk like Gareth
within striking range. God, if those three hundred were
all combrogi! Like Arthur, Gareth would whittle the odds
with quick raids before a full confrontation. I allowed
myself a long bath and a stiff draft of hot wine and lavender and drifted off to sleep in the paradise of the complacent.

Paradise ended just before dawn when Imogen and I
were jarred out of sleep by the pounding at our door.
Lord Bors stood on the threshold, mud-splashed and
haggard.

"Bors! You must have ridden all night."

"Constantine's not two hours behind me."

As we hurried out to the forum the palace woke about
us, already alerted by Bors on his way to me. Penrwd and
Maelgwyn hurried in, then Galahalt, red-eyed and half
dressed, then the staff; finally Regan on Rhian's arm, rattled as myself but a deal more presentable even at this
hour. She fled to Bors with a little yelp of concern.

"What of Gareth?" Rhian pressed the young knight.
"Where's my husband?"

"Well, I hope." He rubbed his stubbled chin. "With a
miracle, he'll here just after the Cornish."

My mouth felt dry. "Just after?"

"They tricked us, Lady. A map; I can show't on the map."

"Imogen, fetch my maps. Penrwd, what readiness on the walls?"

"Manned and the horse alerted. I was on the wall myself when the lad came in."

"Good, there's luck. What happened, Bors?"

Bors laid it out for us as we crowded about the map, his speech slurred with the need for sleep. The road junction east of Bancor was the crux; its right fork was a twenty-five-mile spur that met the road to Eburacum.

"We raided the infantry the night before, rattled them good."

"Yes, I had Emrys' letter."

"This morning before light we moved on the cavalry to hit them and run. They were better defended but we did some damage—horses mostly—then withdrew. Some of them came out after us, mad as hornets. By then it was light enough to see the foot troops advancing from the east, archers to the fore. The ground was marshy, bad for maneuvering. We broke off."

Galahalt asked in all seriousness, "Why did not the Lord-Milite offer combat?"

Bors was too tired to be irritated by the ridiculous question. "Prince, you don't offer anything to that kind of superiority unless you've no choice. You make life generally unpleasant for them and hope you can get close enough to kick them in the arse, then be off before they turn around. Oh, lass." He pulled Regan close to him. "Is the bairn still kicking?"

"Fair knocked me out of bed just now. A lummox like his father."

"Bors, I love you both dearly," I remonstrated, "but do get on with it. What happened?"

They withdrew then to a small wood already selected, from which they could cover the road to Legis and be safe from any attack in force. They watched for the infantry but never saw it again.

"About four hundred of their cavalry gave us a lively chase. But then they just pranced about, half a mile in front of our wood, as if they couldn't decide what to do. We waited at our horses' heads. We thought sure we'd have a battle then, and there's Gareth mumbling to Bed-

ivere and looking like he'd eaten something tainted. Then he just groaned and kicked a tree and turned around to Lord Bedivere—"

"Bedivere? What was he doing there?"

"Gareth brought him from Legis with his guards."

"Why? On what authority? I gave orders to pack him here straight."

Bors didn't know why, but there Bedivere was, and considerably cooler than his Dobunni guards who passionately appealed to Emrys to let them return to Legis before the Cornish decided to attack. Emrys told them they'd just volunteered. They were in his service anyway, and there an end.

Then Gareth enlightened them all, thoroughly self-disgusted. Constantine hoodwinked the lot of them— feinted at Legis, even gave them a false chase and was by now very like running with his main cavalry force up the spur route to the Eburacum road.

Bors was wearily bewildered. "It's as if he *knew* our dispositions, knew we had nothing on that road to stop him. Bloody hell, we're few enough as it is, with fifteen hundred foot ready to jump at Legis."

Bors took the hot wine Imogen poured him and drank half of it in a gulp. "We faded back into the woods a few at a time. Then Gareth bade me mount and get here before Constantine if it was the last thing I ever did. If he could shake off the damned Cornish without a fight, he'd be right on my tracks."

"And you did it." Regan kissed him proudly.

"Only just. When I passed the spur crossing, I could see their banners already. Gareth will have—"

"Lord Penrwd! Where's Lord Penrwd? Lady?" One of the captains from the wall strode into the forum, a vinewood club clutched in one fist. "There's cavalry on the west road."

"Whose? What banners?"

"Too far, Lady. It's just coming light, but we heard them."

The city walls bristled with nervous men, onagers, catapults, bundles of arrows, torches and spears. Captains paced back and forth, worrying at their men like herder dogs, giving unnecessary warnings to stay alert. Rhian

and I peered out over the west parapet onto the still-dark road to Cair Legis. The rumble of horse was louder now.

"Rhian, do they sound like nine hundred to you?"

She listened. "They do not."

Rhian stretched forward through the crenel, eyes on the road where it vanished into ink. She'd only time to do one hasty braid on the way to the wall; the rest of her hair fluttered behind her in the morning wind. Then the sun, rising at our back, picked out a lance point, a flicker of harness stud, a shield bobbing up and down—

Rhian's arm shot out, pointed. "There, the shield! The cross and sun. It *is* Gareth!"

In the growing light and a roaring salute from the walls, Gareth's combrogi rode slowly into the light.

"Open the gate! It's the Lord-Milite!"

By what miracle I knew not, but I breathed a long sigh of relief. "Let's go down to meet him, Rhian."

The street was cold and still barely light when we found Gareth slumped on a mounting block, rationing water to his horse from a bucket. Other combrogi lurched by, leading their horses or merely sprawled in front of the closed shops by the gate. Gareth's fierce, sandy-limbed stallion now looked as if it might topple over on its master, head drooping close to Gareth's knee as he soothed it. Rhian swept down on Gareth in a welter of Irish and wild, inaccurate kisses.

"Ah, poor love, you're entirely destroyed. Did I not say he'd get here first?"

Gareth tried to rise for me, then gave it up. "Lady, I . . ."

"Well done, Lord-Milite. But how in God's world?"

"Well, to this horse's way of thinking, it was neither kind nor Christian. May I never have to do it again."

"Listen to him!" Rhian punched his arm. "Himself who used to ride all night and fight before breakfast."

"We were younger then, *cushla*."

"How close is Constantine?" I asked.

"An hour, two at most. Foot troops tomorrow, I'd say. He's marching the legs off them." Gareth finally managed to rise. "Bors got here, Lady?"

"Yes. A full report."

"Almost fooled us, High Queen. So it will be here, then. I'd rather it were Legis."

"We'll hold. He can't get in and he damned well can't starve us out unless he wants to sit on that moor till spring. There's something I must ask you, Gareth. Why did you take Bedivere from Cair Legis? Why wasn't he sent on to me?"

Gareth toyed with his bridle, evasive. "I brought him, yes. Not his guards, they couldn't keep up and damned if I know where they are."

"I see. Why did you take him from Legis?"

His head jerked to Rhian, then to me. If he'd had the energy, I think he would have snapped at me. "Because *I* wanted to know why he left us."

"And not you alone," Rhian muttered.

"I wanted him with me." Gareth appealed to his wife, confused. "But he wouldn't fight, wouldn't even take the sword I offered him."

"Lord-Milite, he was under my indictment—"

"Just . . . didn't seem to care." Gareth was distant with fatigue. "He told me to go to hell. Me, Rhian. Put him back in irons, says he, he's done with it all, and that's the shape of it."

Whatever, now wasn't the time to debate. "Give him to Lord Penrwd. I'll hear him when there's time."

"Well enough, Lady. What horse is there in the city?"

"A few Parisi squadrons, that's all. Less than two hundred."

"They'll have to do this day, then. My men . . . these poor horses, they've got to rest."

Penrwd's squadrons were already moving west along the narrow streets, threading through the dismounted and disorganized combrogi staggering east toward the stables. Not a man of them would eat or lie down himself until the lathered, limping horses were seen to. I mingled with them, edging along the shop fronts toward the palace. Tradesmen peeked out at the commotion of Parisi horse bustling one way and bedraggled combrogi creeping the other way, and decided to open late if at all. There'd be little business in the streets this day.

By the well in the market square, I saw Emrys standing over the most discouraged horse in Britain. He was trying to coax it to its feet; the poor animal tried to rise, head and neck responding to the halter, but one foreleg was lame and the other three already falling asleep. Out

of sympathy and his own similar condition, Emrys just dropped the reins and sat on the lip of the well, splashing water over his dirty face.

"Emrys!"

He looked up with a wan smile. "God with you, Aunt. Forgive me not getting up."

"The horse speaks for you."

"Poor fellow. But Father bred them to last. You can run them till they drop, but the only thing that will kill 'em is old age. There, boy, just lie there. I'm not in a hurry."

"Good work, your dispatches. I'm proud of you."

"Ah, that Gareth, he's fine. But, Jesus! To look down the throat of nine hundred men who want to kill you. It's a sobering sight. I—I would have liked Mother to know I was there."

"We don't know she's dead."

"To think she wanted *me* to be king." Too tired to laugh, Emrys managed something like a cough. "I could barely keep up with Gareth."

"The Lord-Milite is not too dashing either, this minute. Give yourself time."

Emrys gazed at a squad of horse clattering toward us down a side street. "Penrwd's people. I hope to Christ they can do something today."

"Amen."

My nephew chuckled. "Speaking of God, here comes his little brother."

In full ring mail and helmet, Galahalt swung aside from the rear of the column and cantered across the square to us. His shield was burnished and there was a new lance in his saddle socket.

"Emrys! Are they here?"

Emrys barely nodded. "Coming."

"Really, now." Galahalt appeared shocked. "What's your mount doing asprawl in the damp street? Do you know nothing of husbandry, recreant Prince? He'll catch chill just as you might."

"It was his notion to tarry, and I agreed."

"And the enemy? Speak, man, how many are they?"

Emrys looked up at Galahalt and began to laugh softly, then louder, a weird, hopeless sound, like a man about to be hanged who is asked to speculate on tomorrow's weather.

Galahalt flushed angrily. "Why are you laughing? What is funny?"

"Nothing, Galahalt, nothing at all. . . ."

"Well, then, are you deaf? Quickly, we're going out. How many are they?"

Emrys subsided to a weak giggle, his head wagging back and forth. He made a vague gesture toward the west. "All you'll ever need, my Lord. That way."

"Dolt!" Galahalt yanked the horse around and hurried after the squadron.

"And d-don't trip over the combrogi," I spluttered after him.

"The poor dears are underfoot everywhere," Emrys gasped. We leaned together, laughing so we wouldn't cry.

"Oh, Emrys, you know I'm sorry for everything. Don't hate me forever."

"No, no." He wiped his eyes. "After all, it won't matter that long, will it?"

By the time I reached the palace, it was light in the west. The city's alarm bells started to ring. Our men on the walls could see Constantine's banners approaching.

The banners rippled in the morning breeze, splashing the moor and riverbank with color. They'd straggled into a crescent across the west road, a formidable host but tired. Constantine couldn't manage any squared-off line. We rather counted on that and their slacking off a little.

The captain waited on the other side of the loaded onager. "Now, Lady?"

"Not quite yet."

I watched Constantine ride out to confer with another horseman, probably Aurelius Conant. I'd never met him before: a chunky little man who didn't sit a horse too well. His heavy cloak was wrapped to the fore, doubtless concealing a potbelly.

"Tempting as it is, we'll wait."

The enemy lines grew more and more ragged as the sun climbed higher. Men dismounted, some of them resting on the ground. Constantine had fair run them out; their horses were dispirited as Gareth's and getting less care. The clear sunlight took the chill off the morning. Some of the men began to eat, passing bread and leathern flasks back and forth. After the meal a few walked

out before the lines to relieve themselves (with gestures) as much for insult as comfort. One Silure chief strolled well out beyond the others, nonchalantly loosened his trousers and squatted.

My captain snorted in terminal disgust. "Look at that dirty scut. Please, Lady. Now would be a heavenly time."

I glanced to a spur wood a long bowshot behind Constantine's line, then back to the complacent Silure, and couldn't resist.

"Give the command."

"Light!"

All along the west wall, torches ignited the fireballs couched in the onager bowls.

"Loose!"

A deep stuttering as the onager releases tripped and a dozen fireballs arced up and out over the moor. The enemy was well out of range, but the fire startled their grazing horses and milled them about. Their riders shambled after them, laughing at our pitiful display.

They were still laughing when Penrwd's cavalry shot out of the small wood, a full half-cohort, lances couched, dividing into three tight wedges at full gallop. The surprise was classic. I've never seen so many Cornish run so fast, even he of the dropped trousers who alas bore away what he meant to leave.

That one moment of low but sufficing comedy, then our wedges struck them like slingstones shattering glass. Trampled men and crippled horses went down in their wake. Penrwd's men wheeled tight as a flock of swallows and dashed on toward our west wall.

"Load onagers! Open the gates!"

A few of the enemy managed to mount and pursue. As they came into range, the onagers sent a nasty hail of fire into them and our few archers made themselves felt. My captain was jubilant.

"Nineteen . . . twenty . . . oh, look what they did!"

Nothing fatal but enough to count. Penrwd's prime targets were the horses; every disabled mount lowered the odds against Gareth. Still, we were only harassing them. The difficult trick would be to keep that approaching infantry off our walls. We didn't have the men to repel them.

The day was tense but uneventful, rest for us, not much

for the Cornish, who couldn't be sure what would flash out at them next. I was actually glad to see Galahalt at breakfast which he took in his glory, fully armed, probably regretting that he hadn't at least a scratch or two to show Emrys.

We were merry and confident that morning, Galahalt regaling Sawel with his part in the raid, Sawel nodding in doglike admiration. For the time all the advantages were ours, the situation much like Arthur's at Badon. We were warm indoors, Constantine out in the cold, and he'd made Cerdic's fatal mistake of leaving vital elements of his force unprotected to catch up the best they could. Nor was he eating that sumptuously while he waited. All the trevs close to Eburacum had moved into the city with their threshed grain and livestock. Most of our streets resembled a great livestock fair.

Constantine's lines stretched north to south across the Cair Legis road, just out of onager and catapult range, mounted or ready to mount, not about to be surprised again if they could help it.

The sun slid down in the west, the autumn dark came swiftly. Gareth's force slept all day and into the evening while his horses were pampered like sick babes at the stable. Seriously lamed animals were replaced with fresh Parisi mounts. Near midnight I held a dinner-conference in the large triclinium for my captains, including my princelings who were now considered working soldiers. A most casual supper, food at one table, maps at another, servants plying back and forth between them.

Gareth bent over the maps, chewing placidly, planning mayhem with Dai and Penrwd. It troubled him that he might have done more damage staying behind at Legis to tear at the infantry. But that was spilt milk. Gareth didn't know my situation then, and a force greater than his own was ready to pounce on him the moment he left that small wood. On the odds he made a wise decision.

"But that foot can't have a chance to climb our walls," he said. "The Queen is agreed. We're going out. We'll mount in one hour."

They would leave the city by the east gate, file around the darkened north wall, and wait. A fireball would be the signal: Constantine would hear a great deal of noise at the south gate—buccinas, drums, torches, a show of

archers—and see what appeared to be a sally of horse out from that portal.

"We'll give them a breath to consider that." Gareth nibbled at a piece of cheese. "Then we'll run for the Legis road. And Jesus God, no one stop to say good night."

Emrys groaned. "More soaked oats."

"Try some wild garlic in the water," Bors suggested from experience. "Not bad at all that way."

They would ride in two forces under Gareth and Dai, each two hundred strong. If Constantine pursued, Gareth's element would turn and engage them while Dai pressed on to make contact with the advancing column. Gareth put a blunt finger on the map at a point some forty miles west along the Legis road.

"About here they'll be. Perhaps closer. Strike them, Dai."

"Won't we just, Gareth-fach?"

Not a quick raid this time but a massacre, scything back and forth across the road until the column was no longer an effective force. Depending on the situation, Gareth would join him or at least prevent Constantine's horse from aiding the infantry.

Depending on the situation . . . language can elide so much.

"There'll be a good deal of confusion and a great deal of prayer." Gareth licked the crumbs from his fingers. His glance fell on Galahalt, softening with an emotion the eager boy wouldn't recognize yet. "It will be today, lad. A day for the bards. You can tell Lord Lancelot you were there. Lady?"

So like Gareth to gild the truth with kindness. We would lose many friends tonight and tomorrow. Every mounted knight in Eburacum was committed to this and ultimately expendable. I could at least salute them.

"My good Lords, it is a gallant venture. I drink to the very gallant men who pursue it. May God be with you."

They bowed their heads in acknowledgment as I drained the toast. Then Gareth knelt to me, took up his cloak and left the triclinium. The others bowed and followed one by one. Sawel tucked an apple or two into a pocket of Galahalt's cloak and gave his own blessing in peasant Cornish.

"Oy dew hope yew will be savit, zor, in what falls this day."

"The blessing of my house on you, Sawel. Are we not in God's hand?"

"We are, zor."

"High Queen, if I do not return—"

"But you must, Galahalt. For my sake, be a good combrogus, not a reckless one. Lord Gareth has no use for the foolhardy; he always has to bury them. Go along, God with you."

"Lady, do see Regan stays well," Bors importuned me.

"You know I will. I love the little imp."

"Especially she must be careful on the stairs now. She could hurt herself."

Emrys was the last, cloak and sword belt thrown over one shoulder, a chicken leg in the other hand, no more sense of occasion than his father or uncle.

"Nephew, I refuse to kiss you with your mouth full."

"Oh. Pardon." He tossed the morsel onto the board, wiped his mouth on the back of his hand, not quite ready for it all when I hugged him vigorously.

"Goodbye again, Aunt."

"I'll pray for you, boy. Mayn't I call you boy just this once?"

"Dear Aunt, no one will be praying more earnestly than I. Rest you gentle."

Emrys knelt to me, retrieved his chicken leg and strode off after Gareth.

From the palace roof I saw the signal fire and heard the commotion of trumpets at the south gate. They'd be off then. I returned to my chambers where one of Penrwd's captains was waiting for me, the same fellow who fired my onagers that morning. He was virtually dancing with pleasure.

"Oh, Lady, it was a singing delight! There's the Cornish peering one way and Gareth comes round the other neat as a fox and *swoosh*! right through them onto the road. Oh, lovely!"

"Did the Cornish follow?"

"Don't think so. But 'twas too dark to be sure."

The arrow was loosed. I could control its flight no further and worry would be a waste. Out of habit my mind turned a page.

"Captain, send Bedivere ap Gryffyn to me."

Imogen helped me out of the kirtle into the haven of soft homespun and draped an old traveling cloak over my shoulders. "It's chill in the forum. There's nae fire in there. Gareth's away then, mum?"

"In the captain's words, neat as a fox. Well—Imogen!" I turned to admire her own kirtle, one of my refurbished blues. "You look positively regal. I was right: we're the spit of each other for size. Go to bed, dear. I won't need you more tonight."

Imogen didn't appear anxious to retire. "I can wait and hot up some chamomile, mum."

"You old gossip, you're just panting to hear about Bedivere. There, fetch my tablet and stylus."

Imogen found them and I wrote a memorandum to myself. Morag and my people from Camelot had reached Verulamium and were guests at Maelgwyn's small court, hale and unharmed, but they might need more silver for expenses. I must send it when a courier could get through.

300 denarii to Morag et al, Veru.

"Make sure this doesn't get lost under everything else."

"Shall I hot the tea, then?"

"Yes, yes. If you want, but don't eavesdrop."

"When did I *ever*—?"

"Always. And what I have to say to Bedivere is for him alone."

"Well." Imogen subsided in her dignity. "D'you at least let me know how that strange man takes it."

I lit only two tapers in the cold forum, on the sconces flanking the dais, then withdrew to a shadowed side entrance. I wanted Bedivere there first and waiting in the cold chamber while I decided what to say to him. Sentence and punishment were secondary to me then; the why was what I craved.

The two guards brought him in, his long arms chained and dangling in front of him, plainly dressed as that last night at Sulis in cracked leather tunic and trousers streaked with age.

They waited, shuffling in the silence, breath steaming in the cold air while I took the measure of Bedivere. Morgana used to call him Redhair, nothing else. No more. The copper and fire had long since faded to rust like

mine and Rhian's. Only half-Dobunni on his father's side.
His mother had been Belgae, one of the tribes overrun by
Saxons. They were the last tribe to come before the Romans, and the fiercest: fair-haired worshipers of the sun,
clan-proud men who conquered southern Britain two
hundred years before the first Roman war galley ever
nosed into our shore. When Caesar tried to land, they
pushed him back into the sea—reckless, blue-painted lunatics who danced on the harness shafts of their chariots
as they charged. As this Bedivere once threw himself
alone at Cerdic across a wall of spears at Badon. I could
well believe it.

He inherited the Belgae look and pride but not their
gaudy tastes: that might be one key to Bedivere. He
never wore the gold laurel Ambrosius awarded him. I
managed one for Agrivaine for reasons of diplomacy and
much less merit. He wore it on every possible occasion,
but Bedivere never cared for trappings or even propriety.
More often than not, Myfanwy had to steal his trousers
to mend them. What price would sway such a man to
defect? Gazing at that lank, lonely oak-knot of a man, I
felt less a queen or judge than a woman deserted by a
lover, oddly touched and shamed by the chains I'd put on
him.

*All his life Arthur trusted you more than me. Why did you
run from me, you bastard? Was I less than Arthur or even
Gareth? You'll tell me now.*

The guards nudged Bedivere to kneel when I entered. I
stepped up on the dais and took my chair. "Leave us. Stay
close in the hall."

When we were alone, I let Bedivere wait with his knee
on the hard mosaic floor. He should be uncomfortable,
myself relaxed and unmoving, an image of strength. And
yet, why must I strive for it so? The torches flickered over
us in the sepulchral gloom. Bedivere broke the quiet.

"May I get up?"

"When I say you can. Where's your wife?"

"With my daughter."

"Who is married to a Silure, very pat. Safe behind
the— I gave you no permission to rise!"

He rose anyway. "Get it done with, Guenevere."

"In my own time."

"Is this my trial?"

"It's what I say it is. You owe me an accounting."

"That's why you had me wait, wasn't it?" he said. The image of Owain flashed through my mind, but there was no swagger in Bedivere, only weary contempt. "You want to enjoy this, your right to it."

"Bedivere, my tolerance is thin these days; don't press on it." I suppressed the urge to rise and leap at him. "Why, Bedivere? Oh, I know they're all on your side, Gareth and the rest. They don't have to judge the fact that you probably sold half my country to Constantine. For how much? You never told me."

The chains rattled as he shifted. "Three times my present holding. A place at court when he was chosen."

"Impressive. His Lord-Milite?"

"Not me, I'm common born."

"And he's not as democratic as Arthur."

"I don't know that word."

"You should: you've profited well by it."

"I didn't. I bloody laughed at him."

"I don't think so."

"Woman, I never sold you any more than Blodwen did. But you're not one for large trust, are you? Jesus, it's a wonder you're not hanging the scullery rats."

"I had your word, Gryffyn."

"Not my oath."

"And wasn't that convenient? You planned it from the day he came to Camelot. I saw you together."

"That wasn't the way of it. I told you what happened."

"You're a liar, Lord Bedivere. No, not lord any more. You'll be what you were before Arthur's misguided generosity, a groom's son. A stable boy. I'm not going to hang you yet. I want you alive. An example."

Bedivere gave me a curious look. "For treason? Or because I hurt you?"

"Yes, you hurt me!" Despite my resolve I pounced down on him from the dais, circling Bedivere like an angry shark. "You self-satisfied monument. Because I was harder than Arthur, had to be, you think I can't bleed? You—just like him—I bled more for this country than either of you ever did."

"For your rights in it, that's all."

"Yes, my rights, my prerogatives. How else do you rule?"

How unlike me: I was blustering at him, hurling truths at Bedivere I should have thrown at Arthur himself long ago. And that was the ambivalent truth. Arthur was here now. Bedivere was always a part of him and always closer than me, and I raged at the abrasive fact of that closed male bonding, knowing in the same breath and for the same reason that I could never kill Bedivere, that I'd run from shedding his blood the same as Arthur's even though Arthur stood here with him now, judging and wounding me from an unfair, unattainable height.

"How else, Bedivere?"

"Aye, how else?" I heard something else then behind his contempt. "Then what difference who pulls the sword from the stones or who the tribes scream for? You or Constantine or someone else. You've all got the same teeth and claws, you'll tear the same carcass the same way. That's all we are now, dead meat. This country died with Artos, but you'll have your share of the guts and kill anyone who gets between you and the plate."

I slapped him hard, twice, back and forth. Bedivere rocked a little from the force of it, the red marks starting out on his cheeks. "That's the truth of it, then," he said softly. "That's why I left. Just like the girl."

My voice sounded ragged. "What are you saying? What girl?"

"I didn't think you'd remember. At Sulis. She was a peasant like me."

"The one with the child. I remember."

"Do you really?" Bedivere peered at me. "Do you remember how frightened she was, how she couldn't stop crying? Country folk never see any lords but their own and not much of them. Remember how the priest had to come out first? They're cautious of your kind, and good reason: in the time it takes to think it you could step on them like ants or take everything they own. That girl didn't have much but her dirty bairn, but she wanted it to be safe. And there's the bloody High Queen of Britain herself. God's a word they can't write; *you* were God just then. Just one word, a hand on hers, and she would have told her children and grandchildren about it. 'Na, I was there the night of the troubles when the High Queen herself took me by this very hand and said, No fear, child. It will be well.' And remember to the inch just where you

stood saying it. Well, they'll remember, right enough. She reached out and you knocked her down."

"What?" I had to laugh at it. "Is that your lament, a lack of democracy?"

"I told you I don't know that word."

"It's Greek, but you'd love it. You've always had the vulgarity of your convictions. I remember the damned woman, and yes, I felt for her, but there wasn't time to hold anyone's hand."

"But that was it," Bedivere said. "Not just her, but it was then I saw the whole thing clear, what I've given my life to. You and Constantine and all the lords of your kind. Life and death, thumbs up or down, you're so used to power and your holy right to it, you've forgot everything else. Even Artos sometimes—but he had the truth of you, Guenevere. Don't I remember the night he rubbed your face in your own murder."

"Enough, Bedivere. I'm warning you—"

"He said it then: you're rotten with power. You stink with the habit of it like a wine sot."

"Guards!"

"And your pride, Guenevere. Your stinking rotten pride that had to drag me back the length of Britain to answer to you and bugger the rest."

"You're going to be an example. I can't let this go. *An example must be made, damn you.*"

"Of what?" Bedivere howled back at me as the guards came running. Not just words, he really wanted to know, more bewildered than defiant. "Doesn't anyone understand anything any more? I wouldn't fight for you or even Gareth now. Bloody Christ, what *for*? There's nothing left. Don't come the country-lover to me. You didn't even know when it reached out to you—just pushed it in the mud and walked away."

"Lady!" The guards hovered by Bedivere while I clamped tight on my temper long enough to be coherent, and bless me for that. I might have done something regrettable, but one of the guards spoke as the thud of hurrying feet grew louder in the hall, other sounds rising behind it. Voices . . .

"Lady, there's something happening in the streets."

"What is it?"

Maelgwyn bustled in from the hall, out of breath,

sword in hand. "Get the Queen to horse and quick, for God's sake. They're pouring through the gates."

I whirled on him. "What? Who?"

"Cornish, Silure—the lot."

"What gate?"

"*All* of 'em!" Maelgwyn screeched in his urgency. "Someone's opened 'em."

"No fresher news than that?" Bedivere asked coolly.

"Bedivere." Maelgwyn shoved past the guards to hug his friend clumsily.

"Hello, you old bear."

"No matter what you've done—Guenevere, release him. You'll need every sword you can find tonight, and he's the best."

"Thank you, no," Bedivere demurred.

Who had betrayed me again? Who this time? "Yes, unshackle him."

"No." Bedivere stepped back. "I've got more chance this way. They'll think I'm one of them."

Maelgwyn drew his sword. "Here, take it."

"No."

"Why not?"

"She knows why."

Desperate, Maelgwyn put the sword against Bedivere's tunic just under his breastbone. "You're a friend, Bedwyr, but you'll take this sword or I'll rutting well run y'through with it. We need you."

"My life for yours, Guenevere?"

"*Yes*, you incredible son of perversity. Take the sword."

Bedivere surrendered to liberty. "Hell, give it me."

"A horse for the Queen, for all of us," Maelgwyn ordered the guards. "You'll ride with us, Bedivere."

The sword spun wickedly in Bedivere's hand as he tested the balance. "What's the difference? The kennel won't change. Just the dogs."

"Imogen!" I called. My voice was high and quaverous in the echoing chamber over the growing noise in the streets. "Imogen, hurry!"

IV

Gwenda with the Scar

he hammering at the palace doors deepened into a steady booming. They were using a ram. We didn't have much time. On my order, Imogen fetched my riding boots, our warmest cloaks and the imperial sword from its repository near my bed. White-faced, she was yet able to clamp down hard on her fear; we'd been in peril together before.

Maelgwyn took charge as we hurried down the corridor toward the armory. "We'll nip out the scullery door to the stables. Maybe the north wall's still held."

Bedivere looked doubtful. "If it isn't?"

"Mun, don't even think it."

"Wait." I stopped suddenly. "Regan's in her chambers. And Rhian. I'm going back for them."

But Maelgwyn stayed me with a firm grip. "There's no time."

"Man, the child can barely move now. I promised Bors—"

Maelgwyn only gripped tighter. "No. You're the Queen. You must get safely out of here."

"Let go, old man. You think I'd leave a child who's like my own? Get away."

But now Bedivere restrained me as well. "If she can't move, she can't ride. Come."

Even Imogen tugged me on. "Please, Lady. You are Britain."

And at what price, sold by what wretch? They were right, though. Without me there was no crown save what clumsy rebels made of it. To that end all were expendable, even myself if it came to that.

In the armory our two guards hastily loaded quivers and strung bows. With a grunt of satisfaction, Maelgwyn took down a centurion's vinewood club, thonged at the butt, and secured it to his thick wrist. "This will do me. You guards nock shafts and be ready. Let's be off."

"Oh! There's the door gone," Imogen hissed as the distant boom pitched suddenly higher in the rending of wood. Not daring a taper, we hurried through the chill corridor and down the steps toward the deserted kitchen where one dim lamp sputtered in a sconce. Halfway down the flight, Bedivere halted. "Someone's following."

Maelgwyn cocked an ear. "You're daft."

"And better ears than you. There's someone back there."

"Well, he's damned quiet then. Guards, fall behind, cover the steps. Shoot anything that moves. Quick now."

The foot of the stairs was a pool of feeble light from the single lamp. We bunched there while Maelgwyn warily opened the door an inch or two and scanned the stableyard. "Clear—no, there's someone—gone now. Guards to the fore. Out we go."

The guards moved past us and opened the door. I missed Imogen at my side, looked back for her. She was kneeling at the foot of the stairs, fumbling with her sandal strap.

"Imogen, hurry!"

What happened then? What did Bedivere hear, what did Imogen see? For years afterward when I tried to recall that dim-lit moment, I could remember nothing that might not be imagination: the furtive scrape of a shoe at the top of the stairs. But Imogen heard and saw. She lifted her head to a sight or sound denied me.

"Aye, well met. Come down, give us a bit of hel—"

Yes, that sound I heard: the *thum* of a crossbow as the bolt took Imogen full in the chest. Bedivere lunged toward her. All I could see was Imogen's head lying toward me, the pinkish spray foaming from her mouth; then, far above us, the final rending of the portals and a rising surge of brute voices, a murderous river as Constantine's

men poured into the palace. I couldn't think then, only crouched over my Imogen to hold her.

"Who was it? Bedivere, did you see?"

"No, no one, I told you, Mal—"

"Why?" I grieved. "Why?"

"Look at her clothes," Bedivere said. "The kirtle and robe."

"Imogen, who was it?"

Her eyes were open but glazing as her heart pumped the blood that drowned her even as I watched. Imogen convulsed, reaching for me, for anything to hold life close. Her lips moved but only that obscene blood-froth emerged.

"Your clothes," Bedivere said. "They thought it was you."

"Did they, then?" Through the layers of necessity and circumstance, I felt my true loss now. Loss of crown, of city, the death of friends, Rhian and Regan left at the mercy of Constantine. It all lay before me in the feeble lamplight, blood running from its mouth. A red curtain descended as I stopped thinking. Sweet Jesu, I would kill someone for this *now*. The imperial sword was in my hand. A howl of murder ripped from me as I charged blindly for the stairs, for whoever did this, to cut off his filthy head myself. Not since Morgana had I so needed a death to pay for other deaths. If Bedivere hadn't caught me, I would have gone screaming up through the halls for that one murderer out of hundreds rat-scrabbling over my lost palace, to offer his heart to dark old gods, and Christ this once be damned.

"Let me go, Bedwyr, I want that bastard—"

"Na, come. You've already told them where we are." He spun me around, shaking me hard. "Listen: you're the Queen. You're the one who's got to think. What can you do up there but die? We've a bargain, you and I, and die for you I will if I must, but not for a whim. Your woman's past caring. Pray for her, but move!"

He bustled me out into the cold stableyard behind Maelgwyn and our guards. We crossed to the stable doors as torchlight flickered brighter from behind an angle of the palace wall; then we heard the voices.

". . . tell you I heard a woman. There! There they are!"

About eight of them from the quick glimpse I got. They

hesitated only a moment, hovering against the distant
roar of my dying city. In that hushed heartbeat, Bedivere
thrust me against the stable door and went on guard.
Our two archers drew their nocked bows. Maelgwyn
tapped the club against his palm in lethal invitation.

"Come on, you lovelies. Don't you owe me for my
boys?"

"It's Guenevere . . . get them!"

They surged toward us, dropping the torches. Our two
archers loosed, nocking new arrows before their targets
went down. Only four of them lived to cross the open
space, then Maelgwyn battered into the nearest, roaring
as he swung the club. Bedivere's lithe form was dim between the two men who closed around him, moving in
circles, never still. Then, without a break in his dancing
steps, the sword flashed out. They were no match for
him; no one ever was, not even Arthur or Geraint. One of
his attackers fell back toward me, wounded, dropping
his sword. The murder in me was still hot. For Imogen,
for all the dear ones sold along with me, I put my knife
across his throat with all my hate to drag it.

"Sothach!"

A dull thud as Maelgwyn punctuated the uneven fight,
then the guards hauled at the stable doors. Bedivere
glanced down at the Cornishman twitching at my feet.

"You do it neat when you must."

Constantine's men weren't yet in the north section of
the city, but closing on it. The only impediment in the
streets leading to the north gate were bawling livestock.
Our horses shouldered them aside until we were within
hailing distance of the wall. The men there were not yet
under attack but waiting for it, onagers loaded. I drew
the sword from my saddle straps and held it high.

"This is Guenevere! Is there a captain among you?"

One man seized a torch and held it overhead. "Here,
Lady."

"Is the north road clear?"

"There's some out there. Can't tell how many."

"And the road to Legis?" Maelgwyn shouted.

"Ah, not a prayer, my lord. Closed tight since Lord
Gareth got out."

"Fosse is the only way then," Bedivere said. "We've got
to go east."

"Captain, I'm going out."

"Bless you, Lady."

"And you, sir. Tell them—" The words stuck in my throat, the absolute defeat. "Tell them to lower my standard. There's no point in butchery if I'm not here. But mark this sword and tell them I will return with it. Constantine may have my city, but he'll play merry hell fitting my Britain to his hand."

"Open the gates," Maelgwyn ordered. "And give us what volley you can."

I set my feet firmly in the stirrups, sheathed the sword and wound the reins about my left gauntlet, my little dagger in the right.

"Get ready, they're unbolting."

A hail of stones and fire went up from the onagers. The north gates swung inward to the thumming of bowstrings, and we dashed out into the dark.

Gone four, must have gone four.

The cold grew from inside me, more desolate than the wind off the moor. Four in the morning is a dismal time, a weak time when nothing in life seems worth the breathing. I was a queen in name alone now, my ancestral city taken, my power reduced to a few hundred knights scattered over Brigantia with the enemy between us. All chaos until I could reforge an opposition.

But, Lord, I was run out. My mind turned over and over on the problems with no answers. Knights hooked forward, castles slashed down the board, pawn wedges advanced. White queen surrounded. Black to move, checkmate in one. Defeat is a weight of fact. No, the larger losses were too much for my dulled mind; they shrank all to the picture of Imogen choking out her life at the bottom of a flight of stairs.

Who killed my Imogen? Who took her life for mine? Who this time?

She came to me a young widow before Arthur and I were married, her husband a man-at-arms killed the night Cerdic attacked Eburacum. My first sight of her: arms akimbo in the doorway. My new chamberwoman? What's your name?

"Imogen, mum." She frowned with annoyance at the

clutter of papers on my table. "I've your supper, and it's hot."

She was a constant shadow by my bed during that tortuous childbearing. Unbidden she summoned the priest when she thought I might want him, permitted him his office and clearly signified when he should retire. She nursed a secret passion for modest, married Gareth confessed to none but me, and a liking for Arthur admitted never at all. Imogen responded against her dour will to his easy manner that carried command so lightly. As with Gareth, she was charmed by the music of his lighter-hued soul but never understood it or its occasional savagery.

She firmly disapproved of my affair with Lancelot but as resolutely followed me into prison, matter-of-factly packed us up—"Folly all, but let's get on wi' it"—and marched with me to the house of my detention, through my rescue and all the days that followed, fat kine or lean. You wonder then that for me the image of loss was Imogen? Of all traitors, I most wanted the one who took her.

The east wind was a whip across my eyes. I felt old.

We had to run east, there was no other way. We'd got out the north gate barely opposed and planned to circle west to Cair Legis as soon as possible. After an hour we stopped to walk the horses awhile when our two archers, riding as rear guard, caught us up.

"We're being followed."

In the pitchy dark with the east wind hurling all sound behind us, we wouldn't have known. Then it dropped just enough for our scouts to detect the rumble of horse—eight, ten, they couldn't be sure, but less than a mile behind and coming steadily on.

"We've got to go separate ways," Bedivere decided.

Perhaps, but not yet. We were blind in the dark with only the paved road to guide us. The wild moor stretched away on all sides, full of bog holes to cripple man or horse.

But our pursuers weren't that far behind. If we were still on the road by first light, they'd have us. For now we could only keep running. When we stopped again, east wind or none, we could hear them.

"More than ten," Bedivere judged.

In the gloom Maelgwyn raised his head to sniff the morning wind. "How soon till light?"

"Seven the soonest." In this northern December, I knew there'd be no light at all before then. When it came we'd have no safety this side of Penrwd's Castle Hull.

"We've got to separate now," Bedivere urged. "There won't be time after this."

"Can't make any speed on the moor," Maelgwyn protested.

"It's that or be taken, and we've more chance in the dark," Bedivere pressed. "You take the men, Prince, turn north and west. Find Gareth if you can. He's the only one left to fight, if there's any fighting left to do. I'll take the Queen across the moor toward Hull."

Maelgwyn reined in beside me. "Lady, is that your wish?"

I could hear the horses closer now, closing the small gap. "Yes, leave us. None of us should die for nothing on a wet road. And this to Gareth when you find him. Until he, the tribes and the Church see my body ceremented for the grave or my head on a pole, I am the crown and Constantine is a usurper. And I will return. Tell them that."

Maelgwyn coughed hollowly in the wet wind. Poor old man, he was ages beyond strife like this. "Shall be done. Long life to the Empress of Britain."

"God with you, Prince."

"Good fortune, Bedivere."

The three of them turned their mounts off the paved road and were swallowed in the dark of the moor. I heard Bedivere's laugh, low and scornful.

"Bedivere, we're cold and wet and lost in the dark. What in hell can you find to laugh at?"

"That Artos called me thick. You never learn, Guenevere. We're finished, the whole of us."

"Haven't you learned that much of me? No one takes what's mine."

"They have, lass."

"Not Morgana, not Arthur himself, and not a pup like Constantine. Come on."

We dismounted no more than a bowshot from the highway and led the horses foot by foot, stumbling and falling again and again over the bog-holed moor. When

the dull daub of light began to broaden in the east, we were safely away from Fosse with light enough to see our way. We mounted again and pushed on until, sometime after pale sunrise, we worked our way to the top of a low rise and saw the higher tor beetling over the river eastward, the intricate circle of earthworks, the hall and outbuildings of Penrwd's stronghold, Castle Hull. To see the smoke curling cheerily from morning fires, you'd never think Britain was already a hacked corpse. Closer, a little to the southwest, lay a sizable trev in its own enclosure. Cattle bawled for milking, pigs rummaged for scraps, and a flurry of hens pecked after a small girl scattering grain from her apron.

I'd have to tell Dorcas, Penrwd's wife, what happened. There was hope. He was with Gareth; he might well be alive yet.

Bedivere shifted his cloak against the sea wind that set an edge to the morning air. "There's Hull, no more than a mile. You can do that safely from here."

"What? You're not coming?"

"No. I'll rest in the trev yonder."

"You'd leave me now?"

"Your life for mine it was. You're safe now and I'm acquitted. That was your word."

"I see. And you don't trust that word once inside Hull. I still need you. Britain needs you."

His head wagged wearily. "Oh, lass, no one needs either of us any more. Just Myfanwy, and that's where I'm bound."

The weary pity in his voice stung me. "You have my word."

"I'll need more than that." Bedivere held out his gloved hand. "Will you give me your signet?"

"Why that?"

"Nowadays no one knows who's king of what or for how long. Your ring will quit us. They'll believe that."

I hesitated only a moment, then stripped off my gauntlet and took the signet from my finger. Every prince and commoner in Britain knew its seal, and perhaps Bedivere deserved that much for damages. "I acquit you. Let all men know by this."

"And my lands?"

"You'll have to wait until I've a stylus. Things are a bit pinched just now."

Bedivere slipped the signet into the purse at his belt. "Done."

Neither of us moved to part. There was a drab sense of ending, completion. The cold wind chilled us, and the ghosts of thirty years.

"Where will you go, Bedivere? Where is there to go?"

He answered as if he'd thought it carefully out. "I'll take Myfanwy and find a place no one wants. And when the armies pass, yours or theirs, I'll sit fat in my chair and wave you all Godspeed."

"Unregenerate. A stable boy to the end."

"Is that less than truth? Rest you gentle." Bedivere gave me a crooked smile and turned his horse down the hill toward the trev. My hand went out to him; now truly the last of Arthur was leaving me. I wanted to forestall that loss, wanted something to last me the hard times to come. "Bedivere!"

He reined about. "Lady?"

The words came hard. They stripped me naked, but I had to ask. "You were with Arthur at the end. Did he. . . ?"

The wind blew. Bedivere gave me no help. "You had his letter."

"I wanted to know . . ."

"What, Guenevere?"

"Damn you, you know. You loved him. You knew him even better than I." But there he waited, male and ungiving while I flung away the last rag-end of my heart. "Was it me? Or Morgana?"

Bedivere ducked his head from the question, perplexed, a man plain to Arthur but opaque to me and not matched to this color of thought. "Women, women . . . you make a coil of everything."

"He was with her that last night. My men might have killed him too. You think I haven't flayed myself with that every day since he died. And every night alone?"

"Is it so important now?"

"Yes, it's important! Do you know so little of women? Haven't I lost everything else?"

"She was a part of him I never saw." He said it softly, piecing it out, perhaps understanding more of it than I'd

guess, but not all. None of us ever knew that. "They were *fhain*, blood kin, but even more than that. That's why she came for him."

Bedivere fell silent, rummaging odd moments from old years stored in dusty corners of his mind. He found something. "There it is, then. She came for him, but Artos came for you. Wasn't I there the day he first set eyes on you?"

"So you were." I felt a flush of warmth despite the wind. "I remember."

"That was a sight he never lost, Guenevere. Does that answer?"

Better than any else and simpler. "Yes. Thank you, Bedivere. Whatever happened, I loved him very much."

"Then why did you fight him so?"

"It needed doing."

"And why did you always have to be his equal?"

"Because I was. Must I repent even that to men?"

That above all sins, apparently. That truth and the un-answered questions, the amputated future and all the love unspoken will go with me to my much-delayed grave. But he loved me. He came for me. I'd believe it less from a canonized saint than Bedivere ap Gryffyn.

"We were difficult people given difficult lives. Don't try to understand it all. Lancelot couldn't either. Go home to Myfanwy."

Bedivere saluted me in the old alae fashion. "Long life."

"And to you, Lord Bedivere. Tell them Guenevere will return."

"Artos said that too."

"And some believe he will. Would you put it past him?"

Bedivere walked the horse away from me. "No, lass," he threw over his shoulder in parting, "that I would not."

I watched until he was off the hill and halfway to the trev.

Tell them Guenevere will return.

That was December, anno Domini—oh, that long ago? I hate to think in years, it's depressing.

By the time I dismounted stiffly on the bank of River Hull, the dreary morning was light as it would be all day, a drab vista of gray sky, brown moor, dark slate river, fen

reed stiff with ice, a few stark trees. From here the cart track ran straight along the bank to Castle Hull. I let the weary horse drink her fill at the water, stroking her withers. "There now, not much more and you can feast."

Reflection for a demoralized queen: there's advantage in being a good horse. A blooded mount was boasted and pet-named, bedded and boarded better than ourselves in many cases. This mare would grain and sleep her fill and be spoiled until needed again, where I would merely nibble and nap before turning again to the inevitable letters and orders. The Church and nobles must know my will and I their readiness. Castle Hull, Badon, Legis and every other free citadel must be strengthened, supplied from God knows where, and held. With luck Lancelot would break out of Constantine's trap to join with Gareth and Maelgwyn, especially now that Galahalt rode with them. By a miracle and a mountain of labor, we would rebuild the combrogi.

My feet tingled with the blood returning after hours in the stirrups. I'd walk the mare as long as possible since we were no more than a mile from Hull. I took her bridle and led her up the bank toward the cart track, but she hung back, favoring her right foreleg.

"Ay! Woman!"

Two men slid out of the fen weed and moved toward me. For a sick moment I thought they might be my Cornish pursuers, but they were too unkempt for that vain crew or any British knight. Herders from the keep: thus I judged and dismissed them.

"Are you Penrwd's men? Come see to my horse, I think she's picked up a stone." And I bent again to the hoof—rudely shocked when one of the men, with a scar slash where his left eye had been, yanked me rudely up.

"Now, sweet, let's have a look at you."

I recoiled from the insolence, but in that speechless moment I knew they couldn't be British. Their filthy clothes were of a foreign cut, beards not so much full as the result of sloth, untrimmed or wiped of the last several meals. The taller man, dirty hair in stiff braids, had a huge head with the absurd comment of a tiny nose and eyes of no color or expression but placid purpose.

"Even were your hands clean, you'll keep them off

me." I stepped back from them, but the one-eyed man grabbed at me again.

"Hands off, I said."

My gauntlet caught him across his good eye. He didn't expect the blow. "Keep your place, *servus*. Don't you know Gu—"

Apparently not. His blunt, pummeled face never changed expression as his fist caught me neatly on the jaw, knocking me flat. He peered down at me with mild curiosity.

"What've we got here, Frith. A lady?"

"Hard to say," the big-headed man allowed.

"From the keep yon?"

"Likely. And look at that mare, will you. She'll bring as much as the woman."

But the violence and the strong alien smell of them frightened the mare. She reared back from the hands snatching at her bridle and shied away, snorting, up the bank.

"Get the horse, Frith, she's worth it." The one-eyed little man produced a pair of irons from under his greasy cloak and knelt to manacle my feet. He had just time to block my arm as it came up with the dagger. "Now then." Still detached, quite used to this, he straightened up and kicked me in the stomach. Writhing, struggling just to breathe, I felt the knife twisted out of my hand. Doubled over on the hard ground, mouth bleeding and breath short, I heard them speak in a rapid jumble that contained just enough bad Brit and camp Latin for me to follow.

"Get the horse!"

"No time. Get the irons on her feet. Quick, Leof."

"There. Let's be off. If the Brits catch us here—"

"And for what? Poor culls like this one."

"So's the rest, but they'll sell." Leof took the second pair of irons from Frith and snapped them around my wrists. "Haul her up."

"Is that someone on the road?"

"What? Where?"

"No, nothing."

"Ah, Frith, don't fright me like that."

By now, gasping and bruised, I knew the horse had much more sense than I, bolting when she did. They

were Saxon slavers—too great an absurdity after all I'd been through, as if God tired of ordering the world and let it drift while he napped. In my brain, only self-preservation was still churning. If they'd caught the mare and seen the sword, it would have been all up. They didn't know me, mustn't know me. One hint and I'd be sold to Constantine for a long price and a short future.

While the one-eyed little brute waded out into the fen reeds, Frith turned me this way and that, feeling my palms, noting the scar over my brow. "No, not a lady, not quite. You've worked in your time. From the keep?"

"Aye, chamberwoman. Lady took me in service when I was still bairn."

He seemed to believe it, more luck there and even more that my signet ring was gone. I thanked God for my homespun garments and the years of gardening and riding that roughened my hands, but almost retched as he pried open my mouth with a grimy finger to explore my teeth.

"Uh! Stop that!"

"Easy on," said Frith as if soothing a nervous horse. "You liked lady service. A good life, all the teeth you've left. Well, the Iclingas will work you hard but fair. Come on."

From the reeds Leof uncovered a hide-shelled curragh and dragged it toward us along the water's edge. Frith pulled me toward it, twisting my arm.

"If it's money, Lady can buy me back for twice what I'm worth to you."

"Not these days, not likely." Frith kept moving. "What's your name?"

Name? No, not Imogen, still too painful. There was my old slave-nurse from childhood. "Gwenda."

Frith shoved me into the curragh and swung in nimbly after. Leof pushed us off. My teeth began to chatter violently. I looked back at my mare ambling away toward the keep and safety, far richer than I now.

"Good horse." Frith followed my gaze. "Wish we'd got her too. Iclingas'd pay high for a breed like that." He took up his own oars and heaved. "Pull, we're too close to shore."

The curragh swung out into the stream. I stared unbelievingly at the irons on my wrists.

"They all do that," Frith said, not unkindly. "Can't take hold of it straight off. But you get used to it. Not the worst life these days. Come on, Leof, pull!"

Arthur and I grew up with slaves. He may have had some furtive liberality in outlawing the trade, but our main motives were political. The traders were Saxons and enemies. We would not allow them access to our ports. Times were thin for them now. They ran a high risk in my lands. Some lords executed them out of hand, more for their race than their calling. Men like Frith still slipped by night up our rivers, and the hazards they endured for profit showed the present pinch in the trade.

My captors rowed hard upstream, keeping the curragh close enough inshore to avoid the main current, far enough out to be safe from any bow-armed patrols from Hull. Huddled between them, I shivered in the wind, wondering when and how I could escape. Clear thought eluded me; I'd ridden all night, not slept since the night before and not deeply then, but through the cold and shuddering, two imperatives surfaced again and again. I *must* escape as soon as possible. Until then, I must be a chamberwoman of Castle Hull. These men were brutes but not idiots. They knew that power in Britain meant Constantine or Guenevere, and would joyously sell either of us to the other, given the chance.

When we approached a westering bend in the river, Frith put a small horn to his lips and blew a muted blast. They both listened. Leof begged of the silence, "Come on, where are you? Again, Frith."

Before Frith could blow again, the answering signal came from around the bend.

"Pull hard."

They labored us around the bend. Not far beyond, in the middle of the stream, the merchant craft waited, anchor hauling up, square sail already unfurling, men busy about the foredeck. We swung out to meet her. As the ship moved downstream toward us, they heaved a hemp ladder over the side. A trim craft, though she'd seen better days. Her planks were salt-streaked but carefully scraped so as not to drag at the helm. She was built on the lines of a raiding keel but shorter by perhaps thirty

feet and not much deeper-drafted, able to navigate our silted rivers or outrun anything afloat.

A large tent was rigged amidships, the afterdeck piled with baled wool. The craft looked exactly what its Frankish flag proclaimed it, a coasting trader making for Humber after taking on cargo at Eburacum.

The ship sheared in toward us without slowing. As we bumped along the side, Frith grasped the ladder and me. "Up, Gwenda."

He and Leof shoved me aboard and were over the side after me in a breath while two others hauled in the curragh. I stood swaying on the halfdeck by the forward cargo space, cold and numb with fear. Only one or two of the scrofulous crew even glanced at me. They were an odd-assorted lot. I couldn't lay an origin to any by guess, men born under any of the flags the ship flew when needed.

When Frith pushed me into the tent, I saw his real cargo. Secured by a single chain that ran through heavy iron bolts, eight miserable men with matted hair and beards lay like stalled oxen against the planks. Across from them, similarly chained, were a red-cheeked boy of ten or eleven and a bedraggled woman. She greeted us with raucous cheer.

"Lor, what they won't fetch in next!"

Frith guided me past her to the other side of the boy who huddled against the planks, away from Frith, to make the smallest target.

"Here." Frith fastened me to the common chain. Close to me, I turned away from the stench that issued from his unclean mouth. "No use mourning. You're for it. New master'll be English. Cut above your own, if I say it myself. Got laws and rules for all, even *laets* like you. Extra food in winter, chance to sell what you make or grow." He nudged the frowsy woman with his foot. "Ought to make your fortune, Rat."

She grinned, displaying the remains of teeth. "Gonter."

Frith rubbed his beard and nodded at the men chained across from me. "We work our slaves hard, but we take care of 'em. When we can find 'em. You plowing Brits are always killing someone—yours, ours, no mind—so the holdings want men. Buy anything now. Wish I'd caught your plowing mistress too."

Someone called from the open deck; Frith deftly inspected the security of my chains and hurried out of the tent. In a moment I heard him roar out in Brit to a distant point, probably the watch from Castle Hull.

"Hallo! You can see what we are. Wool! Wool from Eburacum. There it is."

Frith slipped into Frankish gutturals no doubt as easily as he could shape his tongue to half a dozen other argots motley as his flags. They must have believed him ashore. They didn't yet know Eburacum's wool trade was in some confusion since last night.

The planks were icy against my buttocks. I shifted about in the chains. The fatigue of the long night's ride and the day before dulled my fear and awareness of reality, but not the frustration. Mother of God, I was so close to safety. A few more steps ridden before I rested . . .

Ave Maria, Mother of God, intercede with thy Grace in the hour of my need. Hail Mary . . .

The little boy whimpered into his folded arms. I reached to comfort him, but he jerked away. There were bruises on his cheek.

"Sut ma e'r mab, boy-bach."

He seemed astonished someone would speak without harshness in this place.

"He don't talk Brit," the frowsy woman volunteered. "Saxon he is." She grinned viciously at him. "He'll get took by a nice old man, that's the way of it. Sleep wiv his little bum in the air. Won't yer?"

"God's Eyes, what kind of woman are you? He's only a child."

"Serve'm right, too. Cunting barstid like all men. Name's Rat. Raidda to start, but none ent never called me nuffin but Rat. What're you, na?"

"Gwenda."

"Not half the lady."

"Chamberwoman. To Lady Dorcas at Hull."

"Ow. Well, that's the fall of fate, innit? One day snug, freezin yer bum on a barge like this the next."

I caught the corrupted Trinovante dialect. "And you?"

"Up Londin'um."

I might have guessed. I'd been in Londinium once as a child with my parents. It was long in decline even then, its slums a horror, its overpowering smell a rank mixture

of fog and garbage. No one lived there now but human shards with nowhere else to go. Rat was perhaps thirty, but the sorriest, leached-out, poxy thirty on God's earth. Her hair was brown (I suppose) or simply the dominant shade of the dirt that stiffened it. Somewhere in childhood, if she'd been allowed one, it had started to wave, then simply surrendered to dirt and dampness and fell in crinkles about her misshapen face. Her lips were so thin as to be nonexistent, a mere functional slit that receded almost directly into her neck without much digression for a chin. Beneath wide cheekbones and a flattened nose, the whole effect from above was eyes and beak with nothing below it, like a bird. Like Frith, Rat had almost no teeth left and those remaining were stumps which she shielded from the cold air by opening her mouth as little as possible to speak.

The boy whimpered between us. Rat poked him with an elbow. "Belt up."

"Leave him alone, I said. Here, boy. Come by me. Poor child, his mother must be frantic."

He understood my tone if nothing else and shifted close as his chains would allow.

"Not her," Rat sniggered. "Who yer think sold him?"

"You're not serious."

Rat only shrugged. "Happens all the time. When yer got nowt to eat, sell what yer got." She gave me a cunning appraisal as if confirming an impression. "'Course, you wouldn't know that."

"That scum, saying his kind were a cut above us."

"Well." Rat's inventorying glance slid over my homespun to my boots. "It's all in how they cut, innit? Who yer think sold them?" She jerked her frizzy head at the male slaves across the hold. "Some's Brit. Got picked up last night, very quiet like. Penals straight from the judgin, and brought by a Brit chief. Everyone sells something, dunnay? Who'd yer dear old mum pay or bed down to get you in lady service . . . if that's what yer are."

The bright black bird eyes watched me. I came to perceive that Rat was cunning but not overly bright. Her purposes were of the moment, her attention to any stimulus as brief as a child's. One of the men across the hold was scratching at the nomadic inhabitants of his ragged

breeches. Rat forgot me and brayed across to him. "Coo na, can't yer find it?"

The tattered little man clamped a hand over his pride and wiggled it at her. "Want a bit then?"

"Go stuff it up yer froat."

So much for wooing. They both cackled over the sad joke, rattling their chains as a comment on hopelessness.

"Ent that a man for yer?" Rat rasped to me. "Done for'n he still wants it. Yer got a man, Gwenda?"

"My husband is dead."

"Wish they all was. Leave a girl be."

"You don't like men, do you?"

"Not a bit, never did. Just trade, they are."

She said it casually as if waving away food not to her taste. I didn't ponder it but let the motion of the ship lull me toward sleep. The boy and I warmed each other a little; his healthy young body still pulsed with heat. I leaned my head against the planks and dozed. But confused and more frightened than ever before in my life, some part of my mind would not snuff its lamp. Water lapping against the planks mingled with voices from the deck until all blurred down to a meaningless mumble and rumble like the hoofbeats of the Cornish coming after us in the dark—then fainter, more distant until I was somewhere between dream and waking.

There were Rhian and Imogen grumbling by the fire and Regan awkwardly trying to ease her bulk in the cushioned chair. We'd made three little shirts of linen and were working blue embroidery into the hem when Regan vented a mew of annoyance.

"Isn't that just the way. That close to done and we've used the last of my blue thread."

"Lady!" Imogen seemed terribly upset by the shortage. "We're wanting blue thread!"

I told her to fetch some from my chest, but Imogen persisted. There was something important I must understand. "Lady!"

Imogen grasped my leg, shaking it hard, then harder as the pink froth dribbled from her mouth. "Lady!"

I bolted up out of shallow sleep, feeling vile with a dull ache in my skull. Rat had her hand on my leg. She grinned with a kind of low triumph.

"Yer answer to that, right enough. Yer ent no chamber-

woman. I din take nuffin from yer, just looked about."
She turned back the hem of my homespun, exposing the
embroidered shift. "Lor, look at that."

I pushed her away. "Lady handed it down to me."

Rat wouldn't let it go. "Queer boots, too. Seen them
before." She lowered her voice conspiratorially. "Yer
man combrogi, Gwenda?"

I pretended to ignore the question. "Will they feed us,
you think?"

"When Frith puts the collar on yer, don't even whisper
combrogi. Saxons got no love for 'em nohow. And scuff
them boots."

I flinched away from the smell of her and her subtly
menacing intimacy. "They were from my lady."

"Weren't they just. All the same, you scuff 'em round
the heels. Must've looked proper flash fetchin supper in
yer spurs."

The marks were very clear in the buff leather. "I see."

"Right, yer ent all that wet. I knew't when Frith
brought yer in. Stand like yer got a poker up yer bum
like all the rest of 'em. List to me: Saxons hate combrogi,
always have. Always got beat by 'em, dinnay? So you belt
up and so will I." The beady eyes narrowed as Rat made
her point. "If yer straight wiv me, that is. If yer thinks of
poor Rat now'n again."

She reminded me of a slug crawling over a dinner
plate. "You mean you'll tell."

"Me. Not a word. Wouldn't want to, that is. But one
hand helps the other, dunnit?"

By the heavy list of the hull and the rapid spanking of
the water against our planks, we were running down
Hull as fast as sail could bear us, the crew bending to
oars at every slackening of the wind. A little past midday,
or so it felt, Leof came into the tent with a steaming
bucket and a sack of wooden bowls and spoons. All of us
looked hungrily to the bucket. Leof fed the men first,
then the boy. None of the portions were lavish, but
prompted perhaps by some vagrant jot of humanity, Leof
ladled a bit extra for the boy. Rat thrust out her bowl
immediately.

"Na then, I'll take as much."

"I might later. If you're good."

"Randy little goat."

Lcof gave her no extra, nor to me. It dulled the edge of my hunger to find the bowl hadn't been carefully cleaned of its last use. The food routed the rest of appetite: boiled millet with far too much salt, containing foreign lumps that might have started life as fish.

"They expect us to eat this?"

Evidently so. The boy gobbled with starved relish and Rat was already halfway through hers, bolting it messily.

"Shame they din give yer a ewer to pat yer dainty fingers in."

I swallowed some with an effort. The miserable stuff insulted my stomach.

"Eat." Rat scraped her empty bowl, licked the spoon and set them aside. "Yer might fight for the like afore long. Here, gi 'me that."

She yanked the bowl from the boy deft as a cutpurse. He howled and reached for it, but Rat backhanded him across the mouth, shifting away to where he couldn't reach the food. The sight of that lipless mouth dribbling gruel from her first bowl revolted me as she began to gobble again.

"Give it back, Rat."

"He's fat enough. I ent."

"The child is hungry."

"Be the first time, look of him."

"Bitch!" I lunged across the cowed boy to get at her, as far as my chains would stretch, grabbing her wrist. She managed to shake me off but only because my chains barely allowed me the distance. It surprised me: Rat had not half my own small strength, none in her hands or stick arms.

"You're trash, Rat."

She went on eating. "Don't want me to tell, do yer?"

I gave it up in disgust. "You would, too."

"Why not? Sold myself to get here, why not you?"

That required a moment to grasp. "You what?"

"Everyone sells sumfin, dunnee? Like Leof. He'll come round tonight for what he wants. I'll get what I want. Ent nuffin there, been sellin that since I was twelve. Well, then: penny or pound, says I. Go for the lot."

"You sold yourself?"

My innocence amused her. "Happens all the time. Half

pound silver and a full belly's better'n free, cold and hungry."

Too tired and demoralized to pursue it further, I tried another taste of the gruel and gave it up. "Here, boy. With my blessing."

He wiped his tears with a grubby hand and pounced on the bowl, spooning as fast as he could. As I watched him, it struck me that all of them handled bowl and spoon more functionally than I—the bowl close to the mouth, as if too many had been yanked away before they'd had enough, spoon clutched overhand with all four fingers, thumb doubled under like the fist they shook at the world. Furtively, I mimicked them, awkward as it felt, then used my spoon handle to rub at the spur marks on my boots. Silver leaves a distinctive tarnish.

Privacy didn't exist on the ship for anyone. Rat wouldn't care, and I was sent out to the bucket with her and the boy. Afterward the boy and I were kept outside and allowed to warm ourselves by the steersman's brazier while Rat commerced with Leof and others of the crew. At a halfpenny apiece, she made a fair little sum since none of the men overstayed himself. These dogs bolted their rutting like their food. One man tried to get away without paying, and such a howl went up that Frith had to intervene—Rat screeching, the defaulter bawling furious denials, Leof roaring at the bawdy farce of it, Frith's exasperated verdict booming out into the dark beyond the tent—

"Ha'pny it was and ha'pny it is! *Pay* 'er, you mingy little prick."

Outrage subsided to grumbling. Rat was paid, the offender came muttering from the tent that she wasn't worth a Brit minim, bar a whole ha'pny silver. Frith sent him forward. Business was a serious matter to him. For this, rather than sensitivity, he reserved me (and the boy, for all that) from the attentions of his men.

"For Rat it's no more than going to the bucket," Frith told me. "You'd be sick at it, and I don't want you looking death on the block. You're past prime as it is. Got to make something from you."

Once out of Hull into broad Humber, the crew relaxed. The south shore, Sudhymbre, was Saxon country. Frith

hailed each fishing boat as we raised them and spread the news of the coming auction. Sudhymbre was held by Icel's Iclingas, according to Penrwd. From the nigh-deserted villages along the shore, I wondered where Icel would have raised the two thousand mercenaries he offered us.

The anchor let out sometime past noon feeding next day. We were all led out across the deep hatch forward and up to the halfdeck near the prow where Frith sat by an anvil. Nearby, one man was melting lead over a brazier and pouring it into hand-sized oval molds. The male slaves knelt, one by one, while a leather-lined iron collar was closed and bolted about their necks.

"What are those things, Rat?"

"Slave collar. Lead seals is the bill of sale."

When it was my turn, I hung back, pulled away, physically unable to kneel for that damned thing. It took two of them to hold me, a third to force my neck down to the anvil while they hammered the bolt shut. The collar felt cold and heavy. Each of them had a thick ring at the nape for chaining. I felt at it, sick and stunned.

"Only feels tight at first." Frith reached to the brazier. "Mold."

Frith scratched his seal on one side of the still-soft oval, then turned it over and labored even longer with his bent stylus in a kind of Brit-Latin code of his own, no doubt the only one he knew to write.

GWENDA.PARS.F. C/CICAT. I/X

Gwenda, Parisi female with the scar: one pound/ten.

Arthur always jibed at my arrogance. How he'd roar to hear the High Queen of Britain had a starting price of a pound and a half. So much for the daughter of the gods.

My neck was already raw from the heavy collar when we anchored off a river mouth I couldn't identify. The crew broke out oars and rowed us inland past a monotonous stretch of fen until the tidelands gave way to firm ground on both sides. Long before that we were ready to disembark, the men chained two by two, Rat with me, the boy manacled separately. Skillful sailors, the crew brought the craft within ten feet of the bank without

scraping bottom. The plank was thrown out and we were herded ashore.

"What's this place, Rat?"

"Heard 'em call it Wicandaen."

"What's here?"

"Nuffin. We get sold."

Wicandaen would be a dreary place in high summer with a fair in progress. From the fishing boats at river's edge, up the trodden bank to the drying racks and miserable thatched huts, the ground was littered thick with fish offal, oyster and mussel shells that reeked even in the cold. There seemed no particular plan or center to the village; it had simply occurred. The huts straggled close to or far away from the bank as the owner fancied. Where two dwellings chanced close enough together, fishnets were strung between them or along the sides of the salting racks.

From the drab villagers who gathered to ogle and dog our heels, I wondered how Frith expected to make any kind of sale. Then we were led to the rear of a hut larger than the others, and I knew. A sturdy, weathered scaffold stood waiting for us. Several timber trees still dangled frayed rope ends in the wind. The block apparently served for sale or execution, whatever the business at hand. Gathered round it were more than a score of men and women drinking from leathern pouches, stamping their feet against the cold. These were Frith's customers, obviously more affluent than the wretched villagers. Big sword-bearing men in cross-gartered leggings and heavy cloaks of an odd cut fastened at the shoulder with enameled brooches; women bulky as their men in drab-hued layers of tunic, their hair primly wrapped in woolen veils.

A great *ah* went up as they sighted us. The penal slaves were put on the block first. Despite their wait in the cold, the Saxons were in no rush to buy before inspecting the goods. While they frowned and doubted and looked thrice at each specimen, I had my first close observation of the men Arthur broke at Badon—large by our standards, long-haired, thick-bodied, some of them with Phrygian caps pulled about their ears and small gilt axes in their broad belts. There was a different stamp to these people, a peculiar set to the placidly merciless eyes and

unhumorous mouths. They reminded one of winter, as if they'd lived in a chill wind all their lives.

Each of the male slaves was scrutinized, strong or weak points debated frankly between men or husbands and wives before they stepped down from the block. An older man, better dressed than the others, with a great gold chain of office about his neck, climbed wheezily onto the platform, thumped a carven staff on the boards and made a brief announcement.

"Rat, you know these people. Do you understand the language?"

"Bit."

"Who's the old man, what's he saying?"

"Prince's reeve. Told 'em to get on wiv it."

They did. The standard Saxon price for a slave in those days was one pound. Frith's higher prices were supported by scarcity, and if a buyer haggled here and there, he eventually came up to Frith's figure or someone else would. One by one the penals were separated from their fellows, the price stamped on the lead seal. The reeve then put his own sign into the lead, gave it to the new owner, and the transaction was legal. Legality was important to these people, I learned. Even when a slave was freed, the owner had duties and rights of him, such as the slave's inheritance which went to the former master.

The Saxon boy was sold to a nervous little man with nothing assertive about him but his wealth. I managed to embrace the boy before Frith led him away.

"Be all right, he will," Rat allowed with a tinge of envy. "That old cock's a goldsmith."

"Rest you gentle, boy. Grow you into a man." I kissed his cheek.

"What else?" Rat rasped out of her perpetual disgust. She tugged at the chain that paired us. "Right, Gwenda: up we go."

With the male slaves claimed, competition sharpened for what was left. The men and their dour wives crowded in closer. Rat and I huddled in the wind like disconsolate crows on a fence. Weakened by lack of sleep and the first sharp hunger of my life, I didn't want to look at them: hard faces, not mercurial as a Briton's but carved from determination and granite self-righteousness. The

women, flinty as their men, surveyed us with much less optimism.

Two of the crowd pushed to the fore now, two latecomers just arrived in an oxcart, a hulking slope-shouldered woman and a strapping young man. Stiff gray braids poked out from under the woman's veil. The young man was blond as Arthur but bulkier, heavier in the jaw. He wore the gilt ax that seemed more a badge of rank than a weapon. But the crowd made way for them with greetings—

"Hoch, Thegn Gunnar."

"Gunnar Eanboldson. *Vordan har!*"

—and even the reeve vouchsafed a deferential nod. The man and woman came to the foot of the scaffold as if it were their natural place to be first. Mother and son: they could be nothing else, the same set to their mouths, not cruel but implacable, a mirror image in the cut of their narrow heads, deep-lidded eyes and brow.

Eanboldson. The name was familiar.

The mother was plainly furious at being late. She flung out a despairing arm at the last of the male slaves being led away. There! The best already gone, and these leavings are what we may choose from.

Leavings or not, we were hotly contended in the bidding, though it was plain the two newcomers wouldn't haggle. They bettered every offer without hesitation. Frith repeated the bids in rapid gutturals, hands aloft, fingers jabbing the air to sign the price for Rat as it rose. Used to bargaining with Saxons herself, she could follow it after a fashion.

"Lor! I'm up to pound/ten. And I sold to Frith for half!"

Frith's pantomime was eloquent as speech. With some imagination one could follow his drift from the gestures alone. Pound/ten asking. Who'll meet pound/ten? There's a man! Pound/ten and twelve from Thegn Gunnar Eanboldson. Pound/eleven? Anyone? Pound/eleven? Ah, who am I dealing with? Churls? Cottagers? Do I not see men of five hides and more? I hear pound/twelve! Pound/twelve for Raidda (flourishing her as a penultimate work of God's art). A young unmarried woman in her prime, a fine worker for field and hearth—

"List to him," Rat marveled. "Got me down for all but the Virgin Mary."

I shivered. "You weren't even born a virgin."

"Was too, till my cunting da got on to me. That din ever happen to Mary." The point seemed important to Rat. "Thought about that. What was Mary, I ask yer? Plain folk, nuffin much."

"Oh, be still."

"Nor she weren't no piss-elegant bitch like you, neither. Plain folk like me. Makes yer think, dunnit?"

"Oh, dear God, I'm fainting from hunger and you're onto theology."

"Well, it does! Na—if Lor God were lookin out a mum for Jesu—bit late and a bit west—well, it might've been me, mine it?"

"Why not? At your rates, it's a bargain."

"Ow!" Rat gasped at my blasphemy; some holies were not to be flouted. "You got a pro-*fane* mouth, Gwenda."

"God grant me your purity. I'm chilled to the marrow; leave me be."

"Should et yer gruel like the rest of us," Rat clucked. "You'll learn." Suddenly, birdlike, she cocked her head toward Frith. "Coo! Hear that?"

"What?"

Rat's tone waxed sepulchral; she might have been announcing the Nativity itself. "Five bloody pound!"

"For you?"

"Bof'us."

"Who?"

"Young barstid there in front. Ow, I *wisht* I got more outer Frith. Well, give'm a smile, Gwenda. He's yer new master. None'll best five pounds."

None could and none did. Five pounds stunned them all. Even Frith in the wildest euphoria of speculation could have hoped no better than four pounds the pair of us. His arm swooped toward Rat and me, then to Gunnar Eanboldson. Both arms crossed and uncrossed in a decisive gesture of ending, the reeve's staff thumped on the board: sold.

The crowd began to eddy away from the block. With the reeve in their wake, Gunnar and the formidable dame climbed onto the block. They were big, by God. The woman towered over both of us as she snorted contemptuously at Rat.

"He said you were four and twenty," she growled in

bad but understandable British. "Open your mouth—ha! Less teeth than me and all bad. Where do you come from?"

"Londin'um, please yer, mum."

"And a whore in the bargain."

"No, I nev—"

"Shut up. I know a *kotze* when I see one. Mark me, slut. My son is married to a woman of honor and dowry. You even look at him and I'll break your weak little back."

Her Brit had a Midland fall. I wondered where she'd learned it. She turned to Gunnar and said something that evidently struck him funny. He exploded in a laugh that created shape-changing magic. With laughter all the winter went out of Gunnar's face. Spring woke there, kindled its fires and lit him for the very young man he was as he moved off to busy himself with Frith and the reeve.

"And you now." The glowering woman moved to confront me, gimlet glance missing nothing from boots to brow. "What are you?"

"I was chamberwoman at Hull."

"I don't think so." She thrust her red hands into my hair. Searching for fleas or something else. I saw a glimmer of vindication. "You're a liar like all Brits. That hair's been washed this week."

Cold and hunger stung me beyond caution. "As you will. I didn't ask to be here."

She barely drew back her hand but the slap rocked me, jerking my head aside. "Shut—your—mouth."

"*Mor! Nej!*"

Gunnar barely turned from his business. He clipped out a stern order; quite evidently she was not to do that again. But my caution returned. I dropped my eyes and held my tongue. The time for escape would come.

"My son is Thegn Gunnar Eanboldson. He's disposed to be gentle, not knowing your kind or your language as I do. But your lords know his name."

And so did I now. Penrwd had mentioned him in council at Eburacum, a farmer-warrior. He certainly looked soldier enough.

"Your name is Gwenda? Speak up."

"Yes."

"Yes, *mistress*. And you're Raidda?"

"Calls me Rat, mistress."

"No riddle there." Elfgifu sized us up with acrid scorn. "Welshwomen. I could touch hands around your scrawny guts. Useless. Two and a half pounds apiece, and you won't last the year. I'll put you both on the pyre." She loomed over me like an irascible falcon. "Especially you. But you've burned enough of us in your time."

There wasn't the feeling I'd found a friend.

"You look sick, woman."

"I'm hungry . . . mistress."

This was different country from my familiar open moors. West of Wicandaen the forest closed about us. The oxen jolted us along a single track that grew steadily narrower. The damp cold crept first into my feet then through the thick cloak until Rat and I huddled together for mere animal warmth. The forest would have been gloomy at midsummer noon; in this gray winter we passed into thickening dusk as the ox trail dwindled to a footpath, the wet branches and thicket brushing against the sides of the cart and showering us with their residue of mist and rain.

Once Gunnar halted the team and jumped down to worry at the harness. I had a chance to look about at the forest. The gloom and eerie quiet affected Rat too.

"Haunted, feels like. Old trees like that."

Few Britons would pass this spot without reverence. We were in the stilled heart of the forest. Ancient oaks stretched away on either side, obscuring what was left of the afternoon light with their close-crowded upper branches. Some of the trees were of such gnarled age and thickness that I knew this for sacred virgin forest. The oaks, alder and rowan formed a rough square around a small clearing now sprouted with younger trees and numerous saplings pushing up through mossy turf. The vague outlines of an overgrown ditch bordered the clearing, vaguer each year as nature obscured man's work. At the far end squatted a large stone with the features of a human head pocked into it, still discernible under spreading lichen.

"Quiet's death," was Rat's hushed comment.

"Yes." But eloquent to me for all its stillness. In this sacred grove a pair of white oxen, horns gilded and

bound, once waited while the druid climbed the oak and cut the all-healing mistletoe from the topmost branches to fall into a white cloak held by acolytes below. If it were one of the great feast days, Samhain or Bel-tein, the oxen would be sacrificed in fire and divination made from the smoke that rose from it. But my grandmother sacrificed as often to Epona as she prayed to Christ and her mother was a priestess who cut the mistletoe herself. In this neglected place, by this melancholy measure, I could see how far we'd descended by a Roman road to this laudable modern world.

Gunnar and Elfgifu were relieved themselves to move on. They knew it had been a sacred place. Comfortable enough with their own frosty gods, they were not at all sure of those we might have left behind to wreak mischief.

"Damned forest is a waste," Elfgifu vowed. "We'll clear and sow it someday."

The forest fell away abruptly as it had closed in. Through the last of the feeble afternoon light, I saw the place Elfgifu called Gunnarsburh. Before us was a clearing about a mile broad where turned furrows, fallow or harvest stubble, ran within inches of the bordering forest. Freshly cut trees lay at the wood's edge, their thick stumps beside the holes or tilted stubbornly out of the ground, not easily surrendering to Saxons their British grip on the soil.

A small brook wound across the clearing, dividing several tilled fields. In the center, on the highest ground, the stockade of Gunnarsburh brooded in the winter twilight.

"Lor." Rat peered over the side of the cart. "Smoke. Got fires goin. I'm froze to the bone."

We creaked along the rutted track across the clearing for what seemed forever. It was quite dark before Gunnar halted the team at a tall post, rudely carved at the top into semihuman likeness. Gunnar took a horn from its suspending hook and blew three blasts. He listened. Another horn sounded from within the stockade. Gunnar answered with four shorter blasts, then clucked to the oxen and we moved on.

"You. Gwenda!"

I raised my head to Elfgifu, quite gone with hunger and the cold that didn't seem to bother her.

"This is Gunnarsburh. You may have seen larger hold-ings but none prouder. My son is a man of five hides. His father was warrior-born. The *scin-laeca* was seen at his birth. You wouldn't know of such things."

The cart lumbered on through winter dark. At last we passed men on both sides, holding torches, and heard the high wooden gates swing shut behind us. We halted in a square of cheery light from an open door in a small bower near the hall, from which wafted savory odors of rich promise.

Rat inhaled reverently. "Hot food."

Gunnar jumped down and vanished into the dark, call-ing to someone as Elfgifu herded us through the open door into light and blessed warmth. A wizened little woman stood in the center of the tidy kitchen by the glowing firepit, but I scarcely glanced at her. Over the fire a large cauldron steamed, the source of the delicious aroma. Elfgifu pushed me forward. Numb with cold and a little faint, I tripped over a stool, barking my shin. The sudden pain, the slave collar already chafing my neck, all shot through me like a hot knife. Always high-strung, any sudden noise or loss of balance twisted my stomach and poured a moment's unreasoning fury through the humors of my body. I glared at Elfgifu.

"Clumsy. Go warm yourself. Gytha, feed them."

We were given each a generous bowl of the stew, worlds better for seasoning than the millet on the ship. Hearty barley, thick with shredded venison, pork rind, cabbage, turnips and whatever winter vegetables their bins held. Like good pease porridge, the cauldron had likely simmered for days, its character shading with each addition, and nothing in my life ever tasted so good.

"Don't eat so fast, Rat. You'll be sick."

"Bloody starved." She wolfed it down from a lifetime of swallowing as much as she could before someone big-ger and hungrier snatched it away.

At a word from Elfgifu, Gytha the cook unstoppered the bung of a large barrel and poured us brown ale topped with yellowish foam. Curious drink: bitter and strong, it worked with the good food and warmth to stop my shuddering. I felt my eyelids droop as the warmth enveloped my exhaustion like a blanket. My mind

floated, drifted back three days to another world. Constantine in Eburacum . . .

Were they merciful to Regan? Who would tell poor Bors?

And so I drained the cup, drifting with the warmth to another room plain as this. My prison house at Camelot. Arthur back from Badon, come to me on a day of cold winter rain that crinkled my hair so that I gave up any attempt at style and just let Imogen comb it out straight, undone and stringy when Arthur saw me.

His own hair was heavy with damp, limp over his mud-flecked forehead. Arthur absently pushed it back. In empathy, longing to touch him, my hand lifted to my own frowsy mop. We were both awkward with the need to say something in that painful silence, our first meeting since Morgana's death.

I gave the hair a last futile tug. "It's the wet. I can't do a thing with it. . . ."

I blinked. The figure still stood before me, magically younger, the hair not faded to sand but still thick spun gold. At Gunnar's side there was a pregnant woman perhaps a year or two older than my Regan but much soberer of bearing. Blue-eyed as her husband, with the same remote, superior cast of expression. By her belly she'd give birth not much later than Brigid-feast.

We were told that this was Lady Nilse, Gunnar's wife, mother of his children and mistress of his hall. We would address her always with respect.

I bowed my head to her and repeated the mouth-filling word for lady. *"Hlafdian."*

Rat and I knelt to her at Elfgifu's word. Nilse placed her hands on our heads; that inaugurated us into the household. She withdrew with Gunnar, Elfgifu busied herself with the cook and we were allowed to finish our food.

"Wife ent the worst for looks," Rat judged through noisy mouthfuls. "Won't keep 'em long, spittin out one brat after 'nother."

"Hush. The old woman understands most of what you say."

"Don't fancy you much either."

True. Elfgifu's contempt for Rat was perfunctory; toward me, rather purposeful, as if everything about me

justified and stirred a deep resentment. Rat scraped the last of her bowl and asked for more, but Elfgifu refused with a curt no.

"Ow, mistress, please. Din feed us nuffin on that cruel boat, not a blessed mouthful."

Elfgifu was adamant. "It is winter. Food must last. You won't go hungry, but you'll work for it."

Rat set down her bowl in sibilant disgust. "Hope I get full just once afore I die, straight I do." She eyed with predatory intent a half-wheel of goat cheese set out on a table near the wall, but it was too far for stealth. Then she noticed I'd some left in my bowl. "Give us some, Gwenda."

"No. I'm hungry myself."

"Yer shared wiv that little barstid on the boat."

"That was garbage. Had to be starved to get it down. I'm starving now."

"I think yer ought." Rat's wheedling tone took on a sly nuance of threat. "Yer remember me, I'll remember you. Now give me some."

"Learn to eat more slowly. You won't feel so hungry."

"There's things I could tell."

"You'll do that anyway, high-minded as you are." I was too tired, hungry and frustrated to care what she did, needing all my will not to cry or scream. "Go away."

Her whine became a snarl. "Damn yer selfish—gi' me that!"

She made a snatch at my bowl and gripped it a moment before I wrested it back; quick but no real strength in her arms. Only hunger made her dare. As I yanked the bowl away, Rat snarled an obscenity and clawed me across the face. It tripped the rage that had smoldered since Leof first struck me. Even he bled for that, and this piece of dirt was a reachable target. I slammed the bowl into Rat's face and backhanded her with all my body behind it. Rat flew back against the wall from the vicious force of it, her beaky nose and lipless mouth dripping stew as Elfgifu turned on us, startled. I snatched a cleaver from the cook's worktable and lunged at the terrified Rat.

"You little filth, don't you *ever* touch me!"

Rat saw the undiluted murder in my eyes. She slid

along the wall trying to elude me. "Mistress, geroff me! Geroff me, I ent done nuffin—"

She was the sacrifice to a rage that went far beyond her. I raised the cleaver to bury it in her skull with less hesitation than when I sent Brocan to butcher Morgana. This I'd do myself—but then my arm was caught in a grip strong as the manacles, twisting it back. Elfgifu whipped me around like a child; I lashed out at her, blind with fury.

"Let go, Saxon, I'll kill you!"

My free hand smashed its chain across her heavy jaw. Elfgifu merely shook off the blow and twisted the cleaver out of my hand. The next instant I was lifted off my feet and slammed heavily on my back across the lip of the firepit.

"Oh, yes," she hissed. "Your kind kills very easily. I've seen it."

I felt the heat of the fire on my back, still writhing to get at her, face, eyes, anything in reach. Elfgifu hooked strong fingers through my collar, twisting, cutting off my windpipe.

"Just like your men, aren't you?"

"She ent what she said," Rat screeched from the safety of the wall. "Look at her fancy shift'n boots. Horse boots, spur-marked."

"Be quiet," Elfgifu said, holding me down.

"Her man was combrogi, sure as Lor God."

"Shut up, you stupid cow. You think I haven't seen them before?" Elfgifu didn't turn her hard, unforgiving eyes from mine. "I knew what you were on the block, Gwenda." She gave the collar another strangling twist against my futile struggles. "Did your man tell you about the Time of the Smoke, Gwenda? The men left dead in their fields, the women on their hearths? The children cut apart and thrown into ditches? The years of hope and work wiped out in one summer? *Did* he?" She twisted tighter. "Did your drunken harpers make a song of that?"

The breath rattled in my throat, lungs ready to burst. The fight was long gone out of me when Elfgifu opened her hands and let me wilt to the earthen floor at her feet, gasping while she bent over me.

"Don't worry, little Brit. You'll live. You'll pay back what your men burned. Because we'll go back to the

Midlands someday, and you'll walk every step of the way behind me. If you last."

I put up no more fight as she ran a chain through my collar loop and fettered me to a bolt in the wall. The cook did the same with Rat. We were left in the kitchen bower with no light except the fading glow from the fire and one blanket apiece. I dragged mine as close to the fire as I could.

"Yer all right, Gwenda?"

"Leave me alone. Don't try to take from me again. You've got nothing left to sell."

"Ow, it ent all that bad. Just yer got to learn how things are. Girl does what she can in a hard life. Here."

Something plumped lightly on my chest. I groped for it: a morsel of the goat cheese.

"Pinched it when the old bitch was onto yer. Cook weren't lookin."

Rat seemed to have forgotten or simply sloughed aside the fact that I'd tried to murder her a moment before. It was that common in her experience, likely. People did such things. Rat would simply get out of the way.

"Told yer, din I?" She munched at her cheese through the words, smacking her lips. "They don't like combrogi 'tall, and why should they, say I? What yer sweet-smellin lot ever do but kill 'em all, kill each other when yer bloody felt like it? Inferior, that's what you are, Gwenda."

God knows where she learned or how she retained a word so literate or so unnecessary to her perfect round of survival. But Rat said it again, pleased with her choice and quite serious.

"Inferior."

V

English Voices

o escape . . . to escape. To get back, grasp the lost sword, put things right. I was like a blind idiot child without language, relying on the other British slaves to pass me what few motes of news flew on the wind to winter-isolated Gunnarsburh. Rhodri and Gwyneth had been slaves since their youth: of the Lindissi, once tributary to Cador, friendly enough, glad of another Brit for company, one more quick fox in a den of stern wolves, but knowing instinctively as Rat that I was different from them. When I wore away their shyness, they were more open. Brits love to talk, and Gwyneth would gladly spin half an hour's comment from a moment's detail. I pressed her.

"What have you heard of home? What's happening in the west? In the north?"

Any provincial castle is cut off in winter, and Saxons are far less gregarious than we. Gunnarsburh in winter was a hermitage. At long intervals when the forest paths were clear enough, a rider might straggle in with word of some sort from Icel or Wicandaen. Even more rarely a Christian monk might beg hospitality, never refused but offered at arm's length. Saxons are no less superstitious than our own peasants. A shaman of an unknown god might work hostile magic.

But word trickled in, most of it known to me.

"Eburacum's sacked and the old Queen dead. So said the monk," Gwyneth volunteered.

"Do you tell me so?" said her husband Rhodri over his soup. They were distantly interested; the thing touched them not at all. They'd hoped, long ago in the brief glory of Arthur and his combrogi, that they might be free again, part of Britain. Now it was only gossip over food.

"Did I not see her myself when she was young?" said Gwyneth, as if one fact proved the other. "She must have been very old. That was . . . oh, years."

Peasants have no precise sense of time or need of one outside planting and harvesting. From various events in her youth that Gwyneth recounted, the "old Queen" was a year or two her junior.

"Is it not promised the Pendragon will come again?" Rhodri mused. "Aye, and the combrogi, them that can't die, like the mac Diurmuid and the Gryffyn?"

Britons. Dreamers.

"Lord is *hlaford*," Elfgifu snapped at me. "Bread-giver. Lady is hlafdian. Bread-server. You will see why when men of honor visit. Wear this veil to cover your hair. It is more dignified. In time I will speak no more Brit to you, and you'd better know what I say, for I won't say it twice. Bow your head in front of me!"

This obeisance was not required of the others, but Elfgifu sensed my resistance from that first day on the slave block. More than once in those first months I felt the force of her arm as I struggled to learn alien duties in an alien language. Rat thrived as Rat would, of course; the place was heaven to her. She was warm and fed, the frequent cuffings far less brutality than she'd grown up with. Winter was the one cruelty to her. Her weak chest bothered her; she snuffled and coughed continually. Despising her on principle, I was still moved to help her, if only to rid my ears of the sound of it. With gestures and my scanty store of words, I begged of Gytha the cook a few leaves of the downy harhune she used to flavor vegetables, and brewed Rat a strong tea.

"Drink it. I'm tired of listening to you at night."

Rat gulped it down too fast, as she did everything. "'Sgood. More?"

"I'll make you some at bedtime. It will help you sleep."

"Thank yer, love." Rat's black-toothed grin was her

nearest approach to gratitude. "Yer be good to Rat, she'll do right by yer."

Then Elfgifu loomed over us, accusing as usual. "Gwenda, you are not of the kitchen. Why are you in here? Loafing? Stealing?"

"No."

"No, *what*?"

"No . . . Hlafdian."

Elfgifu was good as her word. After all too little time she ceased to give orders in British at all and I had to hang on every word to comprehend the half of it. Correctly spoken English is a stately language, but the barnyard variety of Gunnarsburh was difficult for a Brit used to relishing each syllable.

Rhodri described it best, commiserating with my labors. "Hard at first, that's the truth of it. They get a running jump on the first sound and then just slide through the rest of it."

If Elfgifu's mood was not too caustic, she might repeat for me. More often I bore the brunt of her disgust, and *that* in British.

"Two and a half pounds for a niddering, useless, stupid thing like you. I bade you feed the *geese*, whore. Not the cows."

We were in the byre. Elfgifu shoved me against the stall gate, Rat hovering in the background, afraid to open her mouth, terrified of Elfgifu.

"I'm sorry, I didn't understand you."

"What, whore? I didn't hear you."

"*Jeg . . . Jeg kan ikke . . . forstan sie, Unskyld, Hlafdian.*"

"That's better."

"*Tak, min gud Hlafdian.* And I am not a whore."

"Oh?" She always welcomed another chance to bait me. "All Brit women are whores, bred to it." She patted my cheek too hard. "And the higher born, the lower."

Humility still not learned, I could scathe in my own tongue more efficiently than she ever hoped to. "Christian women quite often hold the same view, but where there's no temptation there's no virtue. And I doubt if many men have pestered you, Hlaf—"

Her fist caught me on the jaw and knocked me against the stall gate. The byre swam in my blurred sight before I forgot all caution and launched myself at her, reaching

to claw her eyes out. She had four times my strength and would have crippled me but for Rat who threw herself between us, whining, wheedling—saving me.

"Ow, mistress, don't hit her, please. Swear I'll teach her to do right, on Cross I will. Lor knows she's stupid'n I don't go combrogi no more'n you do, mistress. I'll teach her good."

Just then someone hailed Elfgifu from the courtyard. God knows what I would have earned but for Rat stopping me. When we were alone, she whispered fiercely through my tears.

"Listen, Gwenda. Yer gonner learn or yer gonner die."

"Get away from me . . ."

But she persisted because it meant something to her. "Make it hard for all've us, yer do. Who's gonner look after me if yer dies? Na, no mind what yer feels about old bitch. Yer smile and bow yer stupid head'n I'll try to help yer get on. If yer good to me, like the tea'n that."

I wilted to the straw on the floor, letting the helpless, beaten tears flow at will. I had no place, no world, no name. Dead.

"God, where've I come to? Where am I?"

Rat squatted close, stroking me as much as I'd allow. Even that was balm in my poverty. "Yer been hittin all yer life, Gwenda. Yer never knew there was them what couldn't hit back. Na yer one of us. Take care. I beg yer, learn t'take care. We're friends na. Women gotter be good t'each other, donnay?"

"Sweet Christ, help me."

"Sod the prayin!" Rat hissed with all the force of her charred soul. "Yer listen to *me*. 'Cause we're all we bloody got."

In time and necessity I resisted less and began to learn the new world I'd come to. How to measure my lessons? By days or seasons, furrows cut and sown, barley scythed and threshed, flax winding on the slow distaff, hands that blistered, then callused, on the spade and hoe? My menses that finally retired, routed by time as I was routed from Eburacum, the rash that disappeared from sun-darkening skin, muscles each a separate and exquisite agony before growing supple and taut?

Perhaps the theme of my life all along has been sur-

vival; certainly it was Gunnarsburh's. The land was poorer than in the Midlands, rain and sun less reliable, more at the whim of the North Sea, but still better than the sandy soil of Jutland whence Elfgifu and her husband had come. They weren't Saxons. That was my first lesson from Gunnar himself. Britons lumped them all under the one name, inaccurate as calling me Pict because I came from the north. Their tribes distinguished jealously as ours: Iclingas were Angles, but here in Britain they called themselves English.

"Eng-lish, Gwenda. Saxons come from Frisia. They live south of us."

"Unskyld, Hlaford. Then I'm not Welsh but British."

"Of course you're Welsh. You were born here, nej?"

"But, Hlaford, so were you." Born to Elfgifu in the Midlands shortly before Arthur's raid. All the English of Gunnarsburh save Elfgifu were born in Britain. Their remembrance of their forebears and gods was less scrupulous than hers, less shadowed with her pious sense of destiny. God, the burden mothers lay on sons! Eanbold was scin-laecen, hero-born. His mother claimed to see the shining warrior-spirit of his destiny just before his birth. Gunnar was Eanbold's last child, unheralded by any miracle. Sometimes in her anger or drunk, Elfgifu would hurl that at Gunnar like bastardy, along with their loss of the Midlands, as if in her unbending mind one were the cause of the other. Gunnar grew up with the millstone of her debt around his neck.

Tutored by Rat and Gwyneth, I learned English quickly in the way I'd mastered all languages and dialects: by accepting it on its own terms and not trying to make it fit British structure. I never acquired the accent, but this is impossible for most Britons.

"I said it rightly, Hlaford."

"Very right," Gunnar chuckled. "But you always sound like you're singing."

If he came into the world without prophecy, Gunnar at twenty-five was not untried. He fought at Badon with Cerdic. Considering the independent ways of his kind, it's a wonder they got there at all. Things were done in a certain way. First Cerdic's earls came to drink and talk at Icel's board, then the prince's men gathered among themselves to mull the undertaking from every possible view.

Efficient Cerdic must have gone nearly mad waiting on them. To the English any important matter is worth arguing twice. At first with the ale flowing so that men's hearts were open and they spoke their true feelings, foolish or not. Then a second time in cool sobriety, that the mind was known as well as the heart, fools and hotheads discounted and a medium struck.

Badon called for careful drinking and thinking. This prince was for it, that lord not. This one would have trouble raising men, this or that *folc-gemot*—the common folk assembly unknown to Britons but a foundation stone of English government—cannily requested their lords ask *precise* assurances of Cerdic. What lands would be theirs when they won and how apportioned? How did they know the half-Welsh Cerdic would keep his promises?

In the end they went and lost. I came to know the survivors well as they gathered about the feast board to reminisce. Cheery-tipsy, they spoke of exploits and heroes until the drink seared the deep places where the wounds of defeat still ached, and they muttered in their stolid way of realities.

"We could fight Maelgwyn's foot troops," Gunnar remembered over his cup. "We could take that plowing hill. We were taking it, a level at a time. It was Arthur . . ."

The heads would nod over their own drinks: Arthur and his combrogi who fought not man to man honorably but from the backs of devil-horses. So believed the English who knew nothing of cavalry or its potential. What natural animal could move so swiftly, even fly? Didn't Arthur and Bedivere and Geraint, astride such unnatural animals, face a hundred of Cerdic's best at Neth Dun More in their youth?

They even had a grim joke about it. A mare is mounted by a Valkyrie's stallion and the foal, too full of hell for anything else, becomes a combrogi horse. Then a troll plows a Welshwoman and the bastard is the rider. Men muttered assent to this, but they never laughed, they'd seen the truth of it. Arthur himself had a Faerie mother, they all knew that. Of the lords about him, what single one was not dark marvel? Gareth could see a hundred miles and remember every tree and path. Bedivere could

stand off a dozen even afoot and laugh at them. Geraint was a distempered wolf without even a wolf's caution, and everyone knew Arthur's queen bedded a dozen men each night and dishonored her husband at the first opportunity.

As we did, the English hung a god or two in the family trees of all their heroes and royalty. They were half-pragmatic and all superstition: how far removed to imagine the only men to defeat them as devil-spawn? Defeat is not easily understood by these people. They call us illogical and emotional, yet their minds are curiously dual in many respects. Methodical, they proceed by method from need to acquisition. Failure therefore cannot possibly be their fault, but (and here the non sequitur) the intervention of sorcery. As for my dozen lovers a night, they overstated my energies with my sins.

Methodical, practical. Glory and honor were much, but the land was everything. To survive you must put deep roots in the earth. You must have good soil like the Midlands. A shame such good fallow should belong to Catuvellauns who worked so little of it and so wastefully. This was another lesson, the constant theme in men and women alike. *We will survive. We will go back.* I heard its diapason in Nilse as we worked our looms, speaking of the day Gunnar came home from Badon.

"His feet were frostbitten and the good new garments I sent him off with hung loose on his back, he was so starven. His poor cheeks and lips were cracked open from the cold wind, and he could barely hobble the last few steps to the hall. I sat him by the fire with hot soup, and thought, Why will not my husband look at me?

"He could not. Just stared into the fire as if he'd never seen one before and said they lost. I wanted to tell him that I'd lost nothing if he was given back to me. Forgive me, Mother, but a live husband is more than a dead hero, even if you disagree. But such words are not easy for me."

Elfgifu bent her head over her sewing. "I sacrificed that he might come home unhurt. We have not lost. We will win next time."

"Yes, next time," said Nilse as if it were already settled. "We will go back together."

"Damned right." Elfgifu's head came up fiercely, searching me out. "Keep your boots mended, little Brit."

If men waited, the land had daily needs like children, and like Gunnar's children, Edytha and Eadward, would wait just so long for spring, only to burst from the confining hall with the first half-warm day, Nilse or myself running after to see they were well wrapped. On such days, all Gunnarsburh felt a stirring. When I walked into the fields behind Gunnar and his steward Beorn, I saw the substance behind the preposterous myths and absurd genealogies of gods and heroes, saw in small the why of the dream. Gunnar and Beorn would take up handfuls of the damp soil and break them to bare the delicate traceries of ice that bound the clods in a weakening grip. I saw Gunnar lift his head to the east wind and sift it with the alchemy of his senses, parting the elements of that air—heat, moisture, treacherous hint of more winter. His fingers, crumbling the soil, were five separate messengers bringing the news that Freya was awake in the ground or should be left to sleep yet. Too soon or too late were equal dangers. The two men would pause with the future in their hands, silent, feeling and listening; then all their tutors came together to render judgment and Gunnar would fling the clod away, grinning at Beorn.

"Time."

"Time," Beorn would grunt.

"Gwenda! Tell Mother to light the altar and yoke the team."

And that chilly day with no surety of spring but what lay in their bones and flesh, they would start to thaw the ground for plowing. A pig or an ox would be burned on the altar at the stockade as an offering to Freya, goddess of the harvest. An old sow long past farrowing or an ox far gone in age and hoof rot. In respect of their gods, the English are practical as they are in all else. They give what's due and stop this side of prodigality.

That evening, Gunnar and Beorn would clump into the hall, joyous and profane, dirt from one end to the other, streaks of it in the sweat they wiped from their faces, grinning idiotically at each other over their ale. Whatever the future, they had *now*, they had it in their hands.

The noise of the children wouldn't bother Gunnar at all on such a night, and he'd sleep well.

To me, the spring wind brought different music of a younger and lost time. Under the Roman of me was a Briton forever singing lost-and-gone.

"Such a sad song for a beautiful day," Gunnar said as we knocked the clods from our tools at the end of work.

"It's the song I felt, Hlaford."

"You people are always rutting or rhyming. What did it ever get you?"

"I don't know. More poets?"

He'd look down at me, shaggy-blond, vital, quizzical as another man most like him, and laughed in the same way—laughter that could forget time, place or troubles, welling out of youth and the full purse of an unspent future—until life crowded back suddenly with the lookout's cry from the watchtower:

"Men at the pale!"

Gunnarsburh was my school, a way of life behind a wall and a warning. The pale post was carved with the image of Heimdall, god of gates and bridges, and fitted with the horn that all must sound to announce themselves. Anyone drawing closer without the answering horn from the watchtower risked heavy penalty or even death.

They were a people ringed with enemies, Britons to the north and west, hostile Saxons to the south, the eastern sea as pirate-ridden for them as us. The customs of their life came from Jutland but were being reshaped by necessity. They hung from the bare edge of Britain as from a cliff. Any concerted and sustained British effort would have wiped them from our country forever. We never knew that, they never forgot it. It set an edge to the iron of their lives.

They honored their gods and their lords; from these they demanded honor and justice in return to the half-pennyworth. An Englishman does or renders what custom expects of him. One jot more and he'll argue with a mountain of law and his courts in support of him, convocations that, for their splitting of legal hairs, make Talmudic scholars seem careless and arbitrary. A difference in a brush stroke: the British lord is defined by blood and tradition, the English lord by what he owns.

Gunnar's rights and duties were a Gordian knot of custom hardened into law, some of it from the old country, some evolved since their exodus. He owed military service to Icel; in turn the men of his holding owed theirs to him. He farmed much of his six hundred acres himself, the rest let out in a complicated system of tenantage to his *geburs* and cottagers for rents in produce and poultry, service, very little in hard money which was in scant circulation. Sheep and their wool were money among Iclingas.

The children of Gunnar and Nilse were their pride and concern. Edytha was five, Eadward a riotous, inexhaustible four, just this year given his first buckler and wooden sword and still tripping over them. They would have preferred a male firstborn; daughters married away and advantageous matches were not that easy to find among the sparse but profit-minded Iclingas. Edytha became, in time, a very valuable asset—not coldly assessed by any means, but these are people who must move upward or perish. And everything, even the lives of high men and low, is reckoned in money.

The heart of Gunnarsburh was the thatched timber hall, a longhouse with two great firepits. In winter it was the gathering point for all within the stockade—family and servants, with attached bowers for the kitchen, one for Gunnar and Nilse and their children, and one for Elfgifu. All the buildings were sturdy. Most ramshackle was the stone-basined wooden altar to Woden near the smithy, which made an English kind of sense. As Elfgifu would not sacrifice valuable animals, neither would she send them off on her best timber. No Grail seekers, these.

Next in rank below Gunnar came his steward Beorn, called a gebur since he owned a hide of his own land and cottaged a few families to farm it with him. A bit older than his lord, he'd been with him to Badon and functioned much as Bedivere to Arthur with many of the Gryffyn's better qualities—steady and dependable—without his blunt pessimism. His wife Ase attended Nilse much as Imogen did me, but with less distinction between mistress and waiting woman. Nilse relaxed in Ase's company. Elfgifu could wear on her (or anyone), too much given to dogmatic judgment to unlace with. A bit of an old bore, especially in her drinking which was too

much and too often. Ase was a friend and sister to Nilse.
She and Beorn maintained a bower within the stockade
as well as the house on their own land.

The shriveled cook I'd seen on my first night was
Gytha, wife to the smith Cynred. Their helpers were
Rhodri and Gwyneth, taken so long ago they scarce re-
membered freedom.

In the early summer, Nilse gave me my own garden. I
thought of failed flowers and Lancelot and tried to escape.

But that was later. Now it was winter still. The fox felt
the stirring of the earth in his lair and padded on the
mating call. The mole burrowing in the hard ground felt
it warm and tunneled faster. Snowdrops appeared. I
trudged with Gunnar and his men through the fields,
manuring, ditching the low fields against spring rain.
Gunnar drafted me for field work as the healthier. Frail
Rat worked in the kitchen, always happy to be near food
and nimble as her namesake in pinching extra for herself. And in truth I had no more talent for cooking than
delight in its result. I could write a treatise on the stages
of a flower, but the mysteries of food from seed to table
were terra incognita. The plain winter fare of the English—turnips, cabbage, rye meal pudding and salt
fish—was dull to the point of cruelty until the field
taught me what real appetite could be.

Winter days are short in the north, nights long. With
the darkness we would all gather in the hall, family at
the high table, servants across the firepits. If food was
plain and rationed, there were always ale and stories to
tell. At Gunnarsburh, Elfgifu filled the bard's place. She
brought from Jutland all her people's genealogies and
hero tales, an oral history that might have been dictated
to a scribe, so precisely she remembered. Her heritage
and destiny, cropped short by Arthur Pendragon. The
world owed Elfgifu three pound/ten and she was not
going to forget.

Gunnar and Nilse heartily wished she would. They'd
never known Jutland and didn't care about it. The future
called them, not the dead past. But of long winter nights
in the fire-flickering hall, Elfgifu's memories flowed from
the deep spring of the past to the same sea-meeting of
wish and destiny. A nagging toothache of a woman,

wounded, querulous, unforgiving, but these memories were her jewels. She would set out and polish each, placing them one by one before you so that in their antique gloss you saw a side of Britain most Britons will never know.

Hard old bitch, she had a decade on me if a day, hunched over her ale, gray braids splayed on the board under the two shields hung in places of honor, Eanbold's triskelion and Gunnar's lion head.

Our young thegn murmurs with Nilse. Beorn and Ase are exchanging riddles. Rat drowses over her drink at my side. The fire crackles up as Rhodri throws another log on the embers. Elfgifu gazes into the rising flame, conjuring the past. The English have a music of their own (when I learned to appreciate it); slower and darker than ours, but a strain even Trystan could admire. Listen to her in her own words, telling of her home. The times were bad, blood feuds costly and destructive, the young men restless for war-employment, nothing to be gained at home. But oversea, the Welsh Vortigern was calling for mercenaries. . . .

Who is this Christ-man of Jerusalem (Elfgifu demands) and why marvel that he was born in a byre? My husband Eanbold was born in a mean place, and as clear a light and prophecy marked his coming. But those were the days when there were still heroes in Jutland and proper respect for custom. And hard by the sea-stronghold of Hjortspring lived Torvald, a *gesith* of Thegn Witta. Now, Torvald's wife Fricka was big with child. On the night before she gave birth, she woke beside her sleeping husband, and there by her bed stood the scin-laeca, the shining spirit, the war-ghost of the ancient Angles in full war proof.

Fricka knew him at once and his purpose. His ring shirt was of gold, his boar-helm of beaten silver and bronze, his sword set with a gemmed hilt. Most stern was his gaze as he drew the sword and laid it across her belly. Then Fricka knew she was blessed to bear a chosen warrior, one marked for honor in life and to feast with Woden in Valhalla after death. And that was Eanbold Torvaldson, my husband, Gunnar's father. Many I know could look to be as honorable a lord.

"Mother, it's late. You've drunk enough."

"Not enough, boy. Never enough. I'm remembering that which better men respect. You don't know how it was in the old days."

That was—oh, let me think and not be distracted. (She searches for the frayed end of her thought in the ale cup.) That was in the days when Hengist and Horsa came here to Britain to aid weak Vortigern against the Picts. A score of years later a good part of the east was ours, even these lands here, and women like myself came to Wicandaen to make homes for the men, for until then they had none to marry but Britons. (Elfgifu makes it sound like death in life.)

And there among the warriors was Eanbold, young but already rich in war booty, a gesith. His wedding gift to me was a harnessed team of oxen, a spear and sword. Mine to him was a like sword that he carried to his last day, and that very shield on the wall which I painted with my own hands. As it was done in Hjortspring among Angles of place and pride, so that a woman knew she was bound to a man chosen for war and would share that fortune with him, however it fell. However it fell. . . .

We had no prince then. Icel was still young in Jutland. We and our chiefs took the Midlands for ourselves. In fray after fray Eanbold and his war companions scattered and plundered Maelgwyn's niddering people and sent them running to Caius Pendragon for shelter. It was good land, a promised land, and we made a new country that would someday be ruled by an Angle king. Hides? Enough for anyone with hands to work them. I bore three children, two sons and a daughter and Gunnar the youngest. No scin-laeca came at the birth of my sons, but perhaps that was too much to ask in one family. My firstborn Wulf was so yelping healthy death dared not come near him. Eanbold was honored among thegns and the sun conjured the grain from the ground, harvest upon harvest.

When I bore Gunnar—you were a small child, easily come—there was a sign of sorts. Ravens flew out of the west over our fields and the sun hid behind clouds, so

that it was death-cold for summer. I took up my rune bones, but they told me nothing. Yet each day for a week the ravens flew over.

Rat would be snoring now as Elfgifu signaled me to refill her cup. But I heard a more familiar music: with the ravens out of the west, Elfgifu's story became mine as well.

By then (she said) Vortigern was gone and Ambrosius in his place, what was that to us? Just another Welshman with a Roman name. I cast the runes again. They hid all meaning from me . . . except that something had changed in the west. There was new magic abroad in the west, and it came of whoring as it always does with the Welsh. There was a Faerie changeling named Ygerna who lay with Uther Pendragon and spawned Arthur, a demon with no human blood but his father's. And Ambrosius gathered this spawn and others like him, got the same way, into the legion of the devil-horses. The combrogi.

We thought that Cerdic would scatter them like chaff at Eburacum. Some of our best went with him. When they came back few and broken, I knew some part of what the runes hid from me. There was a . . . difference. Eanbold spoke less, slept poorly, as if lying awake to see if his scin-laeca would come to foretell his death. Good luck was at an end. The next summer—Wulf was five, Gunda three and Gunnar just a year then—Ambrosius sent Arthur to burn us out of the country we made with our own hands and sweat.

Our men made the best of what chance they had, and that was none at all. Now we saw what broke Cerdic at Eburacum. Even Romans would not fight from a horse. They left that to their rabble Scythians, knowing it dishonorable. I hovered close to the edge of the last battle with Gunnar in my arms and watched Eanbold lock shields with his men and go down under those horses like scythed wheat. After that they were collecting and slaughtering and burning what was left. Nothing looted, not a grain. All burned. Wasted. I tried to keep the children safe, but for three children, you need three pairs of eyes.

They found Wulf and Gunda. I won't speak of that.

Life was still worth the living for Gunnar. We still had one horse, a poor old thing. I took Gunnar and hid under the straw when they came. They fired our barn. The smoke began to choke us. I went lunatic then: by Freya, they'll kill me and my son to our faces. I crawled out of the straw and saw the combrogi-man.

Not much of a demon for looks. A middling man, built like a bull, plain as bread. No armor, just an old linen shirt and breeches dark with grease and smoke. And there was I, Gunnar bawling in my arms, the fire and smoke curling around us, waiting to die from the combrogi's longsword. But he didn't raise it, just stared at me as if the little space was too far to walk, and all he said was, "God's love, woman, come out of there." I'll never forget that.

That was the end of the Midlands for us. Fire and smoke. I'll never know why they let me live, but we never forgot their names, those of us who came back. The one who spared me, that was Lancelot. They say he married Eleyne, the sister of mad Geraint. A strong and virtuous woman, they say, that's a rarity for Welsh. Of course he betrayed her with Gunver the Queen, and that's not rare at all.

The fire would be burned low, Gunnar and Nilse exchanging to-bed glances, Ase yawning and nuzzling into Beorn's shoulder, and Elfgifu very drunk. She drank no better than Rat, but where Rat's general weakness brought quick stupor, the liquor heated Elfgifu, fed the deep wrongs, fired memory with a need for vengeance. Lost in the end of her somber dream, her head would come up, dangerous as a wounded boar. Nilse knew the look better than I, whispering to Gunnar. He would slip behind her, bending close.

"Time for sleep, Mother."

"Time to remember . . ."

"The people need to go to bed."

"Don't tell me of people. I saw them, the men who fell in their own fields. My children, your brother and sister—"

"Oh, enough, Mother."

"—left for the *flies*! Tell them, Gwenda. You were one of their whores."

"I said enough." Gunnar hauls her out of the chair, pointing her toward her bower. "We're all tired of this, the same old story. Go to bed."

"You? You know nothing. You were a babe. How would you know what they were."

"To bed, Mother."

"You'll never know, never have the destiny. You weren't scin-laecen like your father." Shaking him off, stalking with careful drunken dignity to the door of the hall. "You were the poor last."

With age Elfgifu needed less sleep. She rarely went straight to bed drunk or sober. Some fierce protectiveness or memories that could not yet rest set her to prowl the stockade until all slept but the fur-bundled watchman in the tower. One night when she was drunk to the point of concern, Nilse charged me to get Elfgifu to bed. She was nowhere to be found at first. In the mist of the stockade yard, I was about to call up to the watchman when I saw the tall form move slightly by the Woden altar next the smithy. She was speaking in low, earnest tones as to a confidant. Her fist thudded on the altar boards.

"He must. He must!"

"Lady?"

Elfgifu broke off, her profile sharp in the small altar flame. "Oh. You."

"Let me help you to bed."

"Calls me drunk. He doesn't know drunk or the need for it." Still, she allowed me to steady her perilous progress to the bower. Her arm was powerful beneath the sleeve, muscle that broke and husbanded the ground for years before it was taken from her.

"We made a kingdom from nothing. We saw it growing like the grain. Just a few more years . . . a few more men. What would Gunnar know of that? Beautiful child . . . fairest of my children."

Just a fuddled old woman now, maudlin with ale. "No one but you to get me to bed. You've helped us all to bed, your kind. The waste . . . Arthur was mad, they all were. How could my runes read madmen? Oh, leave off,

Gwenda. I'm all right. I'll put you all on the funeral pyre."

The mirror of her kind, losing remained a riddle to Elfgifu. How could it happen? It won't the next time. And although she drove me, even striped my back with the lash, I knew her loss. If desperation drove her folk out of Jutland, hasn't it driven us before them like a sail before the wind, losing all the way? Loss? Listen to our music: you can hear night falling over an earth we couldn't hold and a heaven we can't reach. Hear Elfgifu's lament and see them naked in an uncertain dawn with nothing in their hands but a sword and a hoe, their ancient sagas and our sad music fading in their ears. Unlikely inheritors, but that's what they are.

Winter still, but the sun moved closer to earth. We plodded the new-turned furrows in March to sow the oats and rye from heavy bags slung from our shoulders. Geese and kestrels swept over on their return from the south. Gunnar and Beorn came home each night filthy and content, and Nilse's second daughter was born. They named her Nerta.

There were myself, Elfgifu and Ase to help when her time came. Nilse's labor was nothing to my own for trouble but not easy for all that and a horror to me, new to midwiving and sickened by the blood and mess. I swallowed hard and wouldn't show it to fuel Elfgifu's contempt.

"There, cry out if you must," I whispered to the struggling girl. "It will ease the pain."

She barely responded; crying out would be an acknowledgment of pain, a surrender to it. Nilse would not. "It is not fitting." You could see her plain in this: naked belly distended, body opening, dignity a foolish word, and yet far above all was Nilse herself, bearing pain with the same stoicism demanded of Gunnar. So these women bore themselves when their husbands or sons limped back from Badon or never returned at all. Their fatalism went deep as their sense of justice. They might wash their hair in the blood of their enemies, but they would close about pain and weep alone. Meanwhile there was milking and haying and life to get on with—no nonsense, look sharp, Gwenda.

Only in her final push did the pain triumph briefly. Her neck arched back, something clouded her eyes before Nilse shut them tight against the betrayal. A moment she writhed, just a young woman on the birth rack; then she was hlafdian again, in command, the voice feeble but steady.

"Gwenda, send for my broth."

Which was brought with fawning ceremony by Rat, whose stunted affection went exclusively to women. She presented the cup with a flourish and burbled over the child in my arms. "Ow, mistress, yer got a little girlchild. Ow, ent it the *sweet*est!"

"Yes. Lady Elfgifu will see to your tasks today since I must rest. Go to the fields, Ase. Tell my Lord he has a daughter."

"Of the Woden blood," Ase said proudly.

"But only a girl. Would it were a son."

Elfgifu prodded me. "Wash the child, Gwenda. See the water's not too hot. I will bring grease to rub her."

"Don't just stare at it, Gwenda," Nilse piped reedily from her pillow. "On my word, you're a weird old thing. One would think you'd never seen a child before."

If you'll not show your suffering, Saxon, you'll not see mine. Your child was born alive. Your daughter's mouth opens to feed at your breast, will open to her first word, first kiss. Her hands will hold a needle or a cup, tug at your skirts, clasp a husband and bairn of her own if she lives. They never showed me my daughter, only a glimpse of Imogen bearing away that still bundle before all grew dark again.

Child, why was the mite of you denied me? I would have loved you as much as my crown. Oh, take your hands off my heart. It's old.

Then Elfgifu: "Well, Gwenda! You were told to wash her. I meant today."

"Yes, Hlafdian."

Unlike me but I drank myself to sleep that night, and sleep was tardy in coming. I cursed in whispers and wept on my pallet until Rat worried for me—drunk as Trystan, mourning the lost things, the child who never breathed, the men dead and gone, all of them who touched me once, and perhaps a mislaid destiny or two; raging to kiss or kill in the same breath. Useless of

course, but if you can't understand the need, you're as big a fool as I.

The snow melted and spring was in earnest. All over Icel's land men stirred to visit after winter's isolation, reaffirm their loyalties, drink in fellowship and tend to business.

The watchtower bell clanged in alarm: "Men at the pale!"

In the fields Gunnar, Beorn and the men scanned the visitors who'd appeared from the forest. Nilse called up to the tower.

"What banners?"

"The Prince and Thegn Witgar. Twoscore men."

We heard the distant horn. "Don't answer yet. Let them wait." Nilse spun about and marched to her bower.

"Let their own Prince wait?" I asked Gwyneth. "That's an insult."

"Nae, shrewd it is," Gwyneth lisped in her Lindissi accent. "Not the Aetheling, but there's dispute 'twixt Gunnar and Witgar. Lady'll not sound that horn till Gunnar's snug home."

Gunnar lost no time in gaining the stockade with a dozen farmers in his wake. Before the heavy gates swung closed, I glimpsed other men urging the ox-teams toward us, and Icel's host still crowded about the pale. Nilse met Gunnar just inside the gate, the hint of agitation in the quick motion of handing him the small ax, a weapon with a curious, elongated head. Gunnar thrust it through his belt.

"It seems we feast tonight. Icel's huntsmen have a boar on poles."

Obviously dinner was not the main concern to Nilse. "And?"

"I've called in my men. They'll come armed." His head snapped up to the tower. "Cynred! Sound them in."

Long before the visitors were at the gate, Gunnarsburh was in feverish preparation for war and welcome alike. I plied between hall and kitchen, reminded of Constantine's visit to Camelot, but these English could not dissemble with a fey British flare, only set meager smiles to their lips, mouthed welcomes and waited in their stoic way for fate to decide the outcome.

The entire company was afoot except Icel and Witgar,

who should have been. Neither sat a horse as if they'd ever been introduced to the beast. The long-limbed animals had the Arab look of those Kay bred for Arthur. You bastard, I thought, that's all you took from Badon but a whole skin.

The men who trudged behind their lords bore scars still red from that embattled hill. First after Icel came Bertwold, the old reeve I'd seen at Wicandaen, then the bear-sarks—huge men with faces and bodies so scarred it seemed God had botched them in practice for more finished mortals. They carried swords or heavy war axes on bulging shoulders, and under crested helmets their heads were shaven clean. A mark of distinction: among their kind, hair was only cut after the first slaying of an enemy. Warriors of a special caste, these, dedicated to the honor and glory of their chief and his hall. In theory they owned nothing, disdained property and owed the very meat in their mouths to their sworn lord. So much for theory. In practice they were rich with plunder, swords, ring mail, shields and jewelry, for chiefs must reward loyalty with whatever treasure they asked, and they asked incessantly. Only land was beneath their acceptance. Few now, a dying breed from old Jutland, unfitted for a new time when land was everything. The bear-sarks lumbered through the gates and after them came the real movers of mountains, the common fyrd, the farmer-warriors.

Not impressive at all, bobbing along like the plowmen they were, but these men almost took Badon from the finest archers and cavalry in the world. Sturdy farmers, wind and weather had burnished their skin brown-bronze, much darker than the straw-colored hair that swung in braids down their necks, the battle rents in their short tunics clumsily patched and splashed with mud. Here and there among them the remains of a helmet. Each man carried a spear and a wooden shield covered in ox-hide. With these and little else but a short cloak against the winter, they'd marched from Winchester to Badon in less time than even Arthur had thought possible. And fought without rest through cold that froze the blood on their wounds and spearheads, with few fires for warmth and nothing but downed horses for food. As I watched them then and many times

later, I wondered where common men found such uncommon valor. One must think in English for the answer: each man saw a piece of that trodden mud as his own when they won. And how does one turn them back? You can't, not now. You can only watch those common plowmen as they inch across Britain and turn it into what they presumptuously call England.

Icel's visit was double purposed, his first progress of the year between the holdings of his two thegns and to ease the tensions between them. A prince whose tributaries are at each other's throats doesn't rule much; hence this English way of mending. Bring them together over meat and ale and let the breach be aired under the roof of hospitality where honor forbade fighting.

To Britons like myself, bred to more sedate dining, there wasn't much difference between English hospitality and English mayhem. When the hall was filled and the ale flowing, men wrestled each other in violent friendship or set to with quarterstaves heavy enough to send the contenders back to the board sweating and happy with a few bruises along with a sharpened appetite.

Gunnar's men arrived with dispatch, all knowing the dangers of Witgar's presence. With so many men in the hall, every trestle table was in use, two rows of them the length of the hall, Gunnar's men aligned with his family along the north side, Icel directly across from him in the position of chief guest, Witgar some distance to his right. From my place at the spit with Rat, I could observe them all. Prince Icel's unassuming dignity would have compared well in my own palace, the ease of bearing that stems from a long habit of command, accessible and at the same time slightly apart from men. Big-bodied with gray-flecked beard, answering jest for jest with a booming heartiness that concealed the watchful distance. The public face of a private man. He'd come from Jutland to rule at the suit of these Angles, and so they took their name from his, the Iclingas. Under the long hair that hung over thick brows, Icel never quite relaxed, needing to be one answer ahead of all questions. As for Witgar, perhaps a decade older than Gunnar, his bluff straight-on manner hid nothing. On dismounting in the courtyard, he planted himself square in front of Gunnar,

tawny head tilted slightly to look the taller man in the
eye.

"Am I welcome in your house, Gunnar Eanboldson?
My man Oslac comes in peace to be heard before the
Prince's law."

"Then enter and welcome, Witgar." They clasped
hands.

These, then, were our noble guests. Flanking them
down the torchlit south wall lined with spears and
shields ready to every hand were their gesiths and fyrd-
men, each with a pride and a piece of the land in return
for their service—roaring, guzzling, unshaven and
largely unwashed, shouting lewd invitations to Rat and
me as we turned the spit. Rat responded with her beaky
grin—"Stuff it up yer mum's bum"—without breaking
her rhythm on the spit handle. She enjoyed the attention
and the chance to insult them with a Trinovante blessing
I could barely understand, let alone Iclingas.

On such occasions, Beorn acted as majordomo. He
banged his staff on the dais, waiting for the hubbub to
cease. "The Hlafdian Nilse."

Nilse in best red habit (not her best color) received the
cup from Gwyneth at the ale barrel and carried it the
length of the hall, presenting it to Prince Icel.

"All welcome to our Prince."

Elfgifu set the horn before Witgar. "And all welcome to
Thegn Witgar."

Gunnar stretched his arms forward to his guests. "Let
us be fellows in the feast. May it well become you."

An audible gustatory sigh and bending to the table as
all fell to. I felt sorry for Nilse and Elfgifu; their duty was
to hover behind the guests of honor to see their horns
were never empty or their thick bread trenchers bare of
meat. When the second helpings were carved from the
carcass, Nilse set me to serve the guests myself. I had a
chance to note the subtle wisdom of the seating. Icel was
separated from Witgar by at least ten men, Bertwold
among them, Gunnar across the hall, the distant base of
a conversational triangle. No two could share any
thought not heard by the third. Not that it mattered now.
The hall was awash in good spirits. Men munched and
washed it down, the talk waxed general and reflective.
Passing behind them to serve or pour, I put my trained

ears to work. Amazing what one can learn simply by listening.

". . . Now look! I know—here, woman, fill me up—I know what I heard. The Geats are all over Jutland, there's a war every ten feet. And our folk are getting pushed out. Ask the Prince if you doubt it."

"That means more here if they'll come."

"If? Where else? The Prince'll beg them to come over!"

Won't he just. More bloody Saxons. I passed down the tables. "Meat, sir?"

"Pile it on. Ah, man, what could the plowing priests do but crown Constantine? But what's he rule, *I* say, when every other man's against him?"

"Let them kill each other off. Then we move in."

May he choke on his next swallow, but he was right. I moved down the long table.

"Guenevere? Gott! Old whore must've been eighty if she was a day. Time she died."

"If she did."

"Ah, you're dumb as bread. Where could she be in Britain? Every man knows Guenevere—here, woman, fill me up."

"Right, sir. Here you are."

"Tak, tak. That's right. Saw her myself once in Eburacum. No place in Britain she could hide."

And a fresh serving of meat to the man on Icel's right.

". . . That's what finished Eburacum, Aetheling. No good foot troops. Why did she turn you down?"

"I can't say," Icel admitted. "She was in trouble, mine was a fair offer, service for land. She needed us."

"Two thousand men," the gesith cackled. "What an offer. Where would you find them if she'd said yes?"

Icel rocked silently with the joke. "Where they got combrogi: out of the air. Better the way it turned out. All we have to do is wait."

At the mellowest moment of the feast, Icel signaled Beorn discreetly. The steward rose: "Hear, hear! Bertwold, the scir-reeve of Icel."

Old Bertwold rose creakily, drinking horn in hand. "Let all men attest the deeds of Cuthwine."

At the name a pall fell on conversation like fire doused in water. The hall grew too quickly quiet and men very attentive.

"Cuthwine was bear-sark among the gesiths of Thegn Witgar. Cuthwine was the son of Eafa, the son of Egbert, the son of Ceolward, descended of Baeldaeg, the hero-born son of Woden."

I elbowed Gwyneth next to me. "Well, we know the family now, but who's the man?"

She didn't look very happy about it. "Him that was killed at Badon."

"Oh, what a shame."

"Could be that, lass. Don't be in the middle when things start, that's the quick of it." And she sidled off to the kitchen.

"Great was the renown of Cuthwine," Bertwold intoned to the hushed hall. "His hair was shaven at fifteen years, so soon did enemies feel his might. Many were the battles he fought to add glory to Witgar's hall. Who was it at Badon, when the horses charged, that held the shield wall from breaking? Who but Cuthwine? Who but he in the van when Cerdic took the first strongholds of Maelgwyn?"

This and more in praise of the admirable Cuthwine; yet as Bertwold spoke, I had the uneasy sense it was not mere elegy. Something knotted tighter in my stomach. Nilse's smile was painted on, Elfgifu's eyes everywhere, Gunnar and Beorn polite but wary, no hand very far from a weapon, and not at all reassuring for me to be in the middle of it. Violence was growing like rank weed. My instinct for men I trust without question. Even Arthur said I knew them better than he. Who would ignite the fury? Icel? No, too prudent, against his best interests. Witgar? No, he seemed honest in his greeting to Gunnar. He might break peace in anger, not in craft.

And yet my stomach twisted tighter with the same sick premonition that gripped it once on the field when Agrivaine might have spurred forward to trample Arthur. That was a flash; here it smoldered.

It was late in the feast. I'd gone to refill the cups for Witgar's men when I saw him. Yes. He was the one, a bear-sark stretched lazily on the near side of the bench just across from Gunnar. A man with tight-muscled arms, his shaven head covered with scars. His eyes never left my lord.

The hair rose on the back of my neck.

When I moved to pour for Gunnar and Beorn, I asked. "That bear-sark, the one with the scarred pate."

"I know him," Gunnar acknowledged smoothly, not even looking across at him.

"Oslac," said Beorn. "One of Witgar's gesiths. Brother to Cuthwine."

"Who is more misery dead than ever he was alive," Gunnar observed. "What of him?"

"Don't trust him, my Lord."

"I wouldn't." Something passed between Gunnar and Beorn, the tacit wisdom of squirrels in a convocation of foxes. Neither of them had so much as glanced the while at Oslac. But I was sure now. The man was stillness coiled in the middle of loose movement. If the hall simmered with tension, he was the center.

"See to him," Beorn charged me. "Keep his cup filled."

I made Oslac my special charge thereafter, and I was not Cador's child for nothing. The premonition in my gut was palpable as indigestion.

"What *is* it out there?" I queried Gwyneth in the kitchen. "You can cut the air with a knife."

"Ah, then, part of it's new and part old, and all to do with owning of the land."

The ancient part was familiar, the arrogance of blood and family that ever weakened our tribal unity and even allowed me to turn on Arthur. After the Midlands, it seems, Elfgifu sued to Icel for Eanbold's original lands that Witgar's father wished for himself. A new prince needing no more enemies than he could bar, Icel put the case before the folc-gemot at Wicandaen, the common assembly of his people. The canny gemot awarded the land to Elfgifu outright. I would have called it the weaker course on Icel's part, not knowing the English mind that well. The commons, ever watchful of their own best interests, returned the decision that two thegns were better than one grown too powerful, since each would be check to the other. This was logic a prince could understand, and Icel commended its proponent, young Alfred of Wicandaen, the plump son of a cloth merchant.

At the heart of all this were the cautious English laws of inheritance. War thegns were one thing. Landlords did not become hereditary until the third generation. Ead-

ward would be the first able to pass his land and title alike to his own son in perpetuity. The lands lost to determined Elfgifu would have made Witgar's line the main power under Icel and his sons conceivably elevated to earls; now Eadward looked to those advantages. Like Constantine, Witgar grew up with a sense of destiny crowded aside, though he made the sensible best of it.

In the matter of Oslac, only this need be remembered: as the bear-sark must take up the causes of his lord, so the lord must espouse the grievances of his warrior. It was Badon that cut a new wound and opened the old.

"Gwyneth, this Oslac: what's he in the troubles?"

"Brave as a lion, bright as an ox. But he's no cause to charge Lord Gunnar with shirking."

"Did he that?"

"Did he not!"

"Talk, talk, talk." Old Gytha passed me the pot of lentils I'd asked for the tables. "Get on with your work, Gwenda."

"Aye, we're just out the door now. Don't ask me his cause," Gwyneth tripped on in her Lindissi lisp. "Something in the battle—Rhodri, you lummox! Close the door!"

"Praise the saints!"

Rhodri kicked the door shut, hair wind-tangled over his radiant smile. "Praise Jesu and the saints and any god come to hand. Miracles I've heard and fresh from the speaking of them in the hall."

With Gytha glowering at the mad Welsh jabbering of us, Rhodri capered across the kitchen to sweep up Gwyneth in his iron-mongering arms.

"Ah, sweeting, turn me loose. What is't now?"

"The King." Rhodri glowed.

"What king?"

"What king, says she! *The* King, that was and will be as the songs tell."

Gwyneth went solemn. "Great Arthur?"

"Himself. He's been seen. He lives."

"Gwenda!" Gytha screeched at me. "Mind the pot, it's spilling."

Arthur alive? Impossible. Bedivere saw him die, I buried him at Witrin. There were stories already, there al-

ways are, and I wanted to believe as much as the singers.
I was prompt in seeing to Oslac's wants and listened
carefully to Icel.

"I've seen Arthur," the prince asserted. "I'll see this
new incarnation before I call it sorcery. Where has he
been seen?"

"Cair Legis, they say."

"It must be sorcery. Arthur was troll-born."

"Does he not ride again with Gareth?"

Aye, Gareth. The devil on a horse who destroyed their
supplies at Badon, always a swift shadow behind them
or just where one wouldn't expect him, a hundred eyes
able to see a hundred miles and remember every tree
and blade of grass.

Their fathers knew these demons before they did. To
deny the stories was to say their fathers lied.

"Some of them have been known to," Witgar remarked
dryly.

Woman and wife, I knew Arthur to be marvelously
mortal, but in the bottom drawer of my Christian soul
was the memory of the Faerie girl who menaced me in
the circle of great stones. That terror still haunted reason. Was it true? Could it be?

Think . . . think . . . as Icel turned from hearsay to the
business at hand and men settled to serious debate.
Think: they said he'd been seen at Legis with Gar—

I stopped dead in my tracks. God's Eyes, of course—
Emrys! He had the Pendragon look, more like Arthur
than Kay when I worked the fat off him. The same bearing; at a middling distance even I saw the ghost of one in
the other's flesh.

Then they *did* it. They hit Constantine's infantry and
won through to shut Cair Legis against him. Crowned or
not, Constantine couldn't cage them all forever. His rule
was full of holes as an old cheese and every one of them
seething with my people. I had to get back, give them
something to rally around. In a boiling pride I longed to
confront these goddamned English with the truth of it:
not demons but men, *such* men. Like Gareth, whose vision and memory for detail were no more demonic than
hard work would make them. He laid objects on a table,
studied them, then turned his back and tried to re-

member the nature, shape and position of each. Years of practice.

But listen to the English now, to the reasons and motives of men untouched by sophistication or the subtleties of education, deep-dyed with the conviction that they were pitted against devils whenever they faced Arthur. His name and others dear to me plucked different chords in the English soul that drowned out their plodding common sense. More than one traced his descent from a god as I did (and believed it with less misgiving). Why shouldn't they believe if my own mind still held such unswept corners? If the ghost of Arthur ramped through my own hungry dreams, let him gallop through theirs with all his spectral lot behind him—*I* wouldn't tell.

The feast was done, the firepits down to embers. Rat scuttled into the kitchen with a good chunk of boar and a pitcher of ale as her booty. Once more I refilled Oslac's horn.

"May it well become the ring-shirt winner."

I took my place by the firepit as Icel said, "Now I will hear of division among my Lords that it may be healed."

Witgar rose with an air of formality. "Aetheling, I urge grievance as Lord to Oslac who was the brother of Cuthwine. Against Thegn Gunnar."

"And the charge?"

"Cowardice."

I stiffened. Among my own lords that word would be fire in tinder. Such as Agrivaine have scarred men for even hinting of it, but neither Gunnar nor Beorn even blinked. The hall grew even quieter.

"The particulars?"

"That on the last day at Badon, when my gesith Cuthwine stood in defense of King Cerdic, Cuthwine was sore wounded. Thegn Gunnar might have come to his aid but refused and so let Cuthwine die."

Icel raised his voice to the hall at large. "Who witnessed this?"

Oslac and four of his near companions stood up. "I do, and these with me."

"And the plaint, Thegn Witgar?"

"That on the proving of this charge, Thegn Gunnar be bound to pay the wergild of Cuthwine in silver or land."

Ah, *there* the quick of it. By custom Witgar must support his man. By the same custom he stood to profit from it.

Icel spoke with slow deliberation. "Oslac, you have honor in my court, but I can't allow you as a witness. You are too near in blood and will profit."

Oslac seemed to expect this. "And these with me?"

"They will be allowed to speak."

Oslac dropped back onto the bench, yawning. "Fair enough."

Icel searched the hall. "Who will speak first in the charge?"

Next to Oslac a gross-bodied warrior raised his hand. "I, Offa."

"If you saw what happened, speak truly."

"We formed a square in Cerdic's defense. Bedivere broke through the shield wall alone, calling for Cerdic to come and fight. Oslac killed the horse under him, but Arthur and his Dobunni were just behind, and the whirl of fighting took me away from Cuthwine. It was a mess, Aetheling. No square any more, just men and mud. Cuthwine and two others went at Bedivere. I don't know what happened to them, but all of a sudden it was Cuthwine alone. I fell under a horse myself."

"Did you hear Cuthwine call for Gunnar?"

"Clearly, Aetheling."

The men with Offa repeated the tale with little variety. Brave Cuthwine was pitted against sorcery. "That sword of Bedivere's—half the time you couldn't even see it, like a windmill in a storm."

And no one else could help Cuthwine? Ah, who? Who else was left whole and standing. But they all heard him call for Gunnar. And where was Gunnar then?

"On my hands and knees in the mud," Gunnar answered. "And the mud was a foot deep."

Oslac roused himself, rubbing his eyes. "Sorcery or not, Cuthwine could have felled Bedivere if you'd helped."

Gunnar shook his head wearily. "Your brother was a brave man but never very swift."

"You could have helped. You're niddering!"

"The charge is already made." Icel raised a cautioning

hand. "Offa? You others, is it your opinion Gunnar could have helped Cuthwine and simply refused?"

"It is, Aetheling."

"Thegn, you hear the charge and the witnesses. Will you gainsay them?"

"My Lord, I do." Gunnar frowned over the picture in his mind. "We hadn't eaten much that last day. All of us frozen, not strong enough to keep up the attack, and Arthur hitting us with those damned horses. We had to go to defense. Aetheling, you sent us off the first level to defend Cerdic. The archers and stone-slingers were at us on the way down. I took a stone in the shoulder."

Beorn spoke up loyally: "His sword arm."

And Nilse. "My husband yet bears the mark like a knot under his skin."

"I make no excuse for myself," Gunnar demurred. "No colder or hungrier than any man there. And no less, Oslac. We saw Arthur and the Dobunni forming to hit us again. Right at us, our square. Then Bedivere came charging through the shield wall alone to get at Cerdic. Arthur right after him. We couldn't stop them. Someone—Oslac, he says—knocked down Bedivere's horse."

It caught Oslac in the middle of a yawn. "Uh—I did. Brained it. Got knocked down and my leg twisted under me. That damned combrogi devil landed on his feet."

Of course, Englishman. Gareth drilled that into them day after week after year. The instant a horse so much as stumbled, the rider's feet were out of the stirrups so he wouldn't be rolled on.

"When the Dobunni came through with Arthur," Gunnar went on, "it was all we could do to get out of the way. Beorn went down. I thought he was dead."

His steward nodded with potent understatement. "So did I."

"Then another horse hit me hard and knocked me down. That's when Cuthwine called. My eyes were full of mud; all I could see was Cuthwine trying to back up from Bedivere in that damned sucking mud, and Bedivere's arms just a blur."

As with Arthur, this was the unspoken misery of Badon, a separate hell beyond war. Whatever pictures men recalled, they were all caked in mud, soaked in freezing rain.

"He was too *fast*, Oslac. Cuthwine had no chance, with or without me. I tried to get up—"

"He did," Beorn attested. "On my honor, he tried to get to Cuthwine."

"I couldn't even feel my hands or feet by then. Then . . . it was like thunder and a great spraying of mud—there was Gareth and the combrogi. Don't ask from where, they weren't even on the field before. But they rolled right over us. My helmet's still dented where the beast's hoof hit it. That's all I knew until Beorn laid me down at your feet, Aetheling."

"Not so!" Oslac denied him. "Even wounded, Cuthwine could have defeated him with a little help."

"Oslac—no." Gunnar wagged his head wearily. "Your brother was never swift. He was muscle-bound. You could predict every move he made. Perhaps it's true the Gryffyn has spirit arms. What I could see . . . was not like any kind of fighting I know. He is not made like other men. His arms work in a queer fashion."

It became apparent to me that this awe of combrogi among the English amounted to an unguessed national resource. However, a fish always looks bigger beneath the water. Before laying your skepticism aside, let me lift Bedivere from the distorting waves.

First, his sword was longer, better tempered and balanced than the English *spatha*. Second, from his earliest days he'd developed a style of attack and defense uniquely suited to his lanky, long-muscled body, particularly in the placing of his feet for balance. With those dainty, circling steps, Bedivere moved not merely in response to his opponent but through a planned series of moves. For him it was simply second nature, because he was not only supple but double-jointed.

Oh, you say. If it's only that. Of course: that and thirty-five years of practice.

Icel announced to the hall at large, "The charge has been heard and answered. What else in this matter before we render judgment?"

"This, Aetheling." Elfgifu had possessed herself in patience thus far; more was beyond her jealous sense of rights. "The root of this trial is not battle or bravery. That's a mask over the truth. It's not honor at stake, but

land, our land that Witgar's coveted since you restored it to me."

"That would be a separate cause if I made it one," Witgar argued. "And a fair one. My family were working it two years when you came with your demand."

"Will our prince give me judgment?" Oslac demanded. "Will he reckon Thegn Gunnar accountable for the wergild of Cuthwine?"

"Oh, enough." Gunnar's fist shivered the board, rattling the dishes as he rose, angry. "I now speak as host to this gathering. With respect, Aetheling, my mother speaks truth. Witgar knows what he came for. This charge is absurd, Oslac. You know your brother was never a match for the like of Bedivere. He was lost, a hooked fish. No one could have helped him."

Oslac sat upright, legs coiled under him. The movement didn't escape Gunnar; his thumb hooked casually in his belt near the ax. "Eanboldson, you lie."

"The gods spare me bear-sarks. You were never worth your keep."

Oslac shot off the bench, spear to hand—swift, but as he brought it to his shoulder, he wobbled slightly. In that moment, Gunnar's ax was clear of his belt. His arm whirled, the ax flew and plowed deep into Oslac's shoulder. An eye-blink: I hadn't even time to be shocked. Oslac fell back on the bench, pawing at the ax. There was a general surge of men on both sides of the hall, shields up, spears leveled. And Icel, nimble for all his years, vaulted over the bench into their midst, freezing them with his command.

"Hold! Don't move. Not—one—man." He turned on Oslac with withering scorn. "You witless fool. You have no more rein on your temper than a boy. If this were my hall, I'd hang you. Witgar!"

Poised with his sword, Witgar lowered it. "This was not my wish, Aetheling."

"No one said it was. But take your men hence from Gunnarsburh. I'll leave your gesith to your judgment. Keep him outside my pale or he's dead. And all of you, listen."

Icel turned about the hall, speaking to every man there. "This matter is not ended. I'll make no judgment

among tempers like these. I'll wait a cooler time. Witgar, go."

Among English it was deep insult for a thegn and his company to be dismissed from such a gathering. Their annals, however, are as full of treachery as ours. Icel put one of his men in the tower to watch Witgar's torches out of sight in the west, and I caught a hurried fragment of the prince's concern as I passed him and Gunnar in the hall.

". . . Right about the bear-sarks, they're practical as plowing with bulls, but don't do anything further to provoke Witgar, you hear me? You struck in self-defense, but you walk softly until you hear from me. That's a command."

"Ja, Aetheling."

"I can't take sides in this. I'll put it to the gemot when they meet and set Brand himself to argue Oslac's case. That's fair as can be. Good night, we'll speak in the morning."

With Icel's men sleeping in the hall, we servants were squeezed out into the byre. I was carrying my bedding and a torch to light my way when I almost collided with Gunnar striding in agitation from the tower.

"Who's there?"

"Gwenda, sir. You'll not to bed?"

"Who'll sleep tonight?"

"You think they'll be back?"

"Not with the Prince here. Anyway, it's not Witgar so much as Oslac. Bear-sarks . . . the less wit the more pride."

I saw his strained face in the torchlight, the look so familiar to me: a man who constantly had to think and decide for more souls than his own.

"Then caution, as your Prince commands. Let them be the ones to break the peace. Then all men will know just how much of this is honor and how much profit."

"You're a wise woman, Gwenda. If the ruling's against me, I owe more than I can pay without selling land. Witgar profits either way."

"You think he urged Oslac to attack you?"

"I doubt it." Gunnar grinned sourly. "Oslac's stupid enough for that without help. I was lucky, though. If he

hadn't lost his balance . . . did you see? He jumped up, then it was as if he'd left most of himself on the bench."

"Well, sir, he did—in a manner of speaking. You set me to keep his horn filled. So I did, and every draft as full of lavender and chamomile as could be without him tasting of it. He was yawning when the trial began. When he leaped up his head didn't yet know the rest of him was falling asleep."

"What? Oh, no, no, *no*." As always the laughter robbed Gunnar of his tension, sounding very young in the darkness. "Wait until Beorn hears this: fire-eating Oslac hamstrung by one small woman with a cup. Saved by Welsh intuition."

"British, sir."

"Ja, ja. Good night, Gwenda." And yet he lingered in my torchlight, his amusement subsided to a sputtering. "You . . . you're worth your price."

"I try, sir."

"And I try, Gwenda. I'm not a hero like my father, just a farmer."

"And Lady Elfgifu has a ponderous sense of destiny."

"She does—and she's right. If you don't push forward, you'll be pushed back. She's been pushed all she can take. For myself, sometimes I wonder if I'd care who ruled so long as there was peace—Rome, Arthur, no mind—so I could plow my land and raise my children and to hell with the rest."

"My husband often wished the same." Easily said. Did he really? Did I? We were both ridden by genius under the cruel bit of ambition.

Gunnar moved closer to me. "Your husband must have been very content with you, Gwenda."

"Now and then. War and peace and war again, like most marriages."

"I've never had much to do with slaves. Rhodri and Gwyneth, I grew up with them; they're like family. But sometimes I look at you and I wonder what I've bought. I try to imagine you in that Castle Hull, living with your husband."

I didn't expect the searching tenderness in his eyes.

"I'll speak to my lady about your due. It's time. Good night, Gwenda." He closed strong fingers around my arm in parting. I felt that pressure long after everyone

else snored around me in the byre, restless on my pallet until I bored even myself: you ludicrous antiquity, pack it in. He was just being kind.

The longing surprised me. My body felt better, stronger and tougher ever since letting go of youth and resolving itself to what is called middle age. But it yearned after its old purpose more achingly than ever. And Gunnar's body evoked a sweet, disturbing memory. . . .

Silly bitch, go to sleep.

March rained into April and warmed to May. Earth began to show her reviving spirits in flushes of green, red and blue as grass and flowers put their trust in spring. The earth felt better than we did; our watchmen were tense and vigilant in the tower, an additional rider on a hard-grudged horse picked his way through the fields and forests between Gunnar's land and Witgar's, ready to dash home at the first sign of men mustering to march our way.

The men went armed to the fields, and I felt better with a knife in my belt. Gunnar's shepherds herded their flocks into the stockade in one great bleating multitude that sounded as disagreeable as it smelled, and, dawn to dusk, we sheared those stinking sheep, storing the dirty brown wool in great baskets, eye and ear always cocked toward the forest as the cry went up again and again—

"Watchman, how in the west?"

"All clear!"

Pigs snuffling about the stockade yard, a gaggle of hens lurching about the kitchen door on the small chance of Gytha's benevolence. Little Eadward bedight with wooden sword and buckler, charging the sheared sheep with a shrill battle cry, and the damned gate open for the witless creatures to amble where they would—

"Eadward!"

The charge halted; Eadward turned, jiggling to get on with his war. "Ja, Gwenda?"

"Didn't your father say to leave the sheep alone?"

"Ach, I'm just playing."

"Gwenda?" Elfgifu planted in the entrance to the hall, beckoning. "Stop loafing and come here."

"Aye, mistress. Go practice, Eadward. But spare the sheep. They've not deserved the holocaust of you."

Eadward galloped off to fresh conquests. I went to Elfgifu.

"Lady Nilse will speak to you in the hall. Come here." As usual, not a request but a command. "Let me see your neck. The collar doesn't chafe any more. I said you'd get used to it. Come."

She led me into the hall where Nilse and Ase sat carding some of the new wool with iron combs. Little Nerta slumbered in her cradle. Nilse was still heavy around the middle with loose fat from her pregnancy, barely noticeable under her gown, much fuller than a British woman would think fashionable, but then so was Nilse. And she'd be pregnant again ere the summer was out.

"Gwenda, I have good report of you from my lord. You don't lie abed when called in the morning. You haven't shirked in the fields or stolen."

"She uses too much water to wash with," Elfgifu complained. "Rat says she washes all over every day."

Which was a source of bafflement to Rat but a Roman habit I'd not relinquish. Winter saw some lapses, but the weather permitted it now. Nilse was apparently as concerned as Rat.

"A bad habit, Gwenda. Not only wasteful of water, but it leaves the body helpless against the harm of night air."

Ase bobbed her head over her carding. "Catch your death."

"If not from me." Elfgifu prodded me in the ribs. I flared back at her, tired of it.

"Oh, shit! Leave off me. I work from dawn to dark. I carry my own water. What do you want of me?"

"Enough, both of you. This is useless." Without rising, Nilse's voice turned hard as Gunnar's in the hall with Oslac. "I was about to commend you on your quick learning of our tongue. Save that you favor certain expressions more suited to cowherds than a woman of my household. You are immodest, Gwenda. For that reason, I find it hard to believe, as Mother says, that you were ever a lady in your own right."

I bit back the answer. They should have heard the High King of Britain in an inspired moment.

"If you must curse at something, do it in your own language and not where my children can hear you."

"Hlafdian, I will try to mend that."

"Good." Nilse put it aside as forgotten. "Now, a good portion of the kitchen gardens beyond the wall is fallow. Measure out ten paces by thirty and plant what you will. My lord said that was your wish."

So it was. I loved the earth and the feel of it on my hands and bare feet. I reveled in the warmth of summer and the hardy new strength that supported me all day in the fields. Hard, a punishment to my body at first, but now I felt ten years younger. And God knows, it was better than being under the constant eye of Elfgifu.

"*Mange tak*, Hlafdian."

"No thanks needed, Gwenda. It's the law. Your laet allowance like the *sester* of beans last winter. Rat will take hers in pence and corn and stay in the kitchen. You'll have your measure of ground."

"And sell your harvest in Wicandaen fair. What will you plant?" Ase asked.

What would I not? Already the plot sprouted in my imagination, took fire in blazes of color. "Flowers, Hlafdian."

"You can't eat flowers," Ase said patiently.

"Welsh ninny wouldn't know that." Elfgifu growled her contempt. "Never went hungry in her life."

Ase said it again as to a backward child. "You can't eat flowers."

Nor could I see much beauty in a turnip. I set about cultivating my own jot of Britain, singing to the spade and hoe. I turned the ground, broke and raked it fine, manured carefully, then went to the woods and fields for my cuttings when there was time, searching for what I needed after the long gray months, a feast of color. I parted the grass or thicket and glutted my starved sight on crowfoot and columbine, starwort and weather-glass. My gardens at Camelot were seeded from the islands off Land's End where summer comes early and warm. These small blossoms were not so lush, but they would serve me.

"What've you got there, Gwenda?"

I put the cutting in its linen binding into Gunnar's hands. "A treasure, Lord."

"Crowfoot? They grow all over."

"And how often do folk look to see how lovely they are?"

Gunnar would see: the tiny thread-thin stems, the exquisite sculpture of the small yellow petals. He held them under my chin so the sun reflected their yellow on my skin.

"You like butter, Gwenda."

I clapped my hands at the sunlit memory. "Oh, my mother used to do that! And I'd wonder and wonder where crowfoot got the magic to tell."

His hand touched mine as the flower passed between us. Whatever Gunnar prayed to, this small life was his faith. Then Beorn waved and jerked his head toward the trees and the patrol rider breaking clear of them. Gunnar forgot all else.

"*Hael!* How in the west?"

"All clear!"

Through May into June my little garden took shape. Many of the cuttings died. Then, as the roots quickened in the soil, like sight returning to the blind, I saw the colors come lush and bright in the nurtured soil, until I could stand at the edge of my creation like God admiring Eden, and wallow in color. I made little Edytha a crown of catchflies and weather-glass that she wore until they wilted.

"There, my queen of summer! White for a maiden, red for the woman's blood that'll not be long in coming to you, and yellow . . . for the beauty of it."

Even Rat caught her breath at the unfurled hues of my garden. "Lor God, ent it fine! Give's some for the kitchen? Dark as the inside of an arse-hole in there."

And yet there was one pale ivory flower that wouldn't grow transplanted. I found it in the mulch laid down by a rotted log near the edge of the forest. Only one cutting; nowhere else could I find more. I nursed it like a child and fretted over it in the midst of plenty like the lost sheep of the Hebrew parable.

"Come on. If I can live here, you can thrive in soil better than the woods. *Live*, you little bastard."

But it wouldn't; it withered and died in the rich soil as my own child in my body. All the women of my line could bear, all of us ramped in a riot of getting, queen-god-

desses all. All but me. It reminded me bitterly of my failures. God and Christ, why this to me? Any sow of a peasant woman could lie down and spit out children like apple seeds, why couldn't I? Am I so barren that even my loving hands with all their patience and care can't make this midge of color breathe?

God walked in Eden and saw it wouldn't work.

"It's only a flower, Gwen."

So I looked up in frustration from the rows of color at Camelot to see Lancelot, loyal and adoring, the day he opened his heart to me, the day I needed it so.

"Only a flower? Don't you see? Can't I make anything of my *own*?"

And I turned to him, into him, suddenly confined and cramped by the garden walls, wanting to run naked as seed like Morgana until the grass grew on me and birds nested in my hair and the very pelt of the wild wolf grew between my legs. Turning, hurting, wanting into his arms that had always been waiting for me. And he whispered the things I'd always known he would—tortured, honorable Lancelot—and now I let him because someone had to love me then and give me something of my own.

Faintly from inside the walls: "Watchman, how in the west?"

How in the west? I reached for the failed flower and pulled it out by its dead roots. There are sermons in stones, and any faith that has endured in my island will tell you that all of existence can be read in small wherever you seek it. I breathed deep of the fragrant west wind, felt it beckon me.

No. I couldn't live away from my soil any more than this flower. At least it knew what it needed as birds knew when to fly home. So did I.

I found a time when Gytha was out grumbling among the hens in the yard to draw Gwyneth and Rat into a corner of the kitchen. "Here's the flowers you wanted. Listen, both of you. I need you. I'm going out."

They stared at me. "Out?" Gwyneth wondered.

"Out of here. Home. Across Humber to Castle Hull."

Rat wailed, stricken. "Yer bloody carnt!"

"I have to, Rat. I can't stay here."

"Anyone sees yer, it's right back here."

"You'll not find a better master anywhere." Gwyneth tried to soothe me. "Whoever caught you could sell you to worse."

No use making either understand. To them slavery and life were one inseparable burden. "I'll need food, Rat. Meat, bread, a few of the new carrots. And some money."

"Ow, ent that just your style," Rat recoiled. "Take my last penny'n get me whipped for helpin yer go off."

"You little miser, you had a good half-pound on the block last winter and not spent a farthing of it."

"Well, what'm I gonner have in my age if I frow it away like this?"

"Christ, woman! You'll have it back tenfold. That's a promise before God. Tuppence'll do me. I'll give you back an English shilling or two sesterces Brit, but *help* me."

They both hung unsure, frightened of my audacity. Gwyneth threw a nervous glance at the kitchen door. "I've a few pence, Gwenda."

"God bless, and you'll see it back."

But Rat caught at my hand. "Don't try it, Gwenda. Don't go."

"I've got to, Rat."

"Please."

"What's it to you? Gwyn's money, not even your own food you're stealing. Selfish bitch, what do you lose?"

For an anguished moment, Rat wrestled with something she couldn't articulate herself. Then she flung away my hand with a hiss of disgust. "Right, then. Garn! Garn, if yer want to."

"You'll put my food?"

"Right 'nough," she said to the wall. "And yer can cuntin well choke on't."

Possible or not, the thing was to be done. Not more than thirty miles to Humberside; I could manage that in a day and a half with good weather, avoiding men wherever I met them. From Hull the word could go in secret to Emrys and Gareth and even dear Lancelot: make ready and wait for me.

A horse was out of the question since one of Beorn's men slept in the byre in summer as relief watch for the tower, but it was not unusual for me to go early to the fields. I waved gaily to the tower watch and hurried out, forded the brook where I stopped to fill my flask, then

headed for the forest. As soon as the trees covered me, I made a wallet of my cloak, tied it to my shoulder with a length of cord, tucked up my skirts and began to run.

Months of walking in the furrows had strengthened my legs but I ran more that day than in my whole life. When the forest broke into downs, I moved faster, slowing only when the trees closed about me again. After three miles I was ready to drop, and fell down to rest by a fallen tree. Panting, heart pounding, trying not to panic, to keep my thoughts clear. The sun was still low. I'd gone out a good half-hour and more before Gunnar went to the fields. He might miss me by now but it would be another hour at least before anyone noticed my absence and another after that before their suspicions woke. With best luck, Gunnar might think Nilse detained me at home—no, the rounds of Gunnarsburh were too well fixed for that. I had perhaps an hour, no more.

Up, girl.

Fear smothered fatigue, kept it at bay and drove me on across the few open spaces and plunging back through the woods. Breath began to burn in my throat, then whistle and rasp. When I fell down again, I lay with my face in the cool turf, nothing but a harsh gasping.

I heard the dog then, the deep baying of a wolfhound. Bane, Gunnar's favorite. I didn't have my extra hour. They were on me already with Bane hot on my scent to bring me down. I bolted away through the trees, floundered upstream through a brook before climbing out to pour the water from my boots and hurry on. Behind me I heard Bane belling his discovery of my last resting place, then sporadic barking as he puzzled at the disappearance of the trail by the brook. The sound of him grew more distant, but as I sank down at the edge of a clearing it neared again.

No time for rest, I'd never get up. Only a few deep breaths for my pounding heart, then I launched myself across the clearing toward the trees on the other side. As I hurtled into their cover I threw one glance back to see Bane break out of the forest behind me, high-belling his triumph. Bane was bred for wolves. His long muzzle and jaws could close over and snap the forearm of a large man. Rearing on his long hind legs, his head was high as Gunnar's; in one stride at full run, he could fly over fif-

teen feet without touching ground. He couldn't climb a tree after me, but he'd wait at the bottom, a baying beacon until Gunnar came. When I heard him crash into the trees again, only seconds behind me now, I turned on him with my kitchen knife, readier than him to kill and all the more apt for my terror.

Then Bane cleared the last thicket and in one bound knocked me over. Rolling under him, I put my arm up to guard. His jaws closed on it. I plunged the knife into his underbelly and ripped toward me. Bane's worrying growl tore into a high scream, but he held on. Death instinct made him loose the arm and go for my throat. I felt his hot, meaty breath as the jaws lunged in.

The slave collar saved me. Bane's fangs lacerated my neck but their killing force closed on iron. An instant's grace, no more. Before the dog could grip higher, I drove the knife in again under his ribs. The fury went out of the hound as he fell away, whimpering. He tried to rise as I did, staggering, lurched a few aimless steps, then toppled over on his side. I backed away to run again—

—And saw Gunnar sitting his horse a few yards away. "Don't run, Gwenda. It's over."

"For Bane, not me." Taking a deep breath, I dodged into thicket and bramble, letting them tear at me, but driving on. When I broke out, scratched and bleeding, there was Beorn, mounted and waiting. Neither vindictive nor angry, just waiting.

"No chance, Gwenda. Give it up."

Still I ran, by sheer will and desperation now. I heard Gunnar and Beorn shouting behind me, then a crashing nearer through the brush—and I went down as my legs simply stopped working. I lay there on my face, gasping, run to earth like a fox, not even caring when I felt my fingers opened and the knife taken. I turned over with a huge effort and panted up at Elfgifu, "You'd best kill me now, Saxon."

"You're lucky someone didn't."

Then Beorn came out of the brush and dismounted. Gunnar lifted me up. The force of him was firm but not rough. He saw my tattered condition, the blood, the torn skin under my collar. It troubled his eyes.

"Why, Gwenda? You weren't mistreated. You live as one of us. Why?"

I croaked at him, "Your own kind cut their wrists in slavery. Is it so hard to understand in me?"

"I don't understand you at all," he said unhappily. He went to his saddle and unhooked the small whip as Beorn tethered me to a tree and tore my gown down the back and pushed it clear of my shoulders. I twisted around to see Gunnar standing between Beorn and Elfgifu with a stain of disgust belying his impassive expression. He said something to Elfgifu in a quick murmur, then handed her the whip.

So I'd descended all the way from the day Bedivere brought me news of Arthur's death, through all the loves and loss and betrayal to this tree. I balled my fists tight and tensed for it. When the first blow fell, the world exploded in pain and I screamed in helpless fury. The second cry was mere animal agony, then no more resistance, only a prayer that it would end, as I writhed against the tree. All the gods deserted me, Christ and Epona, and left me in agony, biting my lips, wondering if I could stand one more blow and knowing I couldn't.

It was brief, five or six strokes, maybe more, I didn't know; only that with all their fire they were less than Elfgifu's arm could do.

"You vengeful bitch. You enjoyed this. You've hated my insides since the first day."

Elfgifu cut the thongs that held me. "No, I didn't enjoy it. I thought I might, but no." She understood no more of it than her son. But I saw something in her not there before. Perhaps respect. "Now you know how we felt in the Midlands. All we could do and still it wasn't enough."

They put me up behind Gunnar and tied my hands around his waist, and I wept in silence against the torture in my back, arms and neck with my face tight against Gunnar's tunic and the male muscle beneath.

"Why?" he kept wondering as we rode back. Once he reached back and patted my leg. "Your flowers would miss you."

Rat begged Nilse that she might tend me, which was a surprise. Rat slipped about, did no more than she must, stole whatever was not nailed down and studiously avoided notice. But when they brought me tottering before Nilse, little Edytha mooning up at me like a cap-

tured dragon, Rat pushed forward from the knot of servants and bobbed her frizzy head to the hlafdian.

"Mistress, let me tend her. Got the poultice down kitchen'n I'll be ever so soft wiv her."

And she was. Rat worked the poultice for an hour, stopping whenever she detected my smothered discomfort.

"Poor girl, all scratched up. Shouldn't've put that filthy dog on yer."

"As the English say, Bane's gone to the crow's banquet."

"You could've too. Lor, I'm glad yer back safe."

"I could have made it, Rat. Another hour's start."

Rat lay down close beside me, her fingers moving over my torn back. "No, love."

"I'm not weak as you."

"No mind. Soon's they missed yer, I knew yer wouldn't. They said there was men skulkin round the norf boun'aries what'd sell yer off or worse. Do yer, cut yer froat, leave yer dead. And more now what wiv old Witgar slippin round."

"How would they know which way I went?" I caught her thin wrist and twisted hard. "You bloody little filth, you told them."

"Ow! Don't, Gwenda. No, I never—"

"You told them. What did they give you for that, an extra piece of bread at breakfast?"

"No—"

"How much, Rat? *How much?*"

"Nuffin." Rat twisted away from me, stung by something I didn't yet understand. "Din gimme nuffin. Din ask. Just like you ent never knowed nuffin, never did."

Rat turned away from me, stiff with indignation. I didn't have the strength to hit her, just lay back down on my stomach in misery. "May God strike you dead and not in a hurry."

"It weren't for nuffin, damn you." Rat slammed the cover on the poultice and pushed it aside. "I told yer not to go. Begged yer, din I?" Her voice went suddenly smothered. "Din I, Gwenda?"

"Jesus. Why, Rat?"

When she saw I was quiet again, she stretched out next to me. "I mean—once I had this friend, only friend ever. Cilla, up Londin'um. We had a room down Mifra."

Only half listening, some thought was needed to connect Mifra with the temple of Mithras near Thames.

"Cilla'd work quayside, I'd go out Ludgate Street, but we always come home'n stayed together after, all snugged up in the same bed. Just like you'n me, only better, good blankets'n straw. And I said: Cilla? Yer won't ever go off from me, will yer? And she tooken oath, she did. She took oath on the holiest thing she had what was a magic fingernail from Jesu Christ, that she'd never leave me."

I wasn't disposed to kindness just then. "Holy fingernails! That's a business in Londinium. She could've bought a dozen."

"No mind, she swore on't. And then she run off. Run off wiv a fat miller what said he were gonner marry her."

Rat fell silent while I weltered in my pain.

"Few days later, old dead wagon come down Ludgate like always. Never looked at it much. Almost din see her. Never knew who nor why. They put her in the field outside east gate. That's how Cilla fetched up dead, just like what yer would've," Rat ended her tale, muffled and wounded. "So don't ask what I got, yer mind? Women ent all selfish like you."

Somewhere in misery I found the wisdom not to say anything. We all reach out to someone somewhere. Rat was more giving in that respect than many women I've known. She called me friend, and if I couldn't be more, at least I no longer had the arrogance and stupidity to despise her reaching. That part of me that Arthur always fought was wearing away of itself. Snake sheds skin, flower opens as it grows, wisdom quiets to silence. I learned pity of pain.

The Honored Fellow from Wicandaen and Other Wonders

t was in my mind to escape again, though the will to it lessened imperceptibly as the reasons to stay increased. Nilse conceived again late that summer, far too soon after Nerta's birth. Weak and ill, of course she'd perish before she complained. Gunnar was always considerate, but there'd never before been such a need to leave her untouched. They were young and used to the frequent habit of each other, now curtailed. When bed is good, everything else in a marriage sorts itself out. When not, nothing does. Gunnar was on edge, as much concern for Nilse as deprivation. Sitting next to him on the wagon seat, jolted against him from time to time on the rutted road to Wicandaen fair, I knew it had been a long time for me as well. I was lonely and needed a man, always more the Goddess' child than Christ's in that respect. There was more to it than that. Being clay but Divinely fired, there always is.

Wicandaen fair was the cardinal event of the year among the Iclingas. Folk separated by distance and winter met and passed the homely news that bounded and measured their lives: who was hand-fasted or plighted, who was born, who died. The wool boats were

sailing from Eburacum again, and it was true about the strife in Jutland. More home folk might well be coming over soon. But all tidings paled beside the dispute between Gunnar and Oslac, and at Wicandaen I learned how important it was, wondering in my Brit soul how the doings of lords could be of such moment to peasants.

"Your notion of a peasant doesn't exist among English," Trystan told me once. Quite true.

Prince Icel had a machinery not available to Arthur or myself or any British ruler since the days of the Roman senate. Where we could need wile, diplomacy, personal loyalties and ultimately force, Icel had law that functioned not only from his court down but from the ground up. I couldn't grasp it at first, plying Gunnar for light in darkness.

"You mean the peasants will say how lords must abide?"

"No, not really, but Icel's shrewd."

Shrewd to this extent: rather than rule for one of his client lords against another, he passed the matter to the folc-gemot, trusting them for a decision to the general good, reserving the final word to himself. If the litigant ruled against chose not to abide, he was "unhold," outlawed and subject to penalty. Thus Icel ruled with order rather than a kennelful of dogs at one another's throats.

The gemot was composed entirely of men below the rank of thegn, men from Icel's court, Witgar's and Gunnar's, and tradesmen of no holding at all. As they gathered in their dilatory fashion near the scaffold where I was sold, the outcome seemed foregone to me. Those of Witgar would find for him, Gunnar's for their own lord. The cheapmen of Wicandaen I discounted; they'd only echo the men from court, but I had a great deal to learn yet about the English. The power of verbal persuasion was highly prized among them, as in their popular game of setting each other riddles. The man of wit and potent argument was respected as much as the war leader; this was part of the schismatic nature of their minds. War was a glory and the subject of sagas, but order and profit were more enduring realities.

In the folc-gemot were men whose minds leaned more to trade and the conditions that secured it than to any lord.

Wicandaen stank in winter, in high summer the odor of fish mingled now with the enticement of baked, brewed or roasted wares set out on the rickety stalls. There were bolts of woven wool from my own city, ells of crisp linen and whole-made cloaks, Frankish jewelry, terra cotta from the Middle Sea ports, pungent spices, new leather for boots. With a meat pie in one hand, Gunnar allowed the shoemaker to measure him for a pair and asked my advice on colors for Nilse, who'd stayed at home with Elfgifu this year.

"What think you for my lady? The red?"

"I'd say not, sir. Hlafdian is too fair. It won't do her justice. Blue will better set her off."

So it did, Gunnar taking credit for it with Nilse. "The blue will better set you off, *min elskede.*"

Wicandaen strained at the seams with humanity as the fair progressed. Witgar was there in strength, and Oslac, favoring his hurt shoulder under a rich green tunic and cloak hung with gold chain. Icel's men strode about, in and out of the dingy tavern, guzzling yellow-foamed beer from great wooden bowls, but everywhere the gossip was of the trial.

"All they talk about," Rat mumbled, stuffing cheese into her mouth from a nearby stall. "Lor, that's good. Have some, love? Been down tavern; the men got no mind for nuffin else. Except the usual."

And since the usual was Rat's trade, she'd martyred herself in a thorough bath and crushed herbs and secured Gunnar's absentminded permission to return to the tavern.

"Look at her, will you?" Gwyneth purred as Rat twitched invitingly through the men toward the tavern door. "Won't she buy one bowl, have eight bought for her and come back a shilling richer. Rhodri'd better not moon after that."

"Rhodri? *Ach-y-fi*, the dear man's better taste."

"And not all in his mouth." She bent a last ominous look on Rat. "Just the same . . . oh, see, Gwenda! Hold this."

Gwyneth snatched a remnant of tow linen from a stall kept by a fat, rumpled cheapman and draped it over me, taking a tuck here and there. "I do believe I could make a

grand shift an it's cheap enough. Mine's more holes than linen."

Late in the afternoon the horn summoned from the scaffold, old Bertwold thumped with his staff, and the folc-gemot of the Iclingas convened. Although all three lords attended, they did not preside in this court. Bertwold held that place as "law-speaker" or arbiter on points of legality and protocol. Men sworn to Witgar clumped on one side, Gunnar's on another, separated by the seedy cheapmen from Wicandaen who kept looking about, searching for someone and very relieved when he arrived—portly, genial and shambling—to share some hearty joke with the men around him. I recognized him as the tradesman who sold Gwyneth her linen.

"Alfred the cheapman." Gunnar waved cordially to him.

"Is he important in this?"

"I'd say so."

"Draw near! The gemot will now consider that matter before it: contention of Oslac, gesith to Witgar, in the wergild of Cuthwine to the amount of two hundred silver pence, claimed of Gunnar Eanboldson. Before the folc-gemot assembled. Let the compurgators come forward."

Compurgators—quite a foreign concept to me—are men representing the two contending interests. Witgar's chief gebur swore by his land's value, and relatively liable if he perjured, that Oslac's claim was genuine. In turn Beorn vowed by his own hides that the claim was of no force. Whereupon all the evidence picked over at Gunnarsburh was trotted out and weighed again by these very attentive men.

"Hlaford, will you speak for yourself?"

"I'm not allowed. Nor is Oslac."

"Who speaks for you then?"

"Alfred."

I threw up the case then and there. Sprawled on the scaffold steps, pudgy fingers folded over the paunch that bulged under his tunic, torpid and nodding, Alfred didn't seem fit to take anything but a nap.

When the evidence concluded, Icel raised his hand and stepped into the cleared space in the middle of the gathering—to say what, I'll never know. As he opened his

mouth, Bertwold's staff whacked down again. Hard, peremptory.

"Privilege, Aetheling."

Then more voices from all sides echoed him. "Privilege . . . privilege."

"What's that, Hlaford?"

Gunnar smiled wryly at my confusion. "They're reminding the Prince of a right. He may not speak here any more than myself. But they've got to object for themselves."

"Privilege!"

Object they did, vociferously, and Prince Icel, who'd faced down bristling spears and tempers in Gunnarsburh's hall, sanguinely returned to his place while I gaped at the transgression. These peasants had not requested his abstention, they'd demanded it—but more and subtler wonders awaited me.

A vital young man strode into the clearing, one of Icel's fyrd men. I recognized him from the night of the feast. In the warm afternoon, he'd thrown off his wolf-hide vest and stood before his fellows in stained breeches and a linen shirt that bulged with his heavy shoulders.

"Looks the proper hero," I admired, "lay on a bath."

"He was one at Badon," Gunnar told me. "But mostly he's a blacksmith. Brand's his name."

"Aetheling, lords, law-speaker, honored fellows," Brand began. "We know what's at issue here. I wonder why it's come so far as a trial, a simple matter of one gesith's duty to another under custom. I don't need to say, and you need not be reminded, that Thegn Gunnar came whole out of Badon where many of Oslac's friends did not. We need not speak of that, nor that recompense is claimed by a man who forswears wealth against a lord who owns the lion's share of arable after our Prince, and yet disputes the modest claim of one landless man because he *might* have to sell a fraction of it to pay. This is only the surface of an issue that touches all of us, just the foam on the ale. Will we not demand loyalty of our raised-up lords as they demand it of us?"

For a man forbearing to speak of so many things, Brand managed to speak of many things. Already he'd taken an unspoken issue—land—and turned it against Gunnar and perhaps fairly since Gunnar owned more

land than Witgar. But *listen* to this Brand: hear the language, this English, double-jointed as Bedivere's limbs. It only sounds awkward. In its ability to join one concept to another as with pegs, its dependent clauses, figures of speech and cadenced alliteration, a man can say one thing five ways and yet imply a sixth; can change meaning with an inflection, a pause or a deliberate misuse of a word, can mock, scorn and flay an opponent without uttering one overt insult.

"From what we've heard, the wergild is clearly owed. Yet my good lord of Gunnarsburh refuses on the ground that he was unable to help Cuthwine. He could still manage a nimble retreat from Badon when it was—permitted."

There was delicate malice in the choice of words and the pause. Icel ordered the retreat, but in a sense conducive to Brand's argument, he permitted it and the word transmitted its stain.

"My honored fellows, here is the case in small. Suppose your kinsman were slain at Gunnarsburh. Though it were no fault of the thegn himself, you would still claim recompense of him as responsible for mishap on his land. And yet I sadden at the picture of this impoverished Lord, with barely half of all Iclingas arable to keep body and soul together—"

A roar of appreciation from all quarters of the meeting, even Gunnar.

"—shaking his starven cheeks over a plate filled from forests where he ekes a living from a bare two-thirds of the hunting rights, and saying to the petitioner in tones hollow with hunger: 'A pity, oh, a pity. But I'm not responsible. I owe you nothing.' As he has said to Oslac."

Brand's pace and manner changed, no longer facetious but grave and hard. "We can shrug and say this is a matter of honor among gesiths, and well you know where I've always stood on this matter of privilege outside common law. But it has been put before us, so let us look at it in the light of the law. If Thegn Gunnar will not honor the custom among his peers, how will he honor it in regard to common men?"

The voice suddenly cracked like a whip in the clearing. "We are not Welsh! We do not cringe under our lords. We serve them as they serve and uphold common law. In ar-

guing Oslac's suit, I admit, as Oslac admits, that the
wergild need not be paid all at once. But it is a law, a
principle of fair dealing between men that is at stake
here, and the principle of the pound begins with the
penny. In support of that justice, support Oslac. In support of common law, as we may have need of it ourselves
tomorrow—support Oslac."

His arms were raised to invoke their support. As they
swooped down to his sides in conclusion there was applause from the gemot at large. Icel clapped politely and
those men with weapons beat spear against shield in
token of Brand's eloquence. As he retired to his place, I
was learning at first hand what Trystan strove in vain to
teach me as Empress of Britain: why their poetry is spoken where ours is sung. No language of the north was
ever so made for it.

A lull now. Men shuffled about, whispering. Heads
turned toward Alfred, where he lolled, oblivious, on the
steps. Then the dry prompting of Bertwold, commenting
with its very lack of comment.

"Will someone wake the honored fellow from Wicandaen?"

Another ripple of good-natured laughter. Alfred started
out of his torpor, snorting like a breaching whale. "Did
the law-speaker address me?"

"There was rumor you wished to speak," Bertwold deferred with massive courtesy. "We would not disturb you
else."

"Oh! Yes. Indeed." Alfred lugged his wheezing girth off
the steps and waddled to the middle of the cleared space
to blink at his fellows like a bear just roused from hiber-
nation. "I was not asleep, merely impressed by the argu-
ments of the honored fellow from court and the vigor of
his presentation."

Here Alfred yawned elaborately and broke wind. It
was a crude ploy, but the English wit can be coarse as it
is edged. The gemot roared. Icel hid his smile to preserve
some dignity, and I darkly questioned Gunnar's sanity in
trusting his fortunes to such a clown.

Alfred patted his ample stomach and beamed at
Brand. "I admire the honored fellow most particularly
for his vision, that he can so readily see what is by no
means clear to the rest of us. But then, when I was his

age, so could I. And it much amazed me that my poor father, in laboring to teach me the cloth trade, could put forth only his long experience against the wisdom I was born with. But he persisted in his ignorance and wore me down to it."

Appreciative titters from the assembly.

"And here am I, facing the same young wisdom with the same ancient folly."

The titters bubbled into scattered laughter.

"With, I hope, the same profitable result."

Goaded by the upsurge of laughter, Brand could no longer keep silent. He stepped forward with a sign to Bertwold, his strong young voice cresting over the guffaws. "Isn't it like Alfred to make a joke where he can't make a point of law!"

"My young friend has left me no choice," Alfred returned mildly, "since he has tried so hard to make a point of law out of a joke."

One bettered, as it were, young Brand just reddened among cries from the crowd: "Let Alfred speak."

Alfred attempted to. "The honored fellow from court has valiantly tried to turn this dispute into a debate on general law and the rights of lords. The meat of this seems to be that if we do not thatch the roof at the roof's demand, it will fall on us."

"I said nothing of the sort!" the younger man bridled.

"The fellow from Wicandaen has the speaking place," Bertwold cautioned. Alfred thanked him with an awkward bow.

"I thank the law-speaker. As I was saying—"

"Oh, sit down," Brand scorned. "Sit down, you old tub of guts."

Alfred froze. He bent one wounded glance on the younger man, then lowered his head and went indeed to do just that. Nor would he be enticed to the speaking place again.

"Now he's got them," Gunnar chortled.

Squatting there in blubber and confusion, despairing and shamed, Alfred had no one I could see. The men were turning in appeal to Bertwold, who signaled sternly to Brand. "May I remind the honored fellow from court of proper proceeding? The honored fellow from Wicandaen heard you out. You owe him an apology."

"He may speak for all I care," Brand allowed with careless magnanimity, "if he has anything of importance to say. It will be the first time." And he folded his arms as if to say: There, I've done. Let the ass bray if he must.

Alfred would not rise.

"Apology!" someone near him muttered. The sentiment spread through the meeting, louder and louder. "Apology . . . apology," but Alfred remained a stone on the steps. Bertwold pounded his staff for order. The men were looking reproachfully at young Brand. He threw up his arms in disgust.

"Oh, let be. I'm sorry."

Alfred raised his head like a tired old dog but made no move to take the speaking place, only gazed at Brand from beneath a mountain of injury. Distinctly uncomfortable now, Brand repeated his apology. "Speak, then."

Alfred vented a vast sigh.

"I *said* I'm sorry."

Alfred smiled with the pained benevolence of Christ on the Cross. "Honored fellow, the old tub of guts has already forgiven you."

Accompanied by whoops of merriment and applause, Alfred rose to take his place again, and I saw indeed what he'd done. The opposition afforded him a chance to retire under insult and return in triumph with probably more men sympathetic to his cause. Now I clearly saw what I'd called a clown. Close-set eyes gleaming with quiet satisfaction and purpose over quivering jowls, Alfred was clownish as a hawk.

"I was trying to say—it seems so long ago—that since my honored friend has chosen to see a point of general law in a particular case, I will be happy to answer in kind.

"I cannot help noticing that Oslac and his companion bear-sarks, while presented to us as men of no property, seem queerly prosperous. As a cloth seller, I could ask a good price for Oslac's tunic. The goldsmiths would have to assess the remainder of his poverty and that of his equally paupered friends. In such a way may all poor men rid themselves of possessions that count as nothing to the battle honor they alone cherish. But let that go."

So said Alfred, letting it go as a cat relinquishes a mouse.

"We've heard today our ancient cry of privilege. This is a privilege given us as speakers by law. Yet how can we argue the rights of law confronted by a privilege outside it? The bear-sarks are a relic of the old country and old times, priests of war who swear not to outlive their chief or withdraw from battle until victorious or dead. Since Oslac is here along with his companions to whom honor alone has weight, it follows to my simple understanding that Cerdic is alive and won at Badon. But that, too, I would have you pass by; nor should we consider Oslac's conduct at Gunnarsburh when he chose to argue his suit with a spear. Our lords made reply to this; we need not.

"What we must consider is that the dedicated war-priest who sits at a thegn's board, demanding treasure of his lord, a burden in peace like extra drones in a hive and a questionable advantage in war—this battle-holy priest, above the law in all but murder and not even that in most practical cases *now* dips into the law for recompense against a man bound by it. Can't we see a certain flaw in that reasoning?"

And now the hawk folded his wings and stooped to his prey. No more a shambling clown, Alfred seemed to grow by inches.

"And he asks payment based on so-called evidence that I would not allow in a dispute over a tavern reckoning. Understand me: if this dispute is one of a master masked behind the man, then Witgar and Gunnar are no different to me. Both are ambitious and both want more. For common men like us, it's a choice of which fox guards the henhouse. Though I add they are both foxes of good care and conscience. We would be less without them. But bear-sark privilege has no place where land and the law are so important and so indivisible. If we have no power over these men, at least we have over our own reason. Find for Oslac in this matter of wergild and honor, and you find for a weight on our own necks. You hasten the hardening of their old yoke in a new place where we are still planting healthy new law in new soil. Find for Oslac on this flimsy charge—that a frozen, near-crippled, half-starved peer failed a moment's duty and therefore owes for it to a man who, by custom, can own or owe nothing, *rich as he stands there*—and how much better off are we, are you, are any of us than the Welsh

peasant whose only hope of peace is that his protecting lord will stay far away from his carrot patch? Whose only hope of redress is the mercy and benevolence of that very fallible lord?"

Imperceptibly the easy tone of Alfred's speech had deepened, strengthened until it rang through the village. Women at the fair stalls paused to listen. Men loitered attentively in the tavern door, listening over their ale.

"My honored fellows, it can be said that I too argue from a privilege as old as that of Oslac, old as the country our fathers came from. But the one benefits a few while mine looks to shelter the many. For Oslac's cause, I urge this gemot dismiss it as of no force, to acquit Thegn Gunnar of any man-price—"

Now the hawk sank his talons into larger prey.

"—and that the folc-gemot consider for future meetings the whole question of bear-sark privilege and its fitness under English law. Oslac, by his ancient right, may challenge Gunnar to personal combat." Alfred grinned suddenly, jowls awag at the notion. "And then take it into his privileged head to descend on us. And then who'll mind the shops?"

He inclined his head to Bertwold. "Law-speaker, the fellow from Wicandaen thanks you. I have said."

As Alfred waddled back to his place amid a clash of spears on shields, I pondered the incongruity of what I'd witnessed this day. Here were common men respectfully forbidding their own lord to speak in a court convened by himself, arguing the rights of one lord versus another and calling the very existence of these rights into open question. It smacked of downright anarchy.

These Angles have brought from their forests a machinery whereby men can pass judgment on the very laws that bind them. Not a perfect machine by any means; it creaks, fails, delays, does injury and sometimes injustice, but somehow it moves and serves and grows like a living thing. I was just to my own commons, as I understood justice, but never trusted them for justice or even common sense in return. It seemed to me that in this folc-gemot, the English lords had taken a serpent to their bosom. I've since reflected that, despite Eve's seduction, the serpent was ever a symbol of wisdom.

The gemot decided for Gunnar.

"We the men of the folc-gemot in congress assembled at Wicandaen, on consideration in good conscience of all circumstance in this matter, do find the charge of Oslac to be of no force and Gunnar Eanboldson not liable for the wergild of Cuthwine."

As with Arthur and myself, sometimes history drags you in its wake. Sometimes it merely plucks at your sleeve with the fat hand of a cloth seller.

To compound my confusion, I saw Brand and Alfred drinking together after going at each other with such potent intent. But I thought long on it. They'd taken opposite sides of a question, but both in their way had bitten an ax into the venerated oak of the highborn. Small ax, large tree to be sure, but I've wondered since if they were really opposed after all.

We the men of the folc-gemot . . . in congress assembled . . .

One wonders where such unbridled notions might lead.

War came suddenly to Gunnarsburh and at the worst time, during harvest. Angle chieftains sailed from Jutland that summer, men with all of Icel's problems but only Oslac's notions of solving them. We were working in the fields when Witgar himself brought the news: a gorgeous day for work, warm but not hot, a day prodigal in its colors. No matter how much you wanted, there was always more. Blue, gold, green, umber—I exulted in them.

Work and health have a tang to them on such days, a delicious sauce of sweat and sun and fragrant dust rising from the scythed barley, the appetite for food earned and eaten in the fields. The still wisdom in a rushing world to look about at harvest glistening in the sun and to know, for that breath at least, one is sufficed.

And to know the beauty is not all squandered on you alone. Gunnar felt it, sitting cross-legged in the stubble, watching his people resting over their food where they stopped, while I sponged the sweat from his bare shoulders.

"So damned beautiful, all of it. The hell with everything else, Gwenda. Just give me this."

It was good to hear joy out of him. Nilse was so trou-

bled in this new pregnancy that all of the family wore her illness like a hairshirt, Gunnar most of all. Sometimes he was short with the children, fretting to find a wet nurse for little Nerta, hurling all his pent male energy into the harvest.

I moved the cloth over his skin, careful of the knot where the stone-slinger wounded him. He was hairier than Arthur, a *Y* of crisp light hair across the shoulders and down his back. The body moved with more stolid strength, not at all mercurial. Arthur's passion flashed like light on burnished metal. Gunnar lacked the dazzle, dark polished wood beside the sun-chariot of my husband.

Arthur and I used to make love on afternoons like this when we had time. Night always found us too grimed with government to come really clean to each other. We were ropes braided from many strands; the gem-hard genius that fitted us so well for what we were, never left us, even in bed. I would have made us simpler in that, and all Britain could have gone to hell while we made an art of amor. In love something must surrender. Neither of us could, but it was splendid sometimes, early on, before the child and other losses.

He had a body much like yours, and it surprises me that this gray middle age of mine with its lines and wrinklings is twice the woman I owned before. The only difference is better taste, less of a need to possess and more to know. If still a fool, then one less imperious, needing less and knowing better how to relish it. Why do they call it age? It's only sunlight gone soft without loss of warmth. Where I glutted, now I could pick like an epicure; where once I asked a banquet, now perhaps a poem.

"You've good hands, Gwenda."

"They have a good subject, sir."

He reached back to close his fingers over mine. "You won't run off again, will you?"

How to answer that? My Britain, my old world was so distant just then. "I was feeling the air and the sun and thinking I'm happy this one moment. That's wisdom in itself."

"What have I bought in you?" he wondered softly.

"Among other things, a rare back-scrubber. Look, riders."

The watch rider burst into the clearing from the north and galloped toward us across the stubble, hastily skirting the uncut stand. Behind him came Witgar and one of his fyrd men, working their mounts hard. The other workers around us straightened up from their food as the three riders reined up by Gunnar. Witgar dismounted, sweaty and too urgent for greeting.

"Well, they've come!"

"Who's come?"

Witgar was a man ready to fly apart. "Who? Icel's sweet dream of reinforcement, the dear folk from home. Five longships, three hundred men." The thegn paced up and down in front of Gunnar, sputtering with outrage yet untold.

"And their lord?"

"Port's his name. Two sons, Bieda and Maegla. They bragged about it, Gunnar, they bragged! How they raided at Wight. Oh, nothing big, just to test their mettle and lug off what was lying around loose."

"You're not this angry about just Wight, that's days from here. What's happened?"

"Well, they landed at Wicandaen and did the same thing."

Beorn stepped closer, his face clouded with a particular concern. "Wicandaen?"

"Cleaned it out. A lot of blood, they say."

"When?"

"Early this morning, barely light when they came up the fen. I was breakfasting with Icel when the news came."

The farmer in Gunnar prompted him: "Away from home at harvest time?"

"Ah, mine's in," Witgar snorted. "I don't have your vast hidage. The Prince seems to find that fitting; that's not important now. Anyway, Icel sent Bertwold to greet them. To *greet* them, Gunnar." Witgar paused to wipe the sweat from his face, then plunged back into fresh outrage. "And to escort their lord and his chief men to feast and parley. Then Bertwold saw the spoils they were carrying. Smoke from the village. Brought along some of the women from Wicandaen, too. They hadn't been

gently used." Witgar continued his pacing as if only movement would contain him. "Bertwold's no fool. He demanded their intentions then and there, and all this foreigner said was that he'd see our Prince soon enough."

In the turmoil of it, I thought, What's so surprising? This is how your own fathers got their own land. Now you call their cousins thieves for doing the same thing?

In Wicandaen Port evidently gathered enough information on the lay of Icel's land to know where the quickest, fattest strike could be made.

"He's not going for Icel," Witgar concluded, planting himself at last in front of Gunnar. "He's coming for us, you or me. No, I never liked you or your land-grabbing mother, but this is another matter. Call up your men. Wherever they hit, we'll make a stand together."

Gunnar seemed to be listening to something other than Witgar's voice. "My village," he murmured. "That's *my* village." His hand thrust out to grasp Witgar's. "Let it be so, together. Beorn?"

The steward was gazing out to the north over the barley yet uncut. "They'll waste it all. What a time to come."

"No better," said Gunnar. "They only have to pick up what we've harvested and cart it away. Take your horse and ride to the farms; get the men and their families to the stockade while there's still light."

Beorn nodded his agreement. "Quicker if there's two of us."

"Yes, I need another rider." Gunnar bit his lip, glancing at his horse and the farmers waiting close by. Beorn divined his thought.

"None of them good with a horse, not for fast riding."

"I am."

Witgar laughed aloud at my suggestion. "Where do you buy your slaves, Valhalla?"

Gunnar didn't laugh. He and Beorn were not the best riders themselves and his farmers about as equestrian as hens. "If I gave you a horse, would I see it again?"

"You have my word, Hlaford."

"You ran once."

"Then you needn't trust me, but the host is coming closer while we stand here, and I'm a better rider than any of you. If Beorn goes one way and I the other, I'll be back before dark or not long after." When he hesitated,

searching me for truth, I said, "Port is gambling more than you. It's worth it. And I have my own distaste for treachery."

He shoved me toward the horse. "Get them here. Go."

Beorn held the horse for me. "He means it, Gwenda. He'd kill you this time. If I didn't. My holding's north of here; Port will make free with whatever he finds there before he even shows his face at Gunnarsburh. I've lost it already. I've always liked you, but if you're false and get caught, it won't be pretty and it won't be quick." Beorn let go of the bridle. "I'll go north, you south. Now let's see how well you can ride."

I gathered the reins and brought up the horse's head. "Beorn, there's a saying in the west that a Saxon on a horse is a contradiction in terms. Don't you wish now for half a hundred of those combrogi you've cursed? Ha! Go!"

I lashed the horse into a run toward the forest.

Yes, I could have run and perhaps won to British land, although I doubt it. I can't tell you clearly why I didn't after bolting only months before. Gunnar was part of it and perhaps the leavening of time and divisible loyalties. Greater decisions have come from plainer elements. All through the afternoon I rode, to each cottage and tun, pausing only to give my message and dashing on to the next and the next: bring your families and weapons to Gunnarsburh. Once I rested the horse and allowed her a little water and accepted some bread and cheese from a gaunt farm wife with three dirty children hanging on her. Neither she nor her husband was rattled by the news, but simply went about getting ready. They were used to this. You planted and you bore. If someone burned you out, you came back to plant and bear again.

The sun was low when I left the last small tun and turned north, hurrying back through the long September afternoon toward Gunnarsburh. Sometimes when there was a path to follow, I passed the fyrd men jogging along or groups of families trudging toward the stockade, children laboring to keep up or drifting off to play, weary mothers screeching at them not to *stray*, damn it, she had more to worry about now.

"Children! Stay with your mothers." I lent my voice to theirs. "Don't run off, keep moving."

Now and then a mother would search about with that sudden panic that meant a thoughtless bairn slipped quicksilver into the woods out of sight, and I'd have to go crashing and hallooing through the brush until the lamb was found, brambled and content, cramming blackberries into a small, purpled little mouth.

"Here, you sticky little thing! Your mum's like to faint worrying about you. Up here with me—hold on—off we go."

By twilight the forest path to Gunnarsburh was crowded with families and oxcarts. When the horse began to tire in earnest, I dismounted and led her. "Poor old woman, you're not used to this. Come, we'll walk."

Twilight deepened to soft murk as I fell behind the last stragglers, leading the spent horse. It was full dark when I broke out of the forest to see Gunnarsburh ringed with fires. It frightened me: I thought they were Port's fires since there were men moving in silhouette outside the walls. I started to skirt along the edge of the fields.

"Who's there?"

I froze, one foot in the stirrup, ready to run the mare lame if need be.

The sharp voice challenged again: "Who's there? Speak or you're dead."

I relaxed with a deep breath. "I'd rather speak, Hlaford. It's Gwenda. I thought they were enemy fires out there."

In a moment Gunnar was at my side, sheathing his sword. "In case they come tonight they can't surprise us."

"Your men are inside?"

"And the families. Our riders found Port. He'll camp on the other side of the forest tonight, most like. But I don't like to be surprised."

"He could come on as well."

"He'd be blind, not knowing where to hit or what was waiting for him. Are you all right, Gwenda?"

"Marvelous." Now the fear was past, I felt even jubilant. "No doubt a physician would deem me far too old for this, and certainly your horse thinks so, but I'll probably live forever."

He offered me something in the gloom. "You want to drink?"

"Do I not! Thank you." I took a long drink of the warm, thick ale and then just sank down in the grass at the edge of the field. Gunnar sat beside me. "Why are you still out, Hlaford?"

"Waiting for you."

"You needn't."

I heard the anger in his voice. "No. And I shouldn't have risked you either, and Port shouldn't be doing what he is. The whole thing's insane. Insane! When he could have joined us. We could've gone west again, if we're really going. This way no one wins. Waste."

I thought about that. "Rather full circle, isn't it? Your fathers killed Picts to protect British land, then you killed us to take it for yourself. Now you'll kill to keep it from your own." The rush of bitterness couldn't be dammed. "How does it feel to have your own kind go for your throat? Is Port any different from your own da when he carved a piece out of my country? Was Arthur any different from you in trying to hold it? Full circle—and ask me not about wheels, they just keep turning. To know history is no blessing, Gunnar; one laughs or goes mad. Little men with large appetites and larger fears. How many ever with vision? Even myself. God, when I think of the—"

I checked myself before saying too much, just swallowed more of the good ale. But this night I felt like being *myself;* it was owed me. "Sometimes I'd sell the whole suicidal island for a pound silver. The good thing about a comedy is, it's brief. We just go on, and the laughter strains. Have a drink, Gunnar."

I gave him the leather pouch and lay back on the earth, feeling its cool softness on my back. "Aye, doesn't that have a brave ring? Here am I, about to stand with English to hold English ground. Yes, I hope you have a sense of comedy, Gunnar."

He stretched out beside me, head on his hand. "I love the way you speak. Even when you talk, you're singing. What've I got in you?"

"You've not heard? I'm a goddess."

"No!"

"And the daughter of one."

"Should I kneel?"

"Should you not! The living flesh of Epona, sometimes called Isis or Ashtoreth in places where it never rains."

"There you go, off in fancy again."

"Oh, yes—and the young chiefs would flock to Mother and me to be touched by the Goddess, and the Christian priests would mutter and shake their holy heads, and we'd have to build them another church, like giving sweets to children to make them behave."

"Oh, you can *talk*, woman." Gunnar was always amused and a bit mystified at British whimsy. "I got a bargain for my two pound/ten."

"Bargain? My Lord, it was robbery."

"And I'll have all your riches when you die."

I liked the nearness of him just now, I needed it. "The other gods may contest the will."

"I'd collect. Gwenda?"

Quiet, so quiet there in the dark field with the distant fires and the night sounds around us and he so close to me. I felt an old need, so long starved, rising in my belly. "Yes?"

"You wouldn't try to run again?" He wasn't asking as a master but a man. "Would you?"

"Not without a great deal of forethought, gentle master. You could free me."

"No." I felt a small warm shock as his hand closed over mine, more than it warranted. "Even if you were someone of note like Dorcas of Hull or that woman in Dyfneint, Geraint's sister, what's her name?"

"Eleyne, I think."

"That's the one. They say even though she has a son, she's still a holy virgin. Can that be?"

"With her, yes."

"Even if you were someone like that—no, I wouldn't part with you."

"I think my Lord is paying me a compliment."

In the dark, even in the light at certain angles, how like young Arthur he was. The tightness I felt I heard in his own voice. "Well, I meant good slaves are rare. Wise ones are priceless."

Another silence between us, longer this time. I felt the dark drawing us closer like drawstrings around two coins in a black velvet purse. "Look at our fires in the night."

Gunnar lifted his head; the dim profile was so dearly familiar, I actually reached to touch it. Gunnar accepted the caress, stroking my hand. "I can almost feel that old bastard waiting in the dark."

He moved closer, putting his arm around me. I was surprised at the hot flush that went through me at his touch. "Think of all the nights in all the years men no different from you huddled in their own small light and tried to save their homes from your fathers. They felt a destiny too. One at least would take it ill to be thought a demon. He always wanted to be a priest."

"Your husband?"

"No, just someone close to me once. Thank God, *my* husband was no part of a priest. You would have liked him."

We drank some more of the warm ale. It softened even more the languor flowing through me, charged with the touch of Gunnar's body. "We should go back," I said with no conviction.

"Yes."

And we stayed.

"I've felt these things you speak of," Gunnar admitted. "How insane it all is. So damned *sick* of Mother's everlasting destiny, as if she'd found one of your—churches, you call 'em?—on being scin-laecen."

"What else has she got to hold?"

"Nothing I do is ever enough. Hell, I don't want it for me, Gwenda. I've got enough, but it's like we're all being borne along on a tide we can't stop." Speaking of surer feelings, Gunnar spoke with less hesitancy. "I was eighteen when I married Nilse, she was fifteen. We were already hand-fasted and Edytha was on the way. If I want more it's for the children, but I don't want this new child. Not if it's going to torture Nilse just to be born."

His voice had turned flat and bleak in the dark. "I wish it'd never come. Oh, I know what women say, and men too as far as that goes. Children are the future, children are wealth. But a man's wife—Nilse's my friend, Gwenda. Try to say that to Beorn, he acts like I was suntouched. But she is. Tell her to put her hand in fire for me, it would be burning. That's worth something. No, I don't want this child."

"Born alive or dead, Nilse will come through," I whis-

pered to him. "And she will need you then. Not your hand
in fire, that's easy enough. She'll need it to hold on to." As
I needed Arthur and denied it, turning to Lancelot. "Did
you ever tell her that, Gunnar? About being your
friend?"

"No, we're not—" His body shrugged against me. "We
don't say much. I've tried. Certainly thought of it. There's
never really the time or place."

"Make the time."

"Always something to do. The same with the children:
look how they grow when you're not watching at all. Almost sneaky."

"I lost a child myself when I was young, so heed me. If
she does lose it—if—she may do foolish things, hurtful
things, but she'll never need you more than when she
seems furthest away. My husband was wise as men go,
but even he couldn't riddle that. He let me . . . no, *we* let
us slip away. I'm not sorry where it led me. My taste was
always more reliable than my motives. But you're a different people. Nilse has fewer choices than I had. For her,
there's only you. Be there."

"You're wise, Gwenda."

"Nigh time. I'm old enough."

Gunnar lay very close to me now. "Not old," he murmured. "Not you."

With a rustle of movement his head loomed over me in
the darkness. Yes, I could reach up and take him to me
now, make it happen, and why not? Tomorrow we could
all be dead.

"You're strange," Gunnar confessed.

"There's gallantry. I think."

"No, I mean Mother's old and Gytha and Gwyneth, but
you're not any age. Or all ages, I don't know. Sometimes
when you speak—Nilse thinks you speak far too much
for a woman—"

"Spoiled rotten growing up."

"No, you are . . . magic. And no age at all. Older than
Mother because you can see all the things that still drive
her and weigh their worth. Younger than Nilse because
she's always so serious and can't understand your laughter. It's as if I were listening sometimes to an echo from a
deep place; like your words about goddesses: folly and
fooling, but there's . . . echoes. I hear the sound, and I

can only guess how far down it goes into the place where the words come from. Deep. Perhaps I shouldn't be saying these things. Just . . ."

I knew his meaning better than he did: that having to deny himself Nilse made him look elsewhere if only in need and even, against all male odds actually *see* women as I saw him. There was civilized hope for Gunnar. And if he bent now over the little distance between our mouths, it would be as much an escape from need as a choosing. I chose for both of us.

"Come here to me."

My hand caressed his rough cheek, then curved around his neck and pulled him to me. I felt him hold back just a moment, then answer me in his simple hunger, tentative at first, then desperate as he felt the answering, assenting hunger in me. I let him know there was no reason to hang back, none even to be gentle when we both came starved to the feast.

"Oh, Gott. Gwenda, listen—"

"No, don't talk." I kissed his mouth into silence, rough as himself in my need. The urgency was a pressure between my thighs, a heat that cried for cooling. He buried his face in my breasts, surprised when my hands found and clasped his hardening penis. It was awkward for a breath, trying to undress without letting go of each other, but our clothes were slung this way and that and we closed as naturally as belt and loop. I reveled, exulted in the glory of being held again. With Gunnar in me, shuddering in his released passion, I was forgivably the adulteress again, as we are all passing unfaithful in the dreams that wander between the start and finish of love. So like young Arthur. I let my memories run rampant; for fugitive seconds between kiss and kiss I stroked another face, ran my tongue and thirsty mouth over a remembered throat and chest, clasped and clawed a smoother back. I had been old. In this magic I was young again.

What a marvel our bodies are. Only a year ago I was a worn stump, bitten to the quick with rancor and fatigue, restive, barely able to eat or sleep, covered with rash and waiting with less than saintly resignation for my menses to give up the ghost. I struck more quickly than I stroked then and would have been a poor, distracted partner for

the most perfunctory lover. But now I was astonished at the health and strength in me, the ease and joy of surrender and conquest twined inseparable in each movement of Gunnar and me locked together. I hid against his moving shoulder the secret smile that knew he was unskilled but not innately clumsy, and turned his artlessness to spontaneity, made it all easy for him.

And for me? I've always said love quicker than feeling it, but perhaps a part of it was that. Gunnar was a delight to me, an unfolding of delights beyond working bodies. I'd thought of myself as old for so long, year by year needing more artifice to present a youth to the world; now, somewhere in the lessons of this slave year I'd let go of youth, turned my back and walked on only to find it waiting for me again in these fields, not much older but worlds wiser, the same music suddenly easier to sing; less of an *I* and more of a *we*, the simple, graceful line that was all there was to the melody in the first place recognized by my own simplicity. Was that all there was to be done, a letting go?

Gunnar's dammed need made him finish quickly, but I clasped him in me, held him and let the second visitation of magic be for myself. The first was a starved bolting, the second a savoring. I surprised him; what he took for dark Welsh magic was merely the difference between a woman's acceptance of her body and his scant knowledge of it. His very need of me, wanting of me, set fire to my flesh and seared it until I laughed and cried, triumphant in my own climax; until the shattering cries sank to whispers and the whispers to soft, sufficed laughter. And Gunnar, young as he was, thought it all his doing.

Finally he sat up, looking off at Gunnarsburh like a place or a state of mind forgotten in magically foreshortened time, now too clearly remembered. "We should go back now."

"Yes. They'll be worried."

His hand strayed gently across my breasts. "Gwenda—"

"No. Whatever you'd say now, please don't. It was lovely. For God's sake don't be solemn or English about it."

"No."

"It doesn't change anything, and it has nothing to do with Nilse. There's still your collar round my neck."

That sounded like I was patting him on the head; it shouldn't be so. I twisted about to kiss his mouth. "I know you love her. This was just a beautiful gift."

Gunnar lifted me to my feet. "You have a way of saying hard things simply."

"The simplicity's the hardest part."

"Let's go to the pale post and tell them we're coming in."

The stockade and hall were bursting with humanity sleeping anywhere they could find a space that night. I took my bedding to the kitchen with Rat. We all rose an hour earlier next morning (my best sleep in several years) and even as we set the breakfast fires, Gunnarsburh was a-rattle with spear, shield and sword. Gytha hotted up a huge kettle of porridge, grumbling that we'd be short of oats again come winter. Rat sliced cold pork and chicken onto wooden plates, and I fetched and carried to the hall, shouldering casks of beer that I'd not have been able to lift the year before. The hall was loud confusion, fyrd men eating in shifts, wives milling about, children darting and squealing. Ase frightened them with dire threats if they didn't behave and made a peculiar request of me.

"Go out to your garden and bring three shoots of fox-glove for the Hlafdians and myself."

As I cut the stalks with their lavender bells, I thought, If you'll fight decorated, so will I. And I pinned a new green shoot of leek to my homespun as I'd seen my own peasants do on holidays.

"Look at Gwenda!" Gwyneth trilled with pride. "Lasses of the vale are we! You're not half dashing."

"Our Lady of the Soup Greens," Rat snickered.

I gave them each a leek to wear. "We'll be smashing war-maidens."

"Nilse, Ase and I will be the Valkyries of Gunnarsburh today," Elfgifu told me. "We've sworn it."

The sweaty riders mumbled their story through beer and porridge. Port and his host didn't turn for Witgar's holding. They camped the night on the other side of the forest and gave every evidence of coming on for Gunnarsburh. Witgar was alerted and not an hour behind

the riders. Our two forces combined just equaled Port's, but we'd be inside which doubled the advantage. Gunnar was confident.

"We'll lose part of the crop, but we'll win. With us in front and Icel behind, what can Port do?"

"Sack every open farm around," Beorn said dismally.

"Icel will come, he must. When he does, we'll go out." Gunnar caught the eye of every man close to him. "Not before. No matter how they try to lure us out, we stay snug until Icel's on the field."

"Port could burn everything outside the walls." The notion grated on Beorn. "That's what I hate most, the plowing waste."

Gunnar agreed, that was the worst. "But Port is used to the old ways like Oslac. I'll still try to talk to him."

"What good will that do, Hlaford?" Beorn mourned. "He's got to fight now he's landed; that or run. How long would he be a chief then? What else can he do now?"

"Damn it, does it always have to be the old way? He can treat with us. This doesn't have to be."

"You said it yourself. He's a prince with sons and gesiths to provide for."

"Well, someone's got to talk to someone sometime."

You can't have peace without it. I hoped Port would be reasonable. Much of our harvest was in but as much still waited the reaping. All the threshed grain stored in the mill had been carted into the stockade. Not a sheep, pig or cow still foraged outside the walls—and the walls were where I wanted to be this day.

"Mother and Ase will be on the walls, but we don't ask our laet-women to fight," Gunnar reproved. "You're not frightened?"

"Petrified, but less if I've something to do. And don't you know those bastards will *ruin* my flower beds. Let me help on the walls. I can carry whatever's needed to the men."

He hesitated out of frank concern for me. "All right. But if we're breached, inside. You hear me?"

Prowling the parapet like a tigress ready to pounce, Elfgifu sent me with a message to Nilse in her bower. I delivered it where the hlafdian lay on the wide bed she shared with Gunnar, Nerta in her arms, Edytha white

but composed, Eadward chafing to wreak havoc with his wooden sword.

"Your father needs his bravest here to guard what's most precious to him," I mollified the small hero.

Poor Nilse, wan as her pillow. She'd dressed in her oldest gown but turned the children out neatly. The foxglove was pinned to her breast and a small skinning knife lay within reach.

"Lady Elfgifu sent me to say that if you'll stay abed until needed, she will keep the oath of the foxglove. I hope that's right. I don't understand a word of it."

Her head barely moved on the pillow. "I'll come then, tell her. I am feeling better today. Now I'm sure you have much to do."

No one could dismiss you with such cool finality. Little Edytha took my hand and led me out the door. "Thank you for the flowers," she piped with her best manners. "And don't be afraid, Gwenda. Mother will fix them good." Her eyes gleamed with innocent feral excitement. "And she's going to teach me today."

Witgar was good as his word. With the watchtower keeping a peeled eye on the north and two riders probing the woods for the first sign of Port, we were vastly relieved when Witgar trotted out of the forest to the west, his ax-head banner rippling and the lines of men running behind him, the whole column taking on speed as the long snake of them broke into the clearing. When the stockade gate closed behind the last of them, Gunnar called a hasty council of war. Both thegns agreed they shouldn't go out until Icel was in position and the odds about five to three. Oslac and the bear-sarks were solidly and stupidly for marching out four-square and standing in the open at equal odds; nothing else was honorable.

"We'll go when it's time," Gunnar decided. When Oslac protested to his own lord, Witgar only echoed Gunnar.

"But we are bear-sarks," Oslac sputtered. "We are expected to go out. They'll call us women."

"Remember the combrogi who beat us more than once," Gunnar reminded him. "They moved as one man, never confused, never wasting a second. Demons or men, they knew how to take orders. See to the edge on your ax; we'll be out soon enough. Now, we need our best archers in the tower."

"And the bravest." Beorn lifted his head to the platform where a man would be always half exposed to other archers when he drew to loose. "Port's archers will have the distance with two arrows, and drift in two more. Then—good night."

It was mid-morning when the first elements of Port's host simply walked out of the forest and stood watching us, tiny with distance, but more men joined them and more and more until they were a group, then a mob and then a mass of spears. Three men detached themselves from the others and strolled casually to the edge of our barley stand. Gunnar cursed in disgust.

"I thought so. They'll give us a taste of our own smoke."

"Waste," Beorn ground out, and all the immorality he felt weighted the sound.

A thin ribbon of smoke rose up from the fields, then flame that began to eat its way through the uncut stand as I felt the rage mount to match my fear. They were not just fields to me now, not just rows of wheat or barley to be assessed or taxed. Each foot of that burning ground had my sweat in it as well as Gunnar's and Beorn's. I'd walked behind the plow, sown the grain and hauled water to keep it alive when the rain passed us by. Every bloody sprout of it. We'd be that much short of food awinter now, eating cabbage ends and roots and hard bread doled out by the mouthful. Children still in the womb—Nilse's, if it lived—would die anyway because their mothers weren't strong enough. And in the spring when that black-burned ground was still half frozen, we'd have it all to do again.

I looked at the spear-bristling mob heaving toward us and the helmeted man leading them, his long mustaches fluttering in the morning breeze, and I cursed Port with more virulence than Gunnar and far better authority.

All because of you, you stupid, greedy old man. Because you won't think, only grab. Because taking and killing's easier and somehow more honorable, and you can sit your arrogant rump in a hall and listen to a wheezy skald drone out what a true son of the gods you are. That's the illusion, the tottering vanity that makes pride cheaper than common sense, speaking from some experience. I've been there, old man. I know the despera-

tion you can't show and the determination you must, and how well or poorly you sleep at night. You can burn the earth, but you won't take it. You never sweated over it to make it yours. You haven't earned it.

Lessons.

Sometimes we do learn something. Arthur said it to me more than once when I scathed his peasant blood. *If you lived a year of their lives.* And the contempt from Bedivere when I pushed aside that dreary girl and her unsanitary child. What was it he said at Eburacum before they broke down my doors? *They'll remember you, right enough.* Aye, God keeps tax rolls like a sharp-nosed Roman. They always balance in the end.

And every man and woman on the parapet with me, seeing the smoke rise up, knew the same, that it all had to be done again, good weather or bad, and the lot of us hungry the while. It was a deeper rage than I'd ever felt, and I understood a little more of the flinty set to Elfgifu's mouth.

As Port's mob lumbered close enough to distinguish faces beneath the battered helmets, others hove into view from the forest behind them, hauling a thick tree trunk on a wagon bed.

"Battering ram," Beorn noted flatly.

"And if my eyes are still good, that's our wagon," said Ase. "Have they burned our place, husband?"

"We'd see the smoke. We didn't leave them much to steal."

"Thieves. And we were so ready to welcome them."

They were within hailing distance now, trampling through my flower beds. I couldn't help myself. "Get out of there, you clods! Have you no souls?"

Gunnar nudged the archer next to him. "Put one in front of the old man."

The red-bearded archer licked his lips, judging the distance. "In his shield. Just for the fun."

"But don't miss. I want to talk."

The archer's bow was captured or crafted after the British style, over six feet in length, the arrow three. He sighted and loosed. The arrow went home in Port's shield. The old man stopped with a comic jerk. All froze, shields up. With a rustling rattle, the heaving lot of them

halted. Suddenly it was very quiet on the walls and beyond them as Gunnar leaned out over the palings.

"Port!"

The old prince, a bull for all his years, raised his short sword. "I am Port, Prince of the Varingas whom the Romans call Varini." He swept his sword to the young men on either side of him. "My sons, Bieda and Maegla. We have sent word to your rabbit-hearted Prince whose lands are now mine to give to my sons and gesiths."

One of his sons swaggered forward a few steps. Like Port his speech was differently accented from that I'd learned in Gunnarsburh. "Knowest thou of the Varingas, slave of Icel?"

Beorn winked at Gunnar before answering. "Hey, when the wind is wrong, everyone knows the Varingas. Do you still cook and piss in the same pot?"

The insults told on Port. He was an unsubtle sort after all, jamming his sword into the ground. "Who calls himself Hlaford of this pig-wallow?"

"I'm Thegn Gunnar, old man." Gunnar raised his sword. "But aren't you past this sort of thing?"

Port's other son, the one called Bieda, made an exaggerated bow. "Pleased to sample your goods, great Lord. Are your women worth the taking?"

"If there are men worthy of the name," Elfgifu sniped. "Pity you brought none."

Gunnar patted his mother's shoulder. "Port! Just as you stand there, you are master of no more land than your broken shoes cover. Listen! And let your two puppies heed as well. You're all a disappointment. We've waited for you a year and more. We've looked for you, hoped for you, that you'd swear to Icel and join with us, make us enough to take the good Midlands again. We expected men of honor. We got thieves fit only for *nithings vaerke* who insulted our Prince and raided my own people at Wicandaen."

"We only stopped to eat," said young Bieda with insolent reasonableness, "and greet a girl or two. I hope they're not the best you can offer."

"You'll find our women a bit stiffer." Gunnar nodded to his mother. "They wear the poison flower for you."

"Then perhaps we should deal with your women," Port

roared. "No matter; at home they say the Iclingas are all women."

"You poor old shit-hound, you—" Gunnar paused to laugh as if the whole issue were a mountainous absurdity. His sympathy was scalding. "The Geats ran you out. You're here on bluff and an empty belly. Wicandaen must have been your first full meal in weeks. Port, this doesn't have to be. Icel's men are behind you, my walls in front. Put down your arms. Swear to him when he comes, make peace and I'll ask no unreasonable payment for Wicandaen or the fields you've burned."

The old man roared his laughter. "You *are* women! And your Prince no better than Welsh. He's not behind us but huddled like you behind his own walls. Will you come out or do we come in?"

Oslac fumed his disgust to Witgar: "Now you see the shame this brings us. Will we go out or suffer more of this?"

"It gets us one wounded man to every twenty of them dead," Witgar snapped at him. "If you want to go out, I'll say goodbye now and fetch your body when there's time. Otherwise shut up, that's an order. You'll have a piece of them soon enough."

"Might it be true?" Elfgifu fretted. "Would Icel leave us to such as these?"

"No, Mother."

"But if he comes too late—"

"We'll still win. You've sacrificed to Woden who only waits on a certainty." Gunnar's voice was cold with regret. "It will start now. They won't reason. Mother, I'm sorry I wasn't scin-laecen born."

"I don't care." Elfgifu clasped him tight and kissed her son with a fierce pride. She placed her hand on his bowed head in a ritual I didn't understand. "Bring me the heads of my enemies."

"I swear it, Elfgifu." Gunnar snapped around to his waiting men, an arrow himself loosed from the bow. "Archers—*loose*!"

At his order, Port's mob became a fighting force. The shields in front were raised, those behind flattened over the men's heads. When the arrow flight landed, the host broke apart into disciplined elements. The wagon rolled forward, inching around the west face of the stockade

toward the barred gates, the straining men well protected by shield-bearers among them and alongside. Their scaling ladders and ropes hit our north and east sides at once.

"Putting up a ladder here!"

"More stones. More *stones.*"

Port's men scurried up the ladders or overhanded up the knotted ropes as their hooks flew over and caught on the palings. Where they could our men hacked the ropes and pushed the ladders down, brained the first men to gain the parapet. The deep, steady boom of the battering ram commenced—

—*pouring through the city gates. Cornish, Silure, the lot.* Did it ever change? Could it?

Arthur always said one person sees very little in a battle. Your blood's up, fear and rage pumping you higher and higher. For the first of it, a minute or an hour, I have a hazy memory of running, sweating, trying to catch my breath, passing bundles of arrows and baskets of stones or hot coals up to the frantic men on the parapet. Ase transformed, screeching, as she hurled down a stone herself, her heavy-lidded eyes and placid nun's mouth distorted by a snarl—Elfgifu calm as at worship, reaching for the bundles I passed up, tossing them to waiting hands in the same motion—one man cursing, another surprised by the arrow in his breast, brushing daintily at it like an alien thing before he went down—Gunnar and Beorn everywhere, loping along the parapet with drawn swords, rushing in where needed, running on—Rhodri snorting as an arrow sank into the ground between his running legs—and myself spitting a stream of Parisi obscenities inventive beyond any that ever shocked Nilse—Rat, braver than I'd guessed or mad with fear, much the same, scampering across the courtyard with a called-for bucket of hot coals for my waiting hands.

"Last of the fire, tell 'em."

"Ta, Rat, and God bless."

"Cunting barstids," she moaned. "Oh, the barstids. We ent gonner live out this day. Pray for me, Gwenda." And she scurried away to the safety of the kitchen.

Again and again the heavy thud of the battering ram intruded on my cold frenzy. Beorn guessed right: the tower was the most important point of our defense. The

archers stationed there sent flight after flight into the Varini manning the ram, thinning them out. In turn they were the prime target for Port's archers as well as those replenishing their arrows. Before the end, nine archers skinned up the ladder and nine were hit. As for the carriers, the moment they climbed above the walls into the line of Varini sight, the range and drift by now well in the archers' hands, they were loosed at. Most were hit. A few gained the platform, tossed their bundles onto it and simply jumped from the top of the ladder.

The battering ram again, an altered sound, a note I knew too well. The gate was giving.

"Arrows! Arrows in the tower!"

"Gunnar, the tower's wanting shafts."

"Carrier to the tower!"

No one leaped to obey as he had before. Gunnar whirled this way and that, but the men within earshot looked away, and no one could blame them for that.

"Oh, for—" Gunnar snatched up two bundles of arrows and started for the tower, but Beorn firmly relieved him of them. "I'm smaller and quicker, Hlaford."

It was a flurry, a moment. Beorn dashed for the ladder as someone on the wall bellowed for the thegn. Diverted for the instant, Gunnar didn't see Beorn start to climb. Halfway up he was sighted. The shafts whistled around him. Beorn lurched, slipped, caught his legs between the rungs and fell, clutching frantically at the ladder, trying to break his fall. He landed in a heap at the bottom.

"Arrows!"

The gates heaved inward; already several dozen men were leaping from the parapet, following Gunnar to form against the inward face of the splintering portals.

"Arrows up here! They're breaking through."

The archer's voice was a prayer, a wail, a plea not to be denied. What was it then, what made me move? Animal fear, not cool courage. A Varini shaft grazed my sleeve, not even breaking skin, but it propelled me like a stone from a sling and only by chance toward the tower. The sick rush of mortal fear is like a stone flung into water. The water gives at first, then geysers up in a huge wave. I was so frightened by the arrow I couldn't control the functions of my body. As I reached Beorn where he lay writhing with a broken leg, the answering anger flooded

over me. I screamed with it. Thinking stopped; if I'd thought at all I'd have frozen there by the wounded Englishman, wetting my shift. The scream bent me down, clawed at the bundles, pushed me up the ladder. The archer saw me and bared his teeth in a grimace of relief.

"Come on, girl. Come on . . . quick now, that's it. Come on—"

The first arrows hit the ladder. "Move, woman, *move!*"

I scrambled up the last rungs, threw the bundles onto the platform and the archer hauled me in after them like a sack of turnips. I lay shivering in a wide smear of blood—mine?—next to a long-haired boy with wide, astonished eyes and quite dead. Already the archer was loosing shaft after shaft down into the men on the ram, but too late. A roar went up inside and out as the portals buckled and gave in.

The rest, the scant rest of it was a blur to me. I remember raising my head just far enough over the side of the tower boards to see Icel's banner and the men pouring out of the forest—a dozen, then dozens, hundreds, a different note in the hoarse voices of the Varini, a blare of horns, Gunnar charging toward the gate, legs pumping, sword before him like a lance, and so few men behind him as the Varini poured in against him. Then my archer's shriek as the arrow took him. He fell back against me, knocking me aside. For a sick instant I tottered at the tower entrance, hanging over empty air, twisted about to catch my balance, and then the world ended.

When the arrow hit me it seemed to hit everywhere at once. Jesu Holy Christ Holy Virgin I'm dead I'm dead got to make an act of contrition . . .

Long before I could open my eyes, before I *dared* open them, I was bothered by a smell like burned chicken *Rat, mind the stove!* and a keening of women. The pain in my body throbbed but now at least I knew where it was. Lying on my back, the world a patch of sky and wooden railing, I saw the long shaft sticking out of my conquered body.

It's in my belly. I'm dead. Slow or quick, I'm dead and not a priest anywhere. Sweet God, help me.

Darkness again, nothing.

I didn't wake so much as become more and more

aware of that damned burned-chicken smell and the horrible keening over it all. Shivering, miserably cold in the warm afternoon, I inched my hand over the dried blood that stiffened my homespun to where it still seeped warm, touched the protruding shaft. Not my belly, thank God. Almost but not, a bare inch below the join of the leg and pelvis. Deep—it must be lodged against the bone or through it, the whole thigh swollen with shock.

Somewhere men were screaming, a high animal sound I thought no male throat could utter. Not Gunnar, Lord, you wouldn't let him be that hurt. Stop those damned wailing women—

I writhed feebly to the top of the ladder and looked out on a landscape from hell.

We'd won.

Dry and hard that morning, the courtyard was a red wallow now. Men stood about exhausted from the violent exertion of battle. Some of them were hauling bodies out the gate where greasy smoke rose from a makeshift funeral pyre. A few hacked carcasses were piled by Elfgifu's altar for sacrifice.

The men had left a clear space in the middle of the courtyard. As I rubbed my eyes to clear them, Gunnar moved through his fyrd men to the edge of the space, holding two severed heads by the hair. One was Port's, the other one of his sons, I couldn't tell which from the blood.

And then I found the source of that horrid keening. In the clearing, the hlafdians of Gunnarsburh crouched over a selection of the wounded Varini, their garments neatly swathed in linen aprons and sleeves. They still wore the foxglove, the bells dark and sodden now as they plied the skinning knives expertly, their keening a grim harmony to the screaming that rose under their blades. Edytha watched with intense interest as her mother laid the nearly whole skin on a pinkish pile, then turned again to the flayed thing in front of her.

It still moved.

I have seen battle, but the picture of those three— Nilse, Ase and Elfgifu—will remain in memory until it goes dark for good. Save for that ritual keening they might have been cooks preparing dinner with the absent efficiency of long practice and utter detachment. Their

unbound hair fell about them, stiff with the blood they had washed it in.

Pale and serene, Nilse laid the point of her knife on the belly of the flayed man whose eyes were still open and moving like trapped flies in a glass.

"Only now, Edytha, now you go into the vitals."

She cut two deft incisions in a *T* and pulled the flesh apart. "So. There is the heart."

"Yes, Mother."

"The heart is given to Woden. When you are Hlafdian, this will be yours to do. Watch, now." She might have been teaching the child to clean a chicken for the pot. Nilse grasped the exposed heart, severing the large arteries in a red spray. With two or three sure strokes she had it free, still beating in her hand. She passed it to Edytha. No more squeamish than her mother, Edytha bore it toward the smoking altar.

"Elfgifu!" Wild-eyed and bloody, Gunnar held up the heads for her approval. "My oath, the heads of your enemies."

His mother raised up from her work, resting on her haunches. Not only her hair but her face had been painted with blood, expunging the humanity. "It is well. We are paid."

My empty stomach tried to empty itself further, squeezing sour bile into my mouth. I never grew foxglove after that; the mere scent sickens me. With the last of my breath, I mewed weakly: "Gunnar . . ."

And he looked up.

I couldn't remember much for a while; someone got me down in a sling of sorts, some few carried me to the hall. There were Rhodri and Gwyneth and Rat hovering over me. Thank God for my own around me. In the shock of pain, death coming on me, I forgot even the simplest English just then.

"Rhodri-fach. *Dy clerigwr . . .*"

"She wants a Christian priest, Hlaford."

"Where? There's not one among the Iclingas."

No priest? Is this then the beginning of hell, to die with all that on my soul, still unabsolved, so much of it unconfessed for reasons of state?

"Trugaredd, Gunnar-rix. Dy clerigwr . . . edifeirwch . . ."

"She begs you, Hlaford."

"Get her inside."

The byre was overflowing with wounded. I lay with a dozen others in the hall between the tables.

"Have to cut out the arrow."

"Don't yer die on me, Gwenda," Rat beseeched. "Don't even think of it. I'll bring yer the best soup tonight'n half my own share laid on if yer'll try'n get well."

"Rhodri . . . the priest?"

"Ah, that's the coil, girl. None this side Humber, but you won't need him. Just got to take that filthy arrow out of you. Gwyneth, Rat, hold her down."

I took a deep breath as Gwyneth placed the folded cloth between my teeth. "Bite hard. And here's my hand. Squeeze hard as you like."

Rhodri was deft. I screamed and writhed like the flayed men and went on dying.

The English know less of medicine than our own most backward tribes, which may account for their stoicism. Our wounded filled the stable and hall, the smell of us mixed with the savory odors of the makeshift meals served and eaten around us. The sickness became my world. I was attended mostly by my own who could understand my Parisi croakings. Rat risked a whipping each time she stole an extra delicacy for me that I couldn't even whiff without nausea. The wound in my thigh suppurated and refused to close, so tender that I screamed when Gwyneth washed it in the most lukish water. Then came the fever and the chills, sweating and shivering. The second morning when I woke on my pallet, Gunnar was swabbing my face with a damp cloth. I tried to see him clearly, so far away, so irrelevant. There was no pain. I was going, just drifting away.

"Gunnar, a priest. I must confess."

To my desperation, he appeared rather unconcerned. The whole concept of confession and its urgency alien to him. "No Jesu-people here but you laets. You won't die, Gwenda."

"Afraid I will. Without your permission."

"No, I won't let you." Gunnar bent close over me. "Not a woman who went up that ladder where brave men hung back."

I needed effort to recall the battle coherently, so long ago it seemed. "I was so frightened I wet myself."

"You too?" Gunnar patted the cool damp cloth over my cheeks. "I think there'll be a lot of wash this week. Ach, what a day." Gunnar blew out his cheeks with the immensity of it all. "What a handful of days. Battles, burning—and you. All in a heap. A man knows his world and suddenly it's too big to know."

"Come close . . . can't talk much. Don't mistake being content for something else."

"I know. It's not like that." He strove to make me understand. "I'm not much at words, but I think some of you has gone into Nilse. Part with you? Not even for your Jesu-god. Listen. Perhaps I can say it now, perhaps never again. If I say I love you, Gwenda, it's like the land I touch without needing words. The way we felt in the field before Witgar came that day, the two of us where we belonged. Did I say it right?"

Yes, there was definite hope for a man who could grow up. So few of them can. "That's what I meant . . . by being simple."

Drifting again. Gunnar was there, then suddenly it was Nilse in his place, drawing back the blanket to examine my wound. Had I been stronger the sight of her would have been a surprise: dressed in her new blue gown, the hair so recently clotted with Varini blood now brushed, braided and shining like wheat in the sun. Along with the new gown, Gunnar'd bought her a little terra-cotta vase of Cyprian scent, painted with a comic face. She was wearing it, a relief from the smell of my own sickness. Nilse shone, fresh-scrubbed and radiant for all her illness. If I wondered at the incongruity, the puzzle cleared when Gunnar passed us on some business. Nilse followed the sight of him, even flushing a little. Perhaps I'd done a better deed than I knew. I hoped God would count it so but doubted it. The Word is stiffish about adultery.

Then I remembered her with the knife, the smoke rising from the stinking pyre. "Nilse, don't burn me like those men. Bury me whole."

She smoothed the cover over me, casual as Gunnar. "Now, don't talk about dying."

"You don't understand. I'm a Christian. I must be buried. Don't throw me into flame like an animal."

"Burning is the honorable way. And cleaner."

I began to cry with weak tears, spitting at her like a dying cat. "You . . . animal yourself. I saw you with those wretched men . . . teaching your own daughter . . . you enjoyed it."

"Enjoyed it?"

Something blazed up in Nilse, a force that pushed me physically down on the pallet again. At last I'd touched a nerve, a core in her that was not serene or sure. "Gwenda, a woman with strength enough to curse is strong enough to live. And perhaps learn something, old as you are. I was fifteen when I married into this house. I married a boy ruled by his mother. And I bore him children and watched the boy grow into his own man but always leaving her enough space to be a bully and take her losses out on me. I allow it because I love him and she needs him. Out of loyalty, out of pity he gives her free rein. And I pay for it. A drunken, self-pitying old—"

Nilse's iron control asserted itself. "But there's more, Gwenda. She is too old to start over. And perhaps I will not have any more children. Perhaps *we* are too late to start over in the Midlands or anywhere. So this will not happen again. Men will see what hangs from our walls and know they cannot do it to us. We must hold." She pressed her hands furtively against her belly, underlip caught between her teeth. "You . . . don't know what holding is, Gwenda. You—you stride around like a man, you curse like a man, smug and confident as a man. Wherever you came from, life was good. You don't know what it is to be starting over, starting over, holding on, hoping there's enough and knowing there's not, and nothing ever good enough for that damned mother of his—" Nilse's voice went ragged suddenly. "And this pain in my womb, eating me from the inside . . ."

She'd barely moved or raised her voice. All the tension was in her shoulders and the tight line of her mouth and the two solitary tears that ran like escaped prisoners down her cheeks. "For Gunnar I'd do twice over what I did to those men. They were our own kind. They betrayed trust. It is the custom, expected of me. And one thing Hlafdian Elfgifu will never say is that her son's wife is weak or wanting. Do you understand that, little Brit woman?"

I saw the iron like Elfgifu's, the hardness, the human

breaking through it. The door closed again. I reached for her hand—how brown mine was beside the fairness of hers, and how weak. "I'm sorry. It troubles you, the child?"

Nilse dismissed it in her way as not worthy of mention. "You ought to catch fire more often, Hlafdian."

"It's not meet."

I waited for the energy to go on. "Do a human kindness and send Gwyneth. It's hard to speak English now. And I beg you to find a priest and bury me."

"All right." She gave in, distinctly humoring me. "But it is a poor way to honor a woman of character."

"Jesus God, whose death is it, yours or mine?"

"For a woman dying, you've plenty of pepper left," said the pragmatic Nilse. "And less respectful than ever. I'll send Gwyneth with some soup, and you're to drink it all. Haven't touched a bite. No wonder you feel ill."

There's the phlegmatic side to the English: in the shadow of death when the soul reaches to grasp the edge of eternity, they'll think of food. The ills of the world can be cured with a hearty meal and a trip to the latrine. I was beyond that now. All around me men fought off death or gave in to it, not discovered until they were cold. They were lifted, heads lolling, mouths yawing wide, and carried to the pyre beyond the gates. I saw myself going into that filthy fire, no matter what Nilse promised. That troubled me, a last vestige of vanity, to think of the mess I'd be to carry out. Even that faded as I felt myself going. Plow them all: their problem now, not mine. Someone else could bear out the refuse. But they mustn't burn it, there was purgatory enough waiting, perhaps worse. Not hell. I don't deserve hell. Get me a priest, Imogen.

I called for Imogen down the twisting tunnels of fever, only to find her there when I turned my head, faithful as ever, the blood running from her mouth—

"Imogen!"

"There, it's me," Gwyneth murmured. "Mistress sent you this good soup."

"Yes, give it me." I forced it down, needing the strength. "I want to make confession. Will you hear it and take it to a priest?"

She nodded, obedient. Priest or none within two days'

ride, such things were solemn duty to a Christian, and Gwyneth was always fascinated with other people's lives.

"This too. What I confess—to no one but the priest. Not even Rhodri. Swear on your salvation."

She took some umbrage, knowing her sacraments as well as anyone. "You need not ask that."

"This is not an ordinary confession. Swear."

My sunken-eyed intensity frightened her, hanging as I was over the grave. "I swear on my hope of salvation. Do you not trust that?"

"I was never allowed trust. Give . . . give me some water."

She wet my dry lips, her face blurring in and out of my vision, dotted with dancing points of light as the fever gained on me like the battering ram at our gates.

"Remember all of it. All."

"Not a word forgot, Gwenda."

"My name is not Gwenda. I am Guenevere ferch-Cador."

A stony stare; Gwyneth sat back from me, reproachful. "Shame, woman. Saying you're near death and making mock of Holy Church."

"Will you for Christ's sake listen?" I tried to sit up. "I am . . . Guenevere of Britain. Arthur's widow."

"Nae, an you'll sport with me, I'll go."

"Gwyneth, *please.*"

She was truly shocked that a friend would so play with her. "Don't lie, woman. Mark how easily I can catch you out. Cador was once our own prince. Haven't I seen his daughter with my own eyes?"

My laughter was dry and weak. "Everyone's seen me, even Icel's gesiths. They didn't know me when I filled their own cups. Even you thought Guenevere an old woman without really thinking about it. And Cador came only once among the Lindissi."

About to desert me, Gwyneth paused. "And in what manner?"

"In a chariot decorated with the phalerae of the Sixth Legion."

"And his wife by his side?"

"Yes—no, wait." I struggled to remember myself a day forty years past. "No. Mother rode in a litter borne by your highest men. She was ill and died the next year."

Gwyneth blinked and swallowed. "So it was."

"Remember? I had red hair then, flame-red before it went auburn. It was summer. Mother dressed me in a little Roman gown. White, tied at the shoulders. There was a supertunica, but I'd taken it off and draped it over the side of the chariot. Mother was angry with me for riding through Lindum improperly dressed, but I wanted to show off my jewelry."

Gwyneth stared. "The gold. I remember."

"A golden snake wound on my right arm and a clasp of gold with red enamel work on the other. I kept both for years. The image of Epona riding was stamped on the clasp. And there was music, yes, your bards sang. What was the song? *Dylan mab Aranrhod!* And one of them choked on a bit of dust near the end—"

"And hid his face for shame," Gwyneth finished. "And not two harvests later the Saxon came. Holy Jesus, that's the truth of it."

"I would not dare anything else at God's doorstep. Tell the priest . . . masses are to be said for me in the Brigid chapel in Eburacum. You'll remember that? Brigid chapel."

She nodded, too stricken to speak.

"Since my last confession it has been almost a year."

I couldn't remember in my fever those sins confessed and those reserved for reasons of state. How does a ruler confess? Mary's son was the only king who never lied or needed to.

Lying was the cleanest of my sins. Murder, adultery, fornication, deceit, manipulation of men lay and clerical, the worship of heathen gods—dear, useful Epona—lack of charity, outright cruelty, vanity, pride, lust—all on my soul and so much of it done out of necessity. I croaked it all out, mortal sin by venial weakness to dumbfounded Gwyneth. My throat was parched at the end.

"Give me some water . . . that's all."

"All?" Gwyneth roused herself. "God, I've heard all but gluttony."

"Thank you, Gwyneth. I can rest now."

"Rest? When did you ever rest?" she gasped in cold astonishment. "It wanted seven women all the hours of the day and years of a life to do all that."

"Cover me."

"You are her."

"Cover me, I'm cold again."

Poor Gwyneth: my own age but a mere jot of my experience. Never far from home, to Lindum that one never-forgotten time, she'd rarely seen her own lords. The day we came close enough to touch must have been vividly remembered, like Moses dazzled by the burning bush, fascinated but feeling better when it dimmed.

"You're her."

I could hear the new gap between us. Like all the rest, Gwyneth wanted her deities at a distance. Arthur and Guenevere were legends to her, one resurrectable as Christ, the other a bitch-goddess crowned with glamour and delectable infamy, even my whoring apotheosized. It was too much for her. She wasn't supple enough to reconcile that with the shivering thing on the pallet before her, leaking blood on her verities.

For me, it seemed a lame end, so weak the tears rolled down my cheeks, breaking the feeble voice into a whimper with the last honest truth of Arthur and me to answer her frightened stare.

"We wanted to free you. We were coming back . . . this year. I made Arthur promise. It was the last thing we . . . we did *try*, Gwyneth. We tried so hard . . ."

—And fear the loss of Grace because I fear the pains of the Faerie girl who was part of hell, snatching up my coin, driving me forever from the circle and what Arthur knew as truth.

Already dead, I must be. Dead and damned. Fire and ice, cold and hot, as if Judgment were undecided where to cast me, what pit sufficient to my sins.

In the furnace, but no, not dead yet. I woke once again before the long dark, burning with the last fever, mouth swollen and dry, Nilse moistening my lips and parched tongue so I could swallow a little water. Night and shadow in the hall and the pervading smell of food and sickness. Elfgifu working at my swollen leg, the ugly red mouth of the wound gaping up at life, opening and closing under her kneading fingers, dribbling the last of its corruption.

A scurry of movement: Rat swam into my vision, setting down the brazier of hot coals near Elfgifu's hand. I

felt the heat from a distance. A large dagger protruded from the fire, red to the hilt, whitening below.

"Mistress, I carnt look."

"Shut up, fool. Cloth, Nilse."

A pitiful whine out of me as Elfgifu washed the wound with the scalding cloth. She put it aside and reached to the brazier.

"Hold her legs, Rat. Nilse, take her arms."

The fever thudded in my ears and the rustle of Michael's great wings as he reached into Judgment for the flaming sword, leveled it over me.

"Hold her tight."

Screaming.

Soundless, windless clarity, a picture in glass.

Moonlight on the parapet lighting the courtyard and gardens of Camelot and River Severn beyond. My hands clenched and unclenched around the cold reality of stone.

A scrawny figure slipped through the curtains from the chamber beyond. "The King's gone to bed. He asks for you."

Tell him I will be in soon.

But not before Arthur fell asleep waiting and perhaps wondering, until my absence from his bed became a habit. I'd loved him once and hated him with a sudden virulence as I despised myself, all the more since the why of it fled understanding. Had I that Merlin he spoke of, some voice to answer mine in the silence, perhaps I'd know. But I was alone.

"People like you are always alone."

Not my Imogen but Rat perched on the parapet, grinning at me over her nibbled chicken leg. "Why don't you go to bed with him? Good sort for a man and he misses you."

I can't let him touch me. I don't want to be touched.

"Aren't we precious."

Why are you here, Rat? You weren't part of it.

"You wanted a Merlin. I'll have to do."

Don't I deserve better than that, even dying?

"Not hardly. Merlin was only the best of Arthur, a kind of twin."

And you're the best of me?

"The something of you." Rat picked assiduously at the chicken bone with the remains of her teeth. "All we've in common, that sort of style. We're survivors, you and me. Only gave them what they want when the price was right, not before."

Not true. I loved Arthur more than—that was my trouble. I wasn't used to loving. It caught me undefended.

"Mind now." Rat raised a greasy forefinger. "Even I never used that word till I meant it. You never said it without wondering what it meant. I charged ha'pny. You asked the lot."

Rat hopped off the ledge, licking her fingers. "We all want to be God, but I got over that, got tired of my power over them, working 'em to the finish slow or quick. Not my Gwenda, though."

God? I couldn't even create a child. They owe me for that.

"Oh, sod off, you're owed nothing. You've had it all, yours and half the bloody rest. Even Eleyne's. You knew all the words for love. She knew one. That was Lancelot."

Desiccated woman with a one-candle soul.

"She was sort of a baby in that. A baby hurts without a word for pain, so it howls. Eleyne howled. No one heard her."

You think I haven't howled?

"Don't bleed on me, Gwenda. I'm the only one left to love you, bugger me if I know why."

I loved Arthur's child. Why couldn't I give it to him? I won't take all the failure on myself.

"And an example must be made."

They pounded that into me, starting with Owain. Earlier.

Rat's lipless mouth broke in a wolf grin. "You do have a poker up your arse. Loved Arthur, did you?"

No one else, really.

Rat produced a chunk of barley bread and munched at it. "Then go sleep with him. You don't half need it."

I can't risk that again. I'd break in two.

"Then it's time for the comedy," said Rat.

There was no laughter. I was in hell then as now. Get out of my death, Rat.

"Lancelot," she remembered. "In the garden, wasn't it?"

When?

"When you allowed it to happen. You always knew it could, any time you wanted him." Rat swallowed a huge mouthful. "A little sunlight . . ."

What was the flower I failed to grow? I can't remember except there was a weight of horrible, sane sunlight on the corroded madness of me and the withered plants.

Rat over my shoulder. "There he is, poor cock," pointing down neat rows of my high-summer garden and Lancelot waiting at the end of one. "How old was he then?"

Not yet thirty with only half the scars on his broad frame that he'd carry to the grave. A plain man, not marked like Arthur with any particular light of God, only an ability to suffer; who must suffer for meaning. Not yet thirty years in the world but burned to ash in the center of his own hell. He wanted God. He settled for me.

Rat belched. "It's all one with men. What do you think they're looking for when they stick it in you? An answer. The Grail's always between God's legs or ours. Here he comes, Gwenda. Time to eat him up."

He came down the garden row in his old black cloak and dun robe: Lord Ancellius Falco of Clermont-Ferrand, known to Britons as Lancelot, a modest and uncrowned god of battle. He winced, seeing me so haggard over the flower dead as myself.

"The King says you are better today."

It's dead.

"It's only one blossom," Lancelot tried. "Just one in the middle of so many."

Don't you see? Is it not the principle of evil magic that what you curse in the image is blighted in the substance?

I tore the dead plant out by the roots, rising to my feet as I would rise off the earth to a place of no pain, glaring at Lancelot and the walls that hemmed in my barren self. My mouth opened, no longer able to dam the cry.

Oh, God . . . why am I so empty?

"Don't . . . please." He tried to hold back his hand but it came out to touch my cheek. "Please, Gwen. I never could stand to see you hurt."

Then help me.

Rat prompted then, munching her bread. "Eat the bugger up."

I chose it then, let it happen, melted into his arms, hearing the tumbled whisper against my face as Lancelot poured out the pent desire I already knew.

"God help me, Gwen. It was hard enough to love you in your happiness, but to see you like this . . . like that day in Eburacum when Cerdic came—"

Help me, Lancelot. Hold me tight. Tight.

"So beautiful."

Lie to me.

". . . Watched you day after day belonging to him. I was so empty then. If God couldn't use me, might not you? Why do they call me blessed, people like Eleyne? All my life has been like someone's second-best clothes."

Don't talk, just kiss me. Yes, give me your mouth.

I ate him up, his face in my hands, kissed him hard again and again, ravening kisses like Rat's coarse mouthfuls, and Lancelot must have felt a joy. For a little space he took a need for an answer. I pushed him to it. Nothing could stop it now.

Help me. I've been so alone.

"Gwen. Sweet love . . ." Yes, he was lost in me now.

So good in your arms. I hate him, Lancelot. I can't stand for him to touch me. He doesn't know, doesn't care.

Lies, but he wanted to believe them.

I know you've always loved me. God won't grudge us this, no one could. Not now. Listen, my darling, we must take what we want when it's in our reach. Now or not at all. You can have me or regret, Lancelot.

"You know what?" Rat marveled at my elbow. "You couldn't swill enough holy water to wash that mouth, Gwenda. Get on with it. Tell him where and when. Going to happen anyway."

Don't fight me, Lancelot. I'm naked as you, and shameless now. I love your mouth. It tastes like a safe place. No, you can't come to me. I'll come when I can. Soon, my love. Soon.

Lancelot could only stammer out his assent, stunned, frightened by his own happiness, hands moving over my back and hair.

"We give up all for this," he choked. "We must be all to each other for it."

We will, sweet. I'll come to you soon.

God, I needed something. When I need, I take. It's called living. Of course I went to him, wrenched him open, went through him. For me he was a door out of hell.

"Can't blame the poor sod," Rat allowed. "Not with that sainted sack he married. Never could understand women like that, making a virtue out of a cold arse."

The Lord moves in mysterious ways, and that is one of his most cryptic.

"You were a poor trade for his conscience."

I knew that, he didn't.

"A bleedin jewel."

I was alive, *Rat, more alive than Lancelot or Eleyne or most of them ever were. Their virtue was timidity or a small appetite. I was goddess-sworn by the time I took my first communion. The priests have always hated that joy that joins us. It's the one thing they can't frighten, so they geld us with guilt because an epileptic had a moment of ecstasy on the dusty road to Damascus.*

Rat tore off some bread and offered it. "Hungry?"

No. I'm dying, remember?

"Time for Arthur first."

No, please. Not Arthur.

"Bitch."

Late afternoon in the scriptorium, the time we once used to stop work and steal away to our own chambers, but we hadn't done that in months. Arthur putting down the Coritani tax rolls with a do-it-later finality, raising his blond head to me, a question without words.

Arthur at twenty-six in a bright blue summer tunic that turned the thick yellow of his hair to treasure. For a moment I could imagine those wide-set eyes blue as Bedivere's, not smoky gray. *Her* eyes, Morgana's, were hued and set in the same manner, and thus they glared sullen out of Modred's malicious, beautiful face. An expression quite alien and unsettling, as if they perceived in sunlight and moonbeam a world invisible to me. Faerie scars, her marks on his cheeks. They say his mother Ygerna was tiny and dark. None of her in Arthur but

those eyes. I would have them blue now. I would have all of him different or gone. Like an artist gone perverse, I botched over the lines that completed his beauty and left it meaningless: Arthur in whose driving maleness I could lose myself, go crying mad with him in me, a rut-scented hind in season. A different season was on me now, a winter of corrosive lunacy. I stood aside, wondered at my decline, and went on destroying.

There are horrors under the bright sun. Like flowers grown out of grave earth, love itself has a dark side. The sun goes down, light turns to dark, turns to light again. When I found him again, or rather remembered what my heart never forgot, it was balm to discover we'd reached something surer, something of deeper trust, something to last. But that was years later, days before the end. Now his hair touseled over his brow from the absent furrowing of his ink-stained fingers. He had not shaven since the day before and his mustache needed trimming. A blot of ink—I missed nothing in my gouging—had left its mark near his nose where he scratched it.

"Gwen, why are you so far away?"

It's nothing, Arthur.

"Nothing. You don't even look at me."

So much to do. These people who always try to excuse themselves from taxes.

"Leave it. I thought I'd take a rest now. A walk or . . ."

Yes, that would be lovely, sweet. Go on.

"Come with me?"

No, I'll stay at work. Always more and more of it, have you noticed? In fact I'd thought it might save us time if I had my own chambers as at Eburacum. There's so much I could attend to when you're at something else.

Arthur started to say something, then looked down at his hands. He knew neither of us was talking about work. Arthur reaching out to me, watching me kill something, not knowing why or how to stop it.

"You look so much better today. You've more color. Perhaps this evening we can ride."

Mistress of tact, I never gave myself away in any word, but as he passed behind me, his hand trailed across my back as it always used to before we went to bed. It always set me off; now I flinched away from it, whole denials in the movement.

"I'll be off then," Arthur said, too casual.

Till supper, husband.

How eloquent a back can be. Arthur's vital, swinging stride, those shoulders moving with the power of him. But not then. I could read a bafflement in their set that would turn to hurt, then to resignation. He turned in the doorway.

"What in hell is wrong, Gwen?"

Nothing. I've been sick. I . . . just don't want to be touched just now.

"Touched? It's been ages since I touched you. I'm not a Demetae tribesman to take you willing or not, but a husband—"

Has rights, my lord?

"Has the right to consideration. You could at least tell me what's wrong."

Nothing! . . . is wrong. Can you think of nothing else? No wonder our affairs are such a muck. Go ride with Bedivere and Gareth. You enjoy their company more than mine in any case.

"At least with them I know where I stand."

Oh, thank God for the forthright male. I asked you for my own chambers.

Half out the door, the remark stopped him, stung him. One always thinks of a painful moment in terms of what might have been said, not what was. Arthur hovered there; I could have smiled or whispered a beckoning word and he'd come to me. But I didn't, and his hurt coiled and flung itself at me.

"Aye, take them and be damned! You miserable woman. You will obey your husband in that much, won't you? Jesus, Gwen, there's no reading you any more. Tonight and be damned. I won't have you in my bed if it's too much trouble for the much put-upon Queen."

One more hurt for the man who loved me as naturally as he loved Morgana. I once thought that a contradiction.

"Not at all." Rat was playing at the writing desk, drawing mountains that looked like food piled high on a platter. "Love was always easier for him than you. Look at him there, waiting for you to cry or curse or hold out your arms. One of the once-born, Arthur. He loved easy

as breathing. The only thing he couldn't understand was a lack of it."

And I took my love for that man, up-ended it like a candle at excommunication and ground out the flame on cold stone. Carefully, meticulously, loathing him in my own place.

My Lord, please leave me now.

"There he goes," Rat sighed. "Young, comely, lord of the lot. How long do you think he'll sleep alone?"

I don't care.

"Bloody hell you don't. Me, now: I always liked money. It's pretty and solid. Hated spending the shiny new coins. You collect men, done it all your life. And no one takes what's yours, right? I asked Cilla to love me because it was all I ever wanted. You asked all from all of 'em whenever you got a bit hungry. Arthur's gone? Not to worry, says my goddess-girl, I'll just polish up Lancelot a bit. Always good to have a bit laid by for a lean day, right?"

You would have done the same. Any woman would, given the will and the power. You think I could use the power for myself all that much?

Rat tossed away the quill she was playing with. "Inferior. You've made up all your reasons and Lancelot's waiting. Get on with it."

And so I went to Lancelot who received me like a sacrament, who watched in holy wonder as I stripped off the kirtle and shift and moved to snuff the candle and felt his hands on me, reverent before they turned ruthless with his need. Respect Lancelot but see him in a clear light. He was a man born to burn, needing to immolate himself on some pyre, mine or God's. When he loved me, before the habit of guilt reclaimed him, I saw the man few others even glimpsed, a passionate man who could laugh or cry, be tender and foolish; who could be happy on the pillow with my head on his chest, speaking of his childhood in the villa at Clermont and the things he loved: training an awkward colt from birth to the wind-graceful shape of a thoroughbred, or the wine festivals where the young people still followed the old Dionysian custom and went nude into the treading vats.

Sometimes there were shadows between us, Eleyne or

Arthur. I'd gag my tears thinking, *No, it will never be the
same with you or anyone but him, but I don't care, I won't
care.* Plain hunger and Lancelot's joy would rout the mal-
aise for a while. He glowed in loving me, he shone. For
that little time he was complete. And I ground myself
against him to wear away what I fled from, to rub it out,
and Lancelot took that for passion. A catharsis for me,
heightened by a racking sense of my own cruelty sharper
than Elfgifu's lash across my back. For Lancelot a shattering of life—all he ever wanted, paid for with all he
was. He knew the simple song; I taught him the sweet
variations, the small denials now for greater rewards
later. It excited him as much for its toxic fascination as
for the simple joy. For such men, nothing can be simple.

That's true when you think of it. Good God, he wallowed in the delight of Thou Shalt Not as much as in me;
it worked in him as an aphrodisiac, like the erotic
murals I've seen in deserted villas—Pan with a straining
erection loping after an alarmed nymph. For some of us
it is merely the staff of life. For Lancelot the poisoned
apple was all the sweeter for growing in forbidden
ground. Perhaps for this he cried out at the moment he
burst in me and possessed me fully, as if he were being
torn from the body of Grace.

So the frail ones measure out their careful lives: a *little*
life, if you please, sir. Not too much, thank you. Just a
taste. But I always knew the face value of my actions.

"Did you?"

Rat lounging at the foot of our adulterous couch,
noisily eating her own apple. "Come, Gwenda. He's
breathing regular now. Always sound like they're bloody
dying at the finish, don't they? Ready to go?"

Yes, quite ready.

"How was he?"

Marvelous. Fresh. In love with me enough to dull the
pain for a time.

"Never had it off myself with a man," Rat confessed. "I
mean they did, but I just wasn't there. You?"

Oh, yes, that was always easy. Even I deserved that
much, a moment not to be alone. I found Arthur like a
swimmer touching an island in a storm. For the rest, I've
been frozen in the crystal of duty set down in a desert.
It's my natural state, the way you grow when trust is a

luxury. Perhaps I raged at Arthur because he shattered my prison and dared me to live, *not* to be alone. And though I always retreated into the crystal, the flaw of his mark remained.

"You could always talk." Rat held out her apple. "Want a bite?"

No. Neither of that nor what the sentimental rest of them call sin. Tasteless and dull like cramming your stomach full of dough. Cador carved me a mind, life and Arthur honed it, and that mind has always dragged the rest of me behind it. Life *was* mind, love an afterthought. I'm self-sufficient, that's my hell, but I'll live with it or die guilty of it, whatever the rules say. I accept the way I was made, Rat. Come rack or angels, I'll make no excuses. If I'd lived longer I might even have stopped flaying myself and others around me for what was not ever part of me. The only tragedy would be Lancelot's kind of guilt. That would make me pathetic. I've more style than that.

"Pah!" Rat spat out a seed and looked at Lancelot fallen asleep with his mouth against my breast. "He'll break with it, and be so quiet in the dying, he'll be breathing for years before anyone knows. And me, I'll break. I'm weak. I'll fall by the way. I'll be frightened and want all the help I can find. Won't have a priest any more'n you did. But you'll be there, Gwenda. You'll even care."

Can't, Rat. I've already died.

"Not likely. Bitches like you go on forever."

Am I that strong?

"Aren't you!" Rat tossed away the ravaged apple core and belched with sonorous satisfaction. "No justice at all."

Soaked from sweating all over, the fever broken. Then the cool cloth a benediction on my sodden skin and daylight stabbing my eyes long used to the dark. They blinked open to Rat squeezing out the cloth. The sight of her was like Man amazed at the first morning.

"Yer awake, Gwenda! Coo, it's been days. Natterin out of your head, yer were. There na: got a nice cool cloth to wash yer."

Terribly weak but no longer sick. I wasn't on my pallet

but a large bed. My pained eyes moved sluggishly around the room: Elfgifu's own bower.

"Old bitch had yer brought here. Went down Beorn's to sleep." Rat bounced on the mattress. "Proper *sof*, ent it? Worth gettin sick for."

"Am I . . . all right?"

"Right as bread, my girl. Got a great awful scar but no more. Poor Gwyneth was feared sumfin fierce yer'd die'n she'd have to leg off to a priest." Rat grinned with sly curiosity. "Must've give *her* a proper earful. Not I'd ever ask, mind. Hungry?"

Not awfully, but I could think of food without gagging. Rat reached down to the foot of the bed and held up the crutch. Gunnar had cut it to my exact height and carefully padded the shoulder piece. It took a minute recollection of my form and height to fashion it so that I needn't crouch over it or hang on the excessive length like a limp garment. Perfect.

A few days later I was well enough to give Elfgifu back her bed, pegging on my crutch like a scarecrow on his pole, muffled against the first autumn chill and supported by Gunnar and Elfgifu.

"They've burned half of it, but we've seed for spring." Elfgifu bent her fierce vindication on the half-dozen skins darkening against the long walls of Gunnarsburh. "And they'll think twice before they try *us* again."

Discouraging sight, the blackened fields, the crushed remains of my flower beds shriveled with early frost. I'd barely strength to get out of the courtyard with help, and a crutch takes practice. Creeping back to the hall, the crutch went one way and I another. Gunnar caught me up in his arms and carried me against the safety of his shoulder.

"You must get well," he whispered into my hair. "I need my brave ones for the spring. There's none will try against us now."

"That's good." I nestled into the warmth of him. "No more battles for me."

"You've been sick and not heard. All the war's in the west now. He that's risen, the great Arthur, he's gone after the new King with those damned combrogi again—don't they ever die?—and beat the living starch out of him, so it's told."

"They won back the crown?"

"No, not enough of them for that. Just a battle," Gunnar said easily, "far away and nothing to do with us."

That's all I could feel about it then, so exhausted I fell asleep in Gunnar's arms before we reached the hall. Another battle in the west, far away and nothing to do with me now.

VII

An End to Beginnings

un rose, night fell, seasons passed and then the years. Forest retreated before the ax, oxen lumbered through the fields. Nilse lost the child and bore no others. Edytha bloomed, Eadward practiced in earnest with his wooden sword and buckler now under the tutelage of Beorn. Nerta crawled, stood up, then streaked about full of bubbling energy.

Elfgifu still stalked the courtyard through the night or smoldered in dark prayer at her altar. Rat cooked and filched, plied her trade at Wicandaen fair, and was content. Life went on, except that life leaves nothing unchanged. Season by season the rain fell off, our harvest was skimpier, men less able to afford generosity or tolerate imposition. As I neared sixty, I began to believe I might actually see that advanced age, perhaps even feel it in my field-hardened body. Sometimes I thought of my wedding dress, that little white shift that tied at the shoulders, and laughed to think of wrestling into its slim measure now.

There was only one bronze mirror at Gunnarsburh, Nilse's, and you had to polish it vigorously to see at all. She used it little; vanity was not among her interesting virtues. I burnished it for her one idle winter evening. She barely noted her own reflection, more judicious than concerned, but a hint of fun played around her lips when she turned it on me.

"No, Nilse. I'd bend it."

"Nonsense, you are very comely. British women have such color. As if you might catch fire if the sun shone a mickle brighter. See? You *are* comely."

"Distinguished, as the Romans would say."

"What's that?"

"You've no word for it. You're distinguished when you're too old for anything else."

A long time since my last look. The mirror showed me a thick gray river of hair shot through with swaths of white over a face brown as Morgana's from weather and time, the old scar a pale white line from ear to forehead.

"Definitely too old for anything else."

The hardness had gone out of the face, no longer tight-drawn but open and relaxed. The rest of me was like Elfgifu now. I'd always feel rain or dampness in the indented scar where Rhodri dug the arrow out of me and Elfgifu closed it. But the legs could work all day without tiring, feet thick-soled with callus and rarely clean, the frame of me heavier by a stone, able to lift and carry all day from mill to byre to field and back again, arms wiry as Elfgifu's. My delicate appetite was a pallid memory. I ate with the zest of a horse, doing a horse's work every day, and with a downright English preference for the open air.

I laid aside the mirror and took up a brush to do Nilse's hair. "That's enough distinction for the nonce."

"Ach, du."

I'd become *du* to Nilse over the years, allowed by unspoken warrant to address her familiarly, a sort of menial older sister. Elfgifu still kept her distance, never letting me forget the collar about my neck.

Gwyneth—now that was strange. Since burdening her with my confession, she'd been civil enough but not as easy in my presence, not really knowing how to deal with me. Guenevere and Gwenda refused to meld in her vision. But even Rat and I grew closer inevitably, two peas rattling in the same pod as years came and went and the differences between us rubbed thin. There was a selective and dogged loyalty under the midden heap of her soul. If she was a thief in her own kitchen where she now did most of Gytha's work, she never failed to share or at least offer it to me at bedtime. She stole as a matter

of principle, even when she wasn't hungry. It was a habit of survival.

Nature didn't warp in Rat, it simply never grew. She loved soft things. I saw her once as she passed a fur cloak of Nilse's hung on a peg. Rat ran her hand over it and her homely face lit like a lamp at the sensuous luxury. That's all she wanted, something soft to touch. A child, thrilled and terrified by the bright delights and vague monsters that shadow the edges of a child's life. When summer thunder rolled over Gunnarsburh, she fled to my pallet and squirmed against me, whining with fear until I promised to make it stop.

"God won't get you this time. He'll have to deal with me first."

Not God frightened Rat but Thor, one of Woden's minions, throwing his hammer across the sky. Elfgifu said so, and it was her altar, so nothing would serve but I had to get out of bed and trudge to the altar and stay there long enough to convince Rat I'd discouraged Thor from doing mischief in Gunnarsburh.

She never wanted to go back to her own bed, snuggling up to me. I found her advances tedious rather than offensive.

"Oh, stop it, Rat. Go back to your own bed."

"Fraid ter. Can't I stay wiv yer, Gwenda?"

"All right. But leave me alone."

We always washed each other's hair when there was rainwater to spare, more and more of a luxury as time passed and rain became scarcer. The fields were suffering. But Rat adored fussing over me. Handling the uncut mass of my own hair was a sensual treat for her.

"There's fine! Slides so sof'n crackly through my fingers. Men likes long hair. Ye could've got rich, Gwenda. Maybe tuppence a tumble."

"Tuppence? Me for a shilling, love."

"Garn! What yer got down there, roses?"

"Ow! Mind the snarls."

"Lor, it ent half white since last year only. Yer took on weight too, my girl."

"And you're still a stick. What ails you?"

Rat paused to wave the brush at me, punctuating the problem. "Don't I eat all I got comin and more what Gytha don't know? Nor it ent doin no good I can see.

Then bleedin winter come'n I get the coughin like to die wivout the horehound yer make me." A hollow sigh. "Ent no justice, Gwenda."

"Do try to eat more. I'll mash it up if your teeth are aching."

Rat bent to peck my cheek. "Yer been straight, Gwenda. Cunting bitch when I first laid eyes to yer, but good since." The brush drove through my hair in long, slow strokes. "Call me Raidda now'n again. Yer says it so nice."

"Raidda."

"That's the style." Hiss of the brush, stroke, stroke. "Maybe yer could've got a shillin, girl. Maybe yer could."

In our hard-held tower, the watchmen scanned the forest and the pale carefully as ever. Visitors waited respectfully to be acknowledged on a holding where enemy skins still shriveled in the wind. And Icel sensed a quickening of the times, entertaining priests at his board, men who could write, men who brought news out of the turmoil in places where weed-grown streets still bore Roman names few could read or write now. Such news came thirdhand to Gunnarsburh, clouded as Nilse's mirror, shadows in distant fog.

Watchman, how in the west?

Only a swirl of dust, the clatter of horse and mail. The Welsh King dashes up and down, fights here and there as the red Pendragon comes against him. All the battles are fierce, but none make an end.

Voices from Gaul and the Middle Sea. They doubt this Constantine who reigns but cannot rule. And they doubt as well the aging men like Gareth and the old like Maelgwyn who will not ride forever. They talk of Emrys and see, for all his audacity, he cannot win either. Loyalty and sentiment are nothing to these practical men. They turn east and think in terms of tomorrow and far-ranging results. Britain should not be lost for her lead, wool and tin, and these Angles are more stable than thirty years ago. This Icel is no pirate, one hears, but a prince with well-governed lords. Perhaps they can deal with him. Perhaps it is time to think and speak in English. Who can they send?

Lucullus Aurelianus . . . yes, a good choice for the

watchful men. Knew Arthur personally, knows Brits if anyone does. He could bring facts out of that foggy mess.

The clamor fades in the west, the mail-clad men couch lances and charge, time and mist swallow them up. They will only dim further into the west and the past. They will never come east again.

Far away and nothing to do with me any more. Nothing but the plaintive ghost of a thought that wherever they ramped, Emrys or Constantine, they left ruined fields, sacked granaries and always the dead and the survivors starting over with nothing. An hundred Gwyneths washing the sweat from as many wounded Gwendas, wondering if they can go on at all, and always another generation of young men to do it all over again.

I began to feel as you did, Elfgifu: the arrogance of the Ports and the horsemen alike, all because Someone was Heir to Someone, Someone had a Right, or an Example Must be Made. The stupidity all the more solemn as it receded from sanity, and I can seethe with it even now as you did because of the bloody *waste*. Because it need not be.

Icel began to receive letters from men with Roman names. At Wicandaen, Alfred was once more moving the folc-gemot to his sinewy will.

That was the spring Edytha turned from child to young woman. Where she'd play with Eadward before, now he was a nuisance. She always loved my stories about the fire, but now the swirling dark glamour of the sorceress Morgana and the spell she cast over Good King Arthur, her swift-riding exploits among the Picts—even these paled beside new matter only vaguely understood but suddenly fascinating. She would strain forward, chin on her hands, rapt in the story of Yseult, all the more exotic for time and difference. There are yet no women among the English with hair so black as to glint like washed coal, or skin of a whiteness that looked astonished against such a stygian flood. Nor did Edytha know knights who were poets as well, poets of a passion to throw their life after a mere woman for love alone. The English are not yet players for such a stage, but a marvelous audience for it.

". . . And loving her family she hated the Cornish knight who killed her cousin in battle. Now, Mark of

Cornwall heard of her beauty, and being owed tribute by
Yseult's father, sent to ask for her hand in marriage. And
who should he send but that same knight, his nephew
Trystan, and he all unknowing what he went to."

"Oh-h . . . what happened?"

"Such a knight, Edytha! A gesith like your father but a
bard as well, with the touch of gods in his harp. For in
my country a bard is honored as the druids were, the
companion and equal of kings, and we take to song more
than we do to drink, or almost, and Trystan was learned
in that lore. Beside being handsome beyond the law's allowance. Aye, there was a dash to Trystan."

Dash did not translate well into English, and Edytha
knew no dashing men. Even Icel's handsome son Helmar
did not dash. I dug for an image.

"Such a man as a woman couldn't hate for very long, if
you know what I mean. A fine horseman, a splendid
dancer and a way of making the plainest woman feel
beautiful. Will that serve?"

Edytha bit her lip in excitement. "Tell, tell."

"On the ship carrying them back to Cornwall, they
knew they could hold back this love no longer."

"Ach! What happened?" Edytha darted her glance
about the hall to see if Nilse was out of hearing. "Like the
rams in spring?"

"All of that with magic and music beside. Oh, it was
gorgeous! She was only sixteen and that beautiful, and
Trystan loved her too much."

Far too much, poor Tryst. Arthur's friend, the dear
companion who lightened my hours, he could have had
anything in the world but her. He broke himself on that,
the damned fool. Neither one of them ever understood
the other for a second.

"She was a fever in his blood and he in hers. And one
night on the ship, not even the faith he owed his uncle
could keep his feet from turning to her curtained bower,
from parting the drapes and seeing no surprise in her
face, only a wonder he'd not come sooner. And their
hands had a life of their own, dropping the garments,
seeing each other in the lamplight, the manhood of him
and the white woman-treasure of her. A spell on his
hands that went out to touch her breasts, and her coming
into his arms, drawn by the same magic—"

Then Elfgifu barked from her ale cup at the board: "Gwyneth? Who's come? I heard the horn at the pale."

"Men from the Wicandaen gemot, Lady."

"Come here?" Nilse wondered. "No matter; my Lord will need the hall to counsel with them. Edytha, come away."

"*Nej, Mor. Jeg er kun snarget med Gwenda.* We're only talking."

"Come away. It's not meet for them to be ogling you."

"Go. We'll finish the tale later. It improves."

"You won't leave anything out," Edytha hoped. "Not the good parts?"

"Not a word, though I blush with the truth of it."

Promised, Edytha skipped off to wait the throbbing sequel. The English are not prudish but their attitude toward bed is cut and dried, as their own saying goes. I saw no harm in a little British glamour.

Nilse put me to serve the visitors. It shocked me to see Alfred with his empty left sleeve pinned up. Port's raid on Wicandaen cost the arm, the hard years of rebuilding took Alfred's corpulence. The lazy good nature was gone now. Alfred was a man with a large ax to grind.

Beside him, older but still vital, sat Brand the blacksmith from court. The third man was a stranger to me, a tanner named Haco from Witgar's holding, plump and amiable as Alfred used to be.

My lord smiled at me with his eyes as I filled his cup. Always secure, Gunnar's strength was now benign. The hand that could hurl a lethal ax more often opened wide in acceptance of his life and the world.

"May the fare well become you," he bade in courtesy. "And tell me how is it you come so far in the cold?"

Shrewd Alfred wasn't quite ready to leap into the fire. "Brand? See where Beorn-gebur's shield now hangs beside our Lord's and that of his father."

"And it's seen good service." Gunnar rested his hand on his steward's shoulder. "Beorn is knight to me now. At Gunnarsburh, courage is common as bread and more plentiful lately. Gwenda there fought like a lioness when Port came."

Not so young any more that his sunburst of a smile could still wipe away the years, but it could still warm. "Not to mention the brazen herd of you. What news?

Have strangers touched at Wicandaen, men from Jutland?"

Alfred chuckled over his food; he'd get to business in his own tactful time. "They come and look, most cautiously now. They've heard of the late Varingas."

"And ask only in terms of respect after our lords," said Haco.

"Very respectful," said Brand.

Haco raised a reassuring finger. "We are as courteous to them. We feast them and speak in the most modest terms of Port's raid."

"So modest they know there's more to it," Alfred put in. "We touch in the lightest way on that one war custom of the Iclingas, the keeping of skins for booty."

Brand guffawed. "They tend to lose their appetites after a time. We send them on their way to Bertwold with good wishes. But more are coming from home. Coming to stay."

"In peace?" Gunnar asked.

"If they've got any sense," Alfred said. "Soon, I don't know when. There's nothing left at home. The Geats have it all."

Haco emptied his cup and held it out for me to refill. "We'll be spilling over with foreigners soon, and the old foreign ways. Like the bear-sarks."

The three men slid expectant looks among themselves. Alfred rose, evidently chosen. "Which brings me to our reason for coming, Lord. We have a petition from the whole gemot. We need a firm position in law regarding the bear-sarks."

Beorn whistled softly. "That will take some soft walking."

"And careful words," Gunnar agreed.

"We did have some ideas on that," Alfred confessed. "My Lord will scarce argue conditions are bad and getting worse. Crops poor, last year's rain less than the year before, little this year. In this part of the country years of enough rain are followed by years of almost none. The land will parch before the good rains come again. There's little silver coming in. Even my Lord must feel the pinch of it."

"We feel it. As for bear-sarks, you've never seen one of those shave-headed bastards at my board."

"We can't support them either at court or within Witgar's holding. They demand generosity in the old way: give me this, give me that, when there's nothing to back it up, not that much war any more. And the Lord's generosity is supported by us." Alfred flung out his open hand. "Where do *we* find it?"

Haco nudged Alfred. "We all know that. Tell Thegn Gunnar what we propose."

"My Lord, we propose a new law to the Aetheling. That bear-sarks no longer be above the law in any way."

Beorn nodded, agreeing with himself. "*Very* soft walking."

Gunnar chewed it over with a mouthful of barley and turnip. "How?"

Brand appealed to him. "We thought you might help, sir."

Gunnar dropped his spoon and vaulted over the table to pace up and down in front of his petitioners. He'd grown thicker through the years, though not in the belly, and let his beard grow out to save water. It grew darker under his chin than about the cheeks. "I am for such a law, Alfred. But it must be very carefully put, as Beorngebur says. The words must be thought out and each one weighed, because it could set the bear-sarks on all of us like Port. If it isn't tight, if it leaks at all, we could lose at the start or see another war."

Brand jumped in, eager. "We've haggled the words, spent days on them."

"Let me hear them."

"Not the final words," Alfred hedged. "Just the shape of it."

"That's not enough," said my clear-sighted lord. "We need exact words, words like a fortress that no one can assail."

Alfred threw up his hand again. "What do you ask, Thegn? There's none of us can write. We bring you our thoughts and ask your help."

"Who cannot write myself." Gunnar shrugged. "We need a scribe from court."

In admiring the natural eloquence of men like Alfred and Brand, I'd never considered how shackled it was to memory. Unable to read the thoughts of others or set down their own, each word had to be spoken and trans-

mitted by memory until it hardened into custom. And yet they deserved permanence if anything did.

"Thegn Gunnar?"

The men were surprised that a woman would interrupt. All but Gunnar. "Let your gemot thresh out this law. I will write it for you."

Alfred gaped—a moment only; then he saw the opportunity. "You can write?"

"And you asked if I'd ever part with you?" Gunnar glowed. "Never."

Brand chortled. "The work's half done. Where do the Welsh get such women?"

"Don't ask where," Haco bustled. "Let's do it. Now."

Goose quills would be easy, but ink was a problem and something to write on. I'd put my trust in Gwyneth before, so would I again, distant as she was since my illness. I'd tried to breach the gap several times, but Gwyneth had the snobbery of the downtrodden, as rigid in its way as that of Eleyne or Agrivaine.

I found her alone with Rhodri in the kitchen over soup while Gytha and Rat were about the courtyard feeding chickens.

"The two of you: I need all your wit to help me. Can you make ink?"

Blank stares. "Ink?" Rhodri mumbled. "What needs ink?"

"To write for Gunnar."

"What are we coming to?" Gwyneth looked away from me. "First you here and then a great writing."

Rhodri stirred his spoon in the soup. "We don't know about ink, Lady."

"Oh, Gwyneth—you told him."

"It was too much for just me to carry, Lady."

"Don't call me that. You've told no one else?"

"No." Rhodri seemed unsure whether he should rise in my presence. "Not the half-whisper to a soul. But I must tell you, though we are Christian and 'twas her duty, you should not have put that on my Gwyneth."

"I thought I was dying. I ask nothing but your silence."

Gwyneth nodded, still looking away. "You have that."

"And perhaps your friendship again. I valued that, and you've taken it from me since I got out of sickbed. Is it so hard to give?"

The thing was awkward for them. "Not that, Gwenda," Gwyneth managed. "But you are not like us."

"You've better eyes than that. How different? I've worked and eaten and slept beside you. You've seen me all blood and muck, cut the arrow out of me, washed the fever sweat from my body. How much difference did you find? Britain's forgot me and that may not be a fall from grace. But leave me friends. And help me now."

They pondered their bowls. "It's hard to change," Rhodri said at length. "We'd only heard of you."

"Gunnar is changing things. We're getting rid of the bear-sarks."

Rhodri gasped. "Jesus, that's war."

"Not war. We'll do it with the law, and you can be part of it. Make me something to write with."

"Oh, leave us in peace, go away," Gwyneth pleaded. "You'll bring them down on us. We just want to live."

"Just want to live. And because of that, the lump of you have always been a weight that Arthur and I had to drag because you can't push something without a spine."

"The bear-sarks are not here," Rhodri temporized. "They've nothing to do with us."

"Bloody hell they don't! They demand constant gifts of Icel, who taxes Gunnar, and *we* have to work the harder to make it up. And where's it to come from with the rain failing year by year as it is?"

"True enough. It is hard."

"And it can get worse, man."

Rhodri inspected the thought like poking a toe into hot water. "A law . . . wouldn't that be a joy, the useless louts. By God it would."

"And you part of the making, Rhodri-fach."

"Yes." He decided, bouncing up with the energy of the thought to fling open the bower door. "You, Rat! Go down to the goose pen and fetch me some feathers. Na, did I not *say* feathers? Gwenda needs them."

He turned back to me in the doorway, already composing a way to solve the problem. "There's charcoal at the forge, but it wants grinding."

"The mortar and pestle I make Nilse's unguents with," I said. "Now, what to mix it with?"

Gwyneth jumped up, infected with our enthusiasm.

"Kitchen fat; I've just melted it down. Fetch the charcoal, Rhodri. We'll do it here."

When he hurried off to it, Gwyneth brought the fat to the table and gave me a shy smile. "Well, Gwenda. Aren't you the one."

"Friends?"

"Aye, though it takes a bit of getting used to. It wouldn't be charity to hold back in your need."

"You old silly, I thought it was my persuasive charm."

"Indeed, it was much to bear. I wouldn't think the devil himself had so much to confess . . . Gwenda?" Her lined face was brown leather like mine, but it actually darkened a shade. "Were there really so many men? I mean . . . what was it like?"

I took her hand and nestled my cheek in it. "Shame on you."

"God's truth, I breathed not a word of that part to Rhodri. I mean . . . I've never had anyone but him."

I took a moment to search out a knife to cut my quills, pondering a simile she'd understand. In her way, Gwyneth had led a very sheltered life. "Do you remember yourself and Rhodri when you were first wed?"

"Oh, yes."

"A singing joy?"

"A great joy. Until the children died of pox."

"Then you know the best of it. And you know how this kitchen feels on a hot day when you'd rather be anywhere else."

Gwyneth cast a sour look at the stove where she spent much of her life. "Do I not."

"Now you know the worst of it. Sometimes it was much the same."

I'd put the joy of it into her own frame. And tedium was something Gwyneth knew well.

The ink was lumpy and the quills poor. Rat ravaged the backsides of a gaggle of resentful geese before we were done. Gwyneth volunteered some linen from her laet-allowance and Rhodri attached it firmly to two pieces of wooden dowling to make a scroll. The first drafts were written on clean-shaved shingles, more than a dozen before we had it clear. The saws plied, shavings flew, geese fled for their dignity. That was the easier part. The

clumsy thing about self-government is that no two men have the same idea how to achieve it.

"Subtle?" Brand roared. "What needs subtle? We want them out."

And Alfred despaired. "Brand, a little common sense. If Thegn Gunnar made a law dissolving our gemot, would you just accept it? Why should the bear-sarks not expect some compensation?"

"My Lord and goodmen," I suggested from my scribe's place at the lower table, "when my former Lord needed a bit of legal juggling, he always made it appear to the advantage of the fleeced. For what you take from the bear-sarks, what can you offer in return that you don't really need?"

Haco approved. "That's the way to do it."

"Good business, very good business." Alfred gave a happy sigh redolent of ale and onions. "All right, let's start again."

I wrote it in Latin later translated back into English by the new priests at Icel's court who came and went freely now. Icel might not be able to spell "logic" but he could wield it. Rome and Byzantium were Christian, a faith quite opaque to him, but they were the reality of power and wealth: ergo.

Gunnar and the gemot men took me to court with them. Icel was agreeably surprised—say rather stunned—when Gunnar handed him the bulky scroll, and the sallow priest marveled.

"In Latin? Thegn Gunnar, you have holy men at your board?"

Gunnar's aplomb was gratifying to behold. "Not yet, but you're welcome to come. That was writ by my own scribe. Please you, Aetheling, she will read it to you now. Gwenda?"

A scroll of smudged linen and kindling, marked with lumpy ink, which may be the first written legislation among the English. I'd plunged into it with predatory zest, discovering in the process my own talent for legal interpretation. Which makes sense: if you need someone to frame a law to stand the test of time, choose one who's bruised a few in the past.

TO ICEL, AETHELING OF ICLINGAS,

**We the men of the folc-gemot in congress as-
sembled at Wicandaen send this petition that it be
meet in his judgment and that of his thegns and so
become law among his loyal people.**

WHEREAS
**the ancient privilege of the bear-sarks is of declin-
ing value and increasing burden to men high and
low in the sorely strained conditions of the present,**

AND WHEREAS
**the state of bear-sarks is supported by revenue
drawn in peace from the commons, the burden of
which falls even on the laet-slave—**

(Listen to the sound of history rounding a corner and
men like Cuthwine turning in their graves. So would I a
few years before.)

**We the men of the folc-gemot declare the mainte-
nance of bear-sarks on the holding of any lord to be
harmful to the state of lord and man alike, and submit that such be abolished forthwith.**

(Oslac didn't laugh, he screamed. When it became law,
and that with the terminal speed of a death sentence, I
hear he wept. Time had passed him by.)

**But as we would wield the rod of law, so would we
the guiding shepherd's crook that protects the war
gesith as well as cottager and gebur.**

IT IS THEREFORE RESPECTFULLY URGED
**that each former bear-sark who will abide these
truths be released of his war oath and resworn to
his thegn or prince as knight-gebur; that he be
granted one full half-hide of arable touching on the
unsown weald-forest which forms the extremities
of Iclingas land,**

SO THAT
**each new holding may have the potency to enlarge
to that of a thegn, subject to the laws of land succession and all other laws of the Iclingas, duties,
protection and liability;**

(Never discount the incentive to profit, as quick in

bear-sarks as other men. Lean times they were then, with
harder to come, but the forests were cleared, every ax
stroke ringing with the glamour of wealth to be gained.
"Liabilities" was a hidden barb. In a very short time the
new landlords knew the pride, rewards and burden of
property. Their new status as geburs earned them a seat
in the gemot, wary of Alfred and Brand to be sure, but
part of the machine rather than a stone to break it. As for
the shepherd's crook, we waved it high while keeping a
firm grip on the rod.)

BUT THAT
those bear-sarks who will not abide these reasons,
and their having passed into law, quit the halls of
their former lords—without loss or fine or any pay-
ment to that lord—and look elsewhere for mainte-
nance and increase. Or, breaking the peace
thereafter even in the rights of a laet-slave, such
men to be clept unholden and feel the full weight of
the law.
To these articles we set our marks, lord and men,
for the holding of GUNNARSBURH and the folc-
gemot at Wicandaen.

> **GUNNAR EANBOLDSON, Thegn**
> **Alfred of Wicandaen, freeborn**
> **Brand, cottager to Icel Aetheling, freeborn**
> **Haco, cottager to Witgar, freeborn**

Gwenda, scribe

We are told by the clergy that the earth is the footstool
of God and that each man has his appointed and unchanging place. But the avouch of my senses cannot see
this world as unchanging, not when so much of mine has
been swept away in my lifetime alone. How fixed, what
left unchanged? It moves and grows. The minds of men
grow to clear shape even as Regan grew with child and
Edytha toward womanhood.

And yet the old ways die hard. We falter forward two
timid steps and shrink back three. But something will
not remain still, that quicksilver element of mind. The
footstool will not remain stable under God's foot. There

is a formidable animus in people who generate power upward as well as down.

Icel made our proposal into law since both he and Gunnar were heartily for it, and Witgar subscribed with an alacrity that astonished his bear-sarks. Yet you wouldn't think much had happened. Alfred went on measuring cloth, Brand pounded at his forge, Haco at his tanner's trade, but all of them moved forward by the inch-measure of what they'd done. Commoners but most uncommon men and dangerous as sparks in tinder. I might have feared them myself once.

Sometimes I can still hear the striding cadence of their subversive genius, and I tell you it's a sound to make the trumpet of Gabriel an anticlimax.

Had Icel daughters, Witgar and Gunnar would have scrambled to place their sons within the bonds of royal kinship by marriage, but he had sons, and Helmar the eldest was now of marriageable age. A fine young man, somewhat inclined to take himself too seriously along with his responsibilities. No doubt to his sorrow, Witgar had only sons himself, and since the hegemony of the Iclingas was small, there were not that many suitable brides for a groom-father anxious to keep his son close to home. One of the benefits of our visit to court was a tentative arrangement which Icel would consider with all gravity for the marriage of Aetheling Helmar to Edytha Gunnarsdattir. Visits back and forth between the couple were promising—in an English way, I suppose, Helmar stolid and correct, Edytha blushing and reserved. But they got on, they understood each other in the way of all young people: the thing was viable or it was not. Neither was a fool or at all self-indulgent, each knew to the jot his and her place in society and what was expected of them. In terms of the world and the men she knew, Helmar was as close to Trystan as Edytha would ever find. After a proper passage of time, Prince Icel sent formal word that his son would ask the hand of Gunnar's daughter at the first opportunity.

In the interval you may be sure Icel looked elsewhere and carefully. The East Saxons could offer him nothing much in the way of an alliance, and the British he considered a total loss. Emrys Pendragon might have a

daughter, but his position as a contentious rebel was chancy, and the strange King Constantine was not even married. Thus the underpinnings of a royal love match. Cador had the same misgivings about Arthur before he was crowned and scoured the marriage mart with a gimlet eye before he gave in to the inevitable.

Nilse was beside herself at the prospect, and even grim Elfgifu forgot dignity and went whooping through the hall. "At last! Good fortune at last and come to rest where most deserved. Edytha? Where *is* that girl? *Edytha!*"

We needed some good news in the middle of gloom. The winters grew colder and the springs later and dryer. Good rain falling in the Midlands, we were told, but we saw little. Gunnar and Beorn collected the men in the spring and began the plowing. I went to bed nights with my shoulders aching from the yoke of buckets hauled tediously from the trickle of water in the brook to the fields, and never enough. Even Ase, Nilse and Edytha came to the fields now. Good men and women had been lost in Port's raid. There were barely enough of us to work the land as it was.

Yes, it was good to have something to look forward to. Rat's racking cough lasted longer into the spring and she was thinner than ever, the first wisps of dull gray in her hair and shadows under her eyes. Called from the kitchen to extra work in the fields, the dust of the dry year abraded her lungs. Half-rations became the usual condition as the forest game grew scarcer. We scraped furiously at the bottom of all barrels. For the first time in his life, Gunnar had to enforce his forest rights against poaching by his own and Witgar's cottagers. The whip became more common. The rioting color in my flower garden went dull green with vegetables and stayed so. I no longer wore the leek, I ate it.

One hot summer day a messenger came from Helmar to Gunnarsburh, a sweaty cottager on Icel's best horse, who stopped at the stockade and then rode on to the fields since almost all of us were working there.

"*Hoch*, Thegn," he saluted Gunnar, wiping his red neck with a sodden rag. "Gifts from Helmar to your maid."

It chanced Edytha and I were working a little distance away, breaking clods around the barley and moistening them with water. Ase brought the gifts to Edytha, who

was momentarily awed by the reality of it all, and not a little frightened. The gifts were traditional: a small ring of gold and a short sword of the ancient Jutish type. I hefted the blade. "There's passion for you. What'll you send him, one of the skins from the wall?"

They'd spent enough time together, but now you'd think Edytha'd never heard of Helmar.

"Come, child," Ase prompted. "Answer the messenger properly."

Suddenly Edytha had a glazed aspect. "Gwenda, what will I say?"

"Something coherent, one hopes. Don't gape; the man will think you've never been asked before."

"I haven't."

"Well, *he* doesn't know that. Do you want to marry Helmar?"

"Yes. I think. I don't know. Gwenda, what do I *say*?"

"Oh, dear. Here, give the sword. Put on the ring. Let me speak for you. Follow me and Ase and try to look demure—*demure*, Dytha, not stricken. Come, we will show this messenger how it is done."

The three of us moved formally to the family and the waiting courier, Edytha between Ase and me like someone condemned.

"So please you, Thegn Gunnar, the Lady Edytha finds the gifts of Aetheling Helmar fair and acceptable in plight of his troth."

"And thus to me," Gunnar sealed it. "My daughter will send gifts in return. Goodman, go to the hall and refresh yourself."

Only when the courier disappeared through the stockade gates did the family relax its dignity. Nilse hugged her daughter and took her husband's waiting arm.

"Well, it's done," she glowed. "And it is a pride."

"And our grandson will be a prince of Iclingas. You hear that, Mother? Aetheling Gunnar Helmarson."

Joy was long disused in Elfgifu; she was stiff at it. "It is well. It is well done. I will make sacrifice to Freya."

"Nay, to Venus," I said. "For a good marriage bed."

"Ach, that's Roman."

"That's civilized. And very pretty with doves."

"A chicken," Elfgifu decided. "That's what. We can't spare anything else."

"Just give thanks, Mother," Gunnar decided. "The chicken you can promise."

"That's niggardly."

"That's thrift, Mother." Gunnar wiped his sweaty forehead on a brown arm and squinted at the fields where so much work yet remained to do. "We're wasting the day. Back to work."

Time wasted or not, Nilse would not let so little mark her daughter's betrothal. She framed Edytha's freckled face in her short fingers. I envied the love that could so light her face. "You are not a child any longer." Part of the mother was discovering it for the first time. "You are a woman and can bear children. Bear them proudly that carry such blood."

A small knot of peasants had gathered at a respectful distance, waiting to be noticed. Their spokesman was naked in the summer heat except for a linen clout about his middle. "The gods bless a good marriage, sir."

The sentiment carried a tacit question quite understood by Gunnar. "There will be no extra payments from you on my daughter's hand-fasting. It is a hard year."

The men were grateful. One of the farm wives held out a coronet of wildflowers. "For the young Hlafdian."

"*Mange tak*, goodwife." Nilse went to place the circlet on her daughter's head, but Gunnar stayed her.

"Let me."

The manner in which he lay the circlet over her brow, smoothing down the tousled hair, said more than Gunnar could or would ever have voiced—I should have done something this foolish an hundred times before this. I had a baby girl and now for one moment a young woman, and bare time to look at you with all a man must do, and here someone comes to take you. A young man who makes me feel already robbed, already old. Yes, I am proud. It is advancement for all of us, and yet I should have looked more to you, Dytha. I wanted you to be a son, but the oldest must always grow up too fast. Now I must show my love from a distance, because the distance will always be there. It is a learning, but it is sad as well.

Gruffly, he asked her, "You choose this for yourself, girl?"

"Yes, Father."

"It makes you happy?"

"Very happy."

"I'd return his gifts if that was your will."

Sometimes the youngest girl is wiser than the sagest man. Edytha reached up and kissed Gunnar. "It is well, Father. Helmar pleases me."

"Well." Her father turned away too quickly. "Done then."

"And I appoint Ase to prepare her for the hand-fasting," Elfgifu announced.

"No." Gunnar said it with absolute and final authority.

"But Ase is a married woman of honor, and can teach her—"

"Ase is my knight's wife. She will not regret excuse from one duty where she has so many others. No." Gunnar made an end-to-it movement of his hand. "I will say who attends my daughter."

"This is woman's business, my son."

"My daughter is my business, is she not? Did I not speak with the Prince and arrange it myself? Must I contend not only with worked-out fields but contrary women as well? *I* will say who is wedding matron to Edytha. There are things I may *still* do, aren't there?"

We women were a little shocked at Gunnar's outburst. Always before in matters of the children and house he simply left it to Nilse's good judgment. But he stood intractable now and oddly upset. Nilse sighed and gave in. "And, my good Lord, what is your pleasure in this matter?"

"Just like a man," said his mother. "He'll not give tuppence worth of attention when he should, and when he can leave it properly to women, he's the great law-giver. There are so many women of honor within a day's ride that we can choose among them?"

"Mother, there are times when you're thick as fat in February!"

"That's a fine way to talk to your mother in front of—"

"Damn it, it's true!"

"I'm not the stubborn one, it's *you*."

Then Edytha's quiet determination cut the anger out of mother and son. "I would choose my own matron, Father."

Gunnar nodded somewhat lamely. "Well, I would at least hear it."

"If you please, Father, I would have Gwenda."

Surprise from Nilse, pure shock from Elfgifu, but one glance at Gunnar told me Edytha had anticipated his own choice.

"Damned right you may." He struck his palms together. "That's it. Settled, done, finished. I want to hear no more about it. The day wastes. Everyone! Back to work!" And the Thegn of Gunnarsburh marched defiantly away toward his men.

"Gwenda." Edytha swung me around and set her coronet on my head. "I'm going to be a Prince's wife. I was scared just now but I've just realized it. I'm going to be Helmar's wife! And I'll have none but a beautiful queen of magic for my wise woman. Weeeee!"

And Edytha scampered away to sing through the rest of the day, young enough to know one will never grow old or tired.

"See you attend her well, then," Elfgifu warned. "Not that I approve. She is a maiden. Remember her modesty in the teaching."

Nilse and I shouldered the bucket yokes and started for the brook again. "My back's so sore. Well, Gwenda, I'm not fifteen any more. Whatever took Gunnar to go up in flames like that?"

"I think all men are surprised at love and caring. They think they control it, then it creeps up from behind and changes things without their consent. That's why they all look stunned at weddings. There, I'll rub your back tonight."

At brookside I lifted the yoke from her shoulders. She stretched her back with a hand at the small. "You thought me cold when you first came here."

"You were a different world for me."

"I know you better now. And you me. I'm much happier now. I think it was losing the last child and finally knowing it didn't matter that much; that now there could be us." Nilse spoke haltingly, always reticent in such matters. "It started with the time of the Varingas when we all could have died. After that day Gunnar couldn't be tender enough to me. We are very happy."

I wondered where this tack was leading her.

"I know you've had many men, Gwenda."

For an uncomfortable moment, I misread her intent.

"In spite of that, I think you are a virtuous woman."

"Perhaps because of it."

"Be serious. You know men. I want you to teach Edytha that . . ." Nilse gave much attention to her own stubby feet paddling in the shallow brook. "That marriage can be a pleasure for her as well as her husband. My mother didn't. But you are good with words, even able to write. You have been many places. You can tell her better than Ase or myself."

Her appeal was touching in its incongruity: Nilse, who very efficiently tutored her daughter in the gentle art of skinning an enemy, asked someone else to teach her love. Schismatic, but the English can think two ways at once with neither thought touching. Emotion always troubles them.

"She will be prepared."

"But touching what Elfgifu said," Nilse caught at my sleeve. "You will do it in suitable language?"

"Oh, Nilse!"

"Why do you laugh?"

"You're so—English. I'll do my subtle best, but one can't pick British apples from a ladder in Gaul."

Nilse bathed her feet in the brook. "You know how to put it. I was terrified the first time with Gunnar. We were clumsy. There was pain. So frightened I'd not be able to give him sons, frightened how it would hurt to bear one. Children are a duty. It is sad to learn so late they're a joy as well. There are things I would spare Edytha."

She crumbled the earth in her fingers as she spoke. The clod sifted like powder through her fingers. "I've never seen the earth this dry. No life in it at all."

Following Iclingas custom they were to be hand-fasted before the actual wedding which would not take place until Edytha conceived. All matter thereto was my office. By Nilse's iron and sensible decree, we were to have strict privacy in Edytha's bower, built for her in the last few years when her budding womanhood and her position in the household called for a measure of privacy. On the appointed evening, I took Rat aside and enlisted her help for certain supplies.

"I need a small sharp knife from the kitchen and some fresh linen and a little oil. And clean tallow if there is any."

"Plenty on't. What for?"

"I want to make a phallus."

"Garn, yer nasty old thing," Rat was genuinely shocked. "Yer gonna diddle that sweet child?"

"*No*, you horrible woman. I want her to wear it. To stretch her gradually."

The notion was foreign to Rat whose initiation had been much more direct. "Lady know?"

"No. Nor will she if you don't want your ears boxed."

"Nary word. Won't it hurt awful?"

"Shouldn't. I'm going to get her tiddly first."

"Not on ale yer won't. Child's been pullin on that since she were dropped."

"And some of the uisge Alfred sent me."

"Ow, ent we generous! Wisht you'd give me some. Couldn't half teach the child myself. What I don't know about doin men ent been did."

Now there was a viable thought. Nilse would gasp and Elfgifu reach for her whip if they knew but, properly controlled, Rat might be a master to attend. "All right. Think of her as a work of art, Rat. We must give her the bones before the flesh. Come later when I've got her ready."

There's an artist in all of us; Rat brimmed with the possibilities. "Lor, couldn't I just teach her. What yer bleedin mum never told you, bet."

"Oh? And what will you wager on that, pray?"

"Penny ha'pny to cuppa uisge."

"Done. And not a whisper to anyone."

Rat lifted a hand to heaven. "Quiet's the grave."

"This is not a bawdy joke," I warned. "She chose me to teach her life as my mother taught me. Whatever you learned in Ludgate Street, it wasn't delicacy. If you put a leer on it, if you coarsen it, you'll spoil it in a way I won't forgive, Rat. You understand me?"

Strange: she stiffened, shadowed by an emotion I'd never seen in her. "Coarse. I know what that means. You're the coarse one, Gwenda. Got no heart. 'Cause I don't go men like you, think I got no feelings 'tall. Straight off yer think I'd have a go at the child myself."

"I only meant—"

"Yer ent the only one got old enough to think of some things second. That's a sweet child. Don't yer think I might want to see her blissful bedded? Na, say yer sorry for that, 'cause I won't let yer off wivout it."

"Oh, you . . ." But she wouldn't. Nagging child, she'd complain and sulk until I made formal apology. "Mea culpa, Rat."

"Thank yer. Ow, almost forgot. Look what I pinched. Want some?" From the bosom of her garment, Rat unrolled a length of tow linen containing a slice of venison and some cheese.

"Rat, you've got to stop taking from the larder."

"Work gets harder, I ent gettin stronger."

"It didn't matter when there was enough, but Gunnar's already told his parkers to kill poachers on sight. We're all hungry. Please stop, they'll whip you half to death or worse. Anyone else would tell."

"But not you?" she asked warily.

I wouldn't tell and didn't know why. "Please, Rat."

As with my apology, Rat turned a corner and forgot it all. "Come to the kitchen for yer tallow. And yer can kiss that cuppa uisge farewell."

Alfred's blessed gift of British uisge was in gratitude for my services as scribe. It lent a potent charisma to plain ale and Edytha took to it as a babe to the breast.

"Mmm. What *is* it, Gwenda?"

"Uisge. We make it in the west. Your traders call it whisky."

"It's goo-ood. Tastes like magic."

"It's said in uisge are all truths revealed. You don't need all of them tonight, so don't be a pig. Now, while I build up the fire, I want you to remove your clothes."

"My clothes? All of them?"

"Sweet, there's nothing to be ashamed of. Do you want Yseult to have all the fun?"

With my considerable patience, Edytha eventually lay bare but tentative on her bed, half covered by the blanket.

"Why are you hiding yourself?"

"It's cold."

"Nonsense. Have a touch more uisge in your ale . . . there."

Chatting easily, I waited until Edytha began to beam

dreamily and without sharp focus in my direction, then started in.

"It's easier than you think. When you've touched yourself, you know where the places of greatest pleasure are." I traced a slow finger over her breasts in spirals, ending at the nipple.

Edytha giggled and hiccuped. "How—oop!—how old were you your first time?"

"About your age. See what a little magic can do? You're feeling fine and the fire is nice and warm."

"Mmm . . ."

"You're a lovely girl, Dytha. Do you like Helmar?" I sat down on the bed, stroking her like a contented cat. Her shyness was evaporating quickly. "You like his body?"

"I don't know." She giggled again.

"He's going to be excited as you and probably all thumbs. Don't let him hurry you. One doesn't bolt at a fine banquet. Helmar will likely feel there's a great deal he must prove then and there, as if all his male ancestors from Icel back were leering from the bedpost. This and the pyramids do not change. He may pretend to more experience than he has, to give himself confidence."

"Well, isn't he on top and me on my back?"

"It's not the only way to skin a Varini. Rat will go into that later. More uisge? And . . . one for the tutor. Just remember, veritable satyr though he may be, once you're truly inspired, you can look up much longer than he can look down."

Edytha whooped, spilling some of her drink. "*Gwen*da! Tha's terrible. You're worse than Rat."

"Rat was in the trade—isn't uisge good in ale? Drink up—but there's much to be said for the dedicated amateur."

It caught her in the middle of swallowing. She sprayed again and sputtered, all laughter on a loose rein now. I pounded her back too hard and then we were both caught in a dreadful fit of giggling that cost some time and most of my own composure.

"Oh, dear . . . dear . . . come now. We must be serious."

"Boys are too serious. Helmar can be such a—I don' know what." Edytha stretched her face into a mask of pompous gravity. "He can be so! very! busy! No time! To spare!"

"My husband was like that when he was young. Terribly serious. Well, it is for men. They have it all on their backs. And we have them. Now lie down."

She stretched like a contented cat. I trailed my fingers across her stomach to the tuft of light brown hair between her narrow thighs. Still half a child. Take a little pleasure first, a little love before the children hang from your skirts. Time is endless to you now, nothing seems to go forward, but it's so brief.

"Am I all right? Mor's so plump and beautiful."

"You'll please him. How's your cup?"

She raised it woozily and peered into the depths. "'Nother?"

"There. Don't slop, child, magic doesn't arrive every day."

"Love uisge and magic . . ."

"A woman-magic and secret. Not even your mother must know."

Edytha stretched her arms to the ceiling and yawned. In the fleeting grace of the movement, I saw the supple woman to come. Helmar would receive quite an armful.

"Part your legs a moment. There are falsehoods to be discarded, such as that men know everything. Not about this, they don't. They may think that your own pleasure comes mainly from their entering you. You already know that's not true."

Edytha colored with a tinge of disingenuousness.

"You know what I mean. See? Just a touch and you feel it."

Edytha burbled muzzily, "Tickles . . ."

Her maidenhead was unperforated. In a woman like myself who rode as soon as she walked, the membrane usually tore of itself and shriveled aside long before her first coupling with a man. Edytha winced a little at my probing.

"Will it hurt when he puts it in me?"

"Not a whit. Does the sword pain the sheath?"

Yet it could if she went to her marriage bed as she was. The pain of the tear in such a tender place and the ooze of blood following could coarsen and spoil what should be a delight. There was no need. I didn't suffer it, neither would Edytha.

A light tap at the door. "And that will be our Rat."

It was obvious Rat appreciated the delicacy of the oc
casion, neatly turned out in her holiday-best Englis
gown with a full supertunica and a clean linen veil, he
dignity stiff enough to shatter.

"Mary Virgin bless yer, Lady."

Edytha was now well beyond mellowness into conviv
iality. She flung her arms out to Rat. "*Thank you*
Raidda. Thank you both. You're my good friends, an
I'm—oop!—*so* glad you came, because you're my ver
good friends." With a beatific smile, the bride wilted
back on her pillow.

Rat was alarmed. "Coo, she's bloody snobbled."

"Just happy."

"Just yer remember our bet. Got enough for me if
win?"

"And a taste for now. Drink up."

"Ow, bless! And don't I need it."

For all my dire warning, Rat rather put me to shame
Her only interest in the girl appeared a dignified profes
sional appreciation. Never before had she been called
like a physician to consult from her personal acumen.
think she took a large measure of pride in it.

"A good body," she judged. "Lady will have man
strong children."

Edytha squirmed with lulled pleasure on the warm
blankets. "Oh, I feel so good. Can I have 'nother cup?"

"Raidda, strengthen the magic. Don't gulp, child. No
you," I whispered to Rat. "You know you can't hold it
Slowly. Edytha, don't gulp it down. You're not immor
tal."

"Oh, yes I am." She beamed up at me with bleary radi
ance, and getting on with it took some time with Edyth
kissing us copiously and cataloging our nobler at
tributes. We were her sisters. She adored us with a full
heart. As for Helmar—bring him on.

"Where's my royal husband! I'm ready now."

"God took six days," Rat wondered, beholding ou
newborn behemoth. "And look what yer did in one."

"Bring the knife and cloth. Lie still, Edytha."

"Won't hurt?"

"Less than pricking your finger. Knife, Rat."

"Oh!" The girl stiffened at the first touch of the knife
eyes squeezed shut. "Tell me when it's over."

"I'm finished."

Her eyes popped open. "Done?"

"And that's the worst you'll ever feel." I stanched the few drops of blood from the tiny nick. "Rat, the wax. Now, girl, lie back and let the magic work a bit. I could use a little sorcery myself."

And work it did through tact, patience and judicious dosings of uisge. Edytha lolled between us on the bed, her head on my arm, and *knew* she must have us and no others to her own bower when she married Helmar, as soon as her father could spare us. So she drowsed while I worked the pliant tallow into her body, Rat ready with the oil to ease the passage. Little problem; she was young, healthy and achingly ready for a man. The young thighs were still a bit stiff and narrow, but that would pass and nothing about love would be difficult for her now.

"You must keep the tallow in as much as you can, even when you sleep. It will stretch you. How does it feel?"

"A little tight."

"That will quickly pass. Use the oil freely so it won't chafe, vinegar and water to clean yourself. Raidda, I think we could all use a little more magic."

"I cern'ly could." Edytha held out her cup with an unsure hand. "Oh, it's nice to be bare and clean and soft and . . ."

"Brave girl." I gave her a maternal kiss, lavishly returned. "Now I believe Raidda may have a word to your profit. From here on, it's esthetics."

"My sweet Rat, come talk to me . . ." Rat had to be embraced again with sisterly warmth. "Rat's my good friend. More sense'n Elfugiv . . . El . . . my grandmother."

Rat acquitted herself with laurels, serious as a scholar expounding the Gospels. Not a hint of lechery, not one word that would so much as take the blush off a daffodil. I was proud of her.

With the tallow placed, Rat advised, no one need tell Edytha how and where it felt best—which was a good thing to know since men had different ideas or none at all about what a woman enjoyed, but there *were* different approaches, for a change once in a while, especially

when she was with child, that would greatly enhance the pleasure of it all.

With patient hands, Rat turned the girl this way and that. As she proceeded, I found myself learning a thing or two. A pity Rat had no interest in men. She certainly knew what to do with them.

"Let'm know yer all for him. But make him wait a bit. Don't throw it all at once, like. Let him—oh, Gwenda, what'm I tryin ter say?"

"Discover."

"Let'm discover, that's the style. Are yer rememberin all this, sweet love?"

Edytha nodded, fuzzy but fascinated.

"And there's times when yer can make yer own weight work for yer both. Up on yer knees now . . ."

And on through an instructive hour, master and apt pupil, bringing our bride through theme to variation to the very capstone of ars amor. Edytha had never even heard of it.

"No mind: men likes that best of all and no mistake."

Edytha grimaced in distaste. "Well, *I'd* never. *Eck!*"

"Well, that's a lane what goes two ways. And a very nice lane for a girl if I say't myself."

Our initiate appealed to me as final authority. "Really, Gwenda? 'Zat the way Christians do it?"

"Some, the enlightened few. Many have a niggling suspicion women shouldn't enjoy it at all."

"Eck."

"Din I say that about oysters," Rat mused, "afore I tasted my first. Makes it better, love. Like salt on meat."

"Adds a little imagination."

"And not lettin him do it all."

"Think of music," I offered, letting the mood take me.

"Good food," Rat savored.

". . . Love oysters." Edytha drowsed on her pillow. Then, her head groaning full of our clandestine teaching, she fell peacefully asleep between one breath and another.

"Ent she a sight?" Rat admired tenderly. "Who couldn't love her? How about my cuppa? Din I win?"

"Not a rout but a definite victory. You are a master, Rat. Fill up."

Rat measured a brimming cup and settled on a stool,

satisfied. "I helped her, Gwenda. I do think I really passed on some what I learned."

"You were noble, Rat. Beautiful. By God's Eyes, *we* were beautiful. We are Magi, Rat. We have brought wise gifts to a very holy child."

"Din we just." After a killing swallow of uisge, she wobbled to her feet and went to smooth the blanket over Edytha. She staggered a little returning to her stool. "Wisht I was that young again," she said in a maudlin, thickening tone. "I hate gettin old."

"Don't drink so fast. That's the last of it."

"It's just I hate gettin old. Gray in my head and my flux stoppin so soon."

"Once that's past, you'll feel much better."

"No," she whimpered, inconsolable.

"Oh, what are you on about now?"

"I'm 'fraid of dyin, Gwenda. Gettin old is the start of it."

"Rot. You're not getting old, you're getting drunk. You never could hold it, and you always—now, Rat, stop!"

But the cup tilted up, her head canted back. She lowered the empty cup with a strangled gasp of pleasure, weaving a little, peering across the space between us, trying to find me in it. Then, with ponderous dignity, Rat slid to the floor and oblivion.

"Oh . . . God's truth." I waited a few minutes, relishing the quiet and warmth, the last of my uisge and a heavenly touch of privacy. Rat twitched once and lay still. A soft snore issued from the bed.

Lifting Rat, she was a mere wisp in my arms. I hauled her erect, let her wilt over my shoulder, and carried her to bed.

Edytha and Helmar were hand-fasted in the harvest month—such harvest as we could wrest. Elfgifu's altar hulked in disuse. We had nothing to thank Freya with or for. Gunnar doubted the use of prayer now anyway.

"The gods stayed in Jutland. They had better sense than our fathers. Nothing here but Welsh devils."

That winter was the hardest any of the English could remember, unrelenting cold but very little snow. The earth froze, thawed and cracked into deep ruts. The pigs and chickens were slaughtered one by one as feed ran

out; when the poultry was gone, Gunnar's own horse was butchered. He regretted the necessity but didn't consider it a weeping sacrilege as Gareth would. The thing simply needed doing.

Payments in food from his peasants were not asked. If Beorn and Ase could barely stretch their substance through the winter, lesser men were in worse condition. My lord and Beorn were drawn in those bleak months with worry they tried to hold back from the women who knew too well their predicament in any case. Over our spare meal in the hall one night, we heard the family at the high table discussing the inevitable in tones they no longer lowered against our hearing.

"Beorn, share out the sheep. Tell the men to come for them. But they'll save the wool for me."

Elfgifu was against it. "Foolish, son. Sheep are money. How can we replace them?"

Gunnar gave her a look she might have taken for warning. "I don't know. Perhaps the Aetheling will help in the spring. We are kinsmen now."

"And if he can't?"

"I don't know!" I heard the jagged edge of anxiety in his voice. "Must I have answers for every—Eadward!"

The squeal of the children was a barb to Gunnar's worn temper. They were running about the hall, shrieking high in their play, too young and heedless to feel the true edge of hunger yet. Eadward chased Nerta with his wooden sword, swinging the flat of it too hard against her small rump. She howled with the sting. Gunnar shot up out of his chair. "Boy! Come here!"

When Eadward obeyed, Gunnar flung the wooden sword across the hall and tore the buckler from his son's arm. "You've been told and told to be quiet in the hall, haven't you? *Haven't you!*" He shook the boy back and forth, turned him over and spanked him hard.

"Beorn, no more wooden sword for this one. Tomorrow take my old one and start him on it."

"It may yet be too heavy for him, Thegn."

"I don't care if his arm drops off. It's time he learned what a sword is for beside frightening his sister. Eadward, you'll listen to Beorn and do what he tells you. With luck you *may* grow up to be like him. And *don't cry,*

damn you. I've raised you better than that. A boy doesn't cry."

With each command he shook the boy savagely. Verging from childhood to youth, verging on tears, Eadward choked them back, edging away from his father.

"Now, get out of here. Nerta, be still."

Nerta only wailed louder in Nilse's arms, shrinking away from her father. Even across the hall I could see how pity colored the fury in his eyes; but manlike, it was out now and something would pay for it.

"Leave the child be, husband. Eadward hurt her. She's tired and hungry."

"I know what she is! Take her to the bower, I don't want to put up with her now."

"It would not have been so in the Midlands. The land is good, the rain falls gentle and often."

It was the wrong thing to say and the worst time for Elfgifu to brandish once more the memory of her husband and her standard of a lord. These values were fixed. They gave her no understanding of men, only impeded it. Corroding over her dreams and ale, she felt herself growing older to no profit, no repayment of the ancient debt. She loved Gunnar, but for such bitter dreamers, nothing is ever enough. There was perfection once, gone now, and all of it fading away with the cold night and the last of the food. She glared at her son.

"Men like Eanbold were making a kingdom. But he was scin-laecen."

"Oh, yes. My noble father." In the tight-coiled desperation of Gunnar turning on her, I remembered Arthur with dead Morgana in his arms. A lethal attention; it would have blood. "You foolish, drunken old woman. I'm sick of you most of all. Get out of my hall. Go to bed. *Get out—*"

Gunnar quivered with rage, looming over his mother. Like a lord must, from his eighteenth year he'd tried to be all to all. As with all such men, there'd been some victory and much failure, battles won and lost, failing land, and always the image of his father held out as an impossible ideal enlarged by an old woman's regret.

He was no hero, not in her sense. He was lord because he was strong. Because he was just a man, he could break and run away in one human moment before the strength

of him checked the tide of defeat. While the rest of us sat frozen, Gunnar hauled Elfgifu from the bench and pushed her around the table.

"Well, it is *not* the Midlands and *not* Eanbold, and there are no more heroes and no more gods, you old fool. It is here and now and there's just me. You chew on *that*, Mother mine, and you damned well swallow it, because that's all there is."

Elfgifu tried to preserve some dignity, eye to eye with her son's fury. "Remember who it is you speak to. And whom you speak of, boy."

"Remember?" Gunnar seethed. "There's been too much remembering." He leaped onto the high table in two bounds, grasped his father's shield and tore it from the wall. In two more strides he was down from the dais and at the firepit, the shield high overhead. Elfgifu flung out her arms to prevent it.

"No—"

"Yes!" Gunnar flung the shield into the fire in a shower of sparks. "Done, damn it. Done!"

"Pull it out. Oh, son, please, pull it out."

"Get away!"

"I beg of you, don't dishonor us this way."

"Dreams, old woman." Gunnar caught her, spun her about, shoved her toward the door. "That's all I burned, just dreams. My children can't eat dreams. Out!"

He pushed her too hard. Elfgifu lost her balance and fell to the earthen floor. She huddled there, shaking, gray braids hanging about her face, frightened now of her son's white rage.

"Go on, go out and pray. Go babble to Woden at your altar. Go cry to hero-father. Tell him how nithing his son turned out. Go on!"

He jerked Elfgifu to her feet and thrust her brutally toward the door. She hunched there with her hand trembling on the latch.

"You think I'd tell him that? We were stronger than that. We would not put a knife in what we loved."

"Not true, Mother," Nilse said quietly. "He shouldn't do this to you, but you've had that knife in Gunnar for thirty-four years. It is well ended."

Elfgifu turned to her son, both of them naked to each other on the dark side of love. Elfgifu saw the burning

shield, the black spreading over the blazon painted with
her own hands and hope. Gunnar might have been right,
there was no more place for dreams, but for her it was a
death.

"I should have smothered you in that burning byre and
run myself on Lancelot's sword."

Gunnar glared at the door that closed between them.
Then his eyes squeezed shut. His words broke on something larger.

"Let no one speak. Don't say anything right now.
This . . . this was not to dishonor my father or the gods. I
used to have many words for honor, but now I tell you
all—if I could find a lord to help us, be he Welsh or English, an Arthur, even a Constantine, I would go to him
on my knees and place my hands in his to give us a living. Listen, all of you. We will not fail. We will . . . go
forward somehow."

Gunnar pointed to the burning shield. "Only that is
ended. Like the bear-sarks, we don't need it any more.
There's none of us but my mother who wouldn't trade it
for a good rain. We have the seed at least. We can carry
the water. We will plant again. As bad years come, so
they must go. That's . . . that's all I can promise you."

Gunnar lunged out of the hall, banging the door, leaving a heavy silence behind him. Nilse carried tearful
Nerta to the bower, Beorn and Ase left for theirs. One by
one we servants left the common table. Only grizzled
Cynred mourned over the lost shield.

"Hlaford should not have done that."

"None too soon," I said.

"Not that, it's the waste. Eadward would've been
proud to carry it. Take out the coals before bed,
Gwenda."

One more tedium on bitter cold nights. The watch
quartered in the byre needed fresh coals for his brazier
that warmed him and our remaining stock. Muffled in
my cloak—old when Frith took me, threadbare now—I
filled two scuttles with fuel and fought my way to the
byre, head bent against the dry razor wind, pushing in
the door and grunting to shut it against the blast.

"Ay, watch! Here's for the fire."

"Don't wake him," the muffled voice bade me. It came
from one of the stalls. Most were empty now.

"Who's there?"

"Just feed the fire, Gwenda."

He sat in the shadows of the stall on a pile of straw, wrapped in his cloak, his back against a post. "Glad it's you. I can't go to Nilse now, not like this."

"How is't, Gunnar?"

"How should it be?" He let me see the tears he'd show to no one else; I was even trusted with his shame. "A brave night's work I've done."

"You cleaned a wound that needed it."

"I wish I could be sure of that."

"Be sure." I pulled his head to my breast, stroking his hair. "You're a man. I doubt your father was more. It's only her love that paints him so."

"I've tried, Gwenda. What with my father and the plowing gods, she never let me be much of a boy, not that long. We never had much, now we're losing that. And because I'm *miserable* inside, I shame my son just for being a boy, shout at my little girl just for crying, because I know she's hungry and I can't do anything for her, and still young enough to play for all that. Then I break my mother's heart. Yes, a brave night's work."

"Let me hold you."

"No, stop—protecting." He shoved me away. "That's my place. Need you remind me like everything else how unfit I am for it?"

"Gunnar, don't."

"Have I hurt you too?"

"Only yourself."

"I said stop it. You've eyes; you see what's happening. My parkers are hanging men because they have to steal to feed their own. Even here there's thieving. Gytha is missing food she knows was stored away. Mother's watching, there'll have to be punishment. I'm sick of punishing. What will it be like in spring? What do we start over *with*, Gwenda?"

"We will plant as you said." I tried to sound convinced.

Gunnar drew me close to him. "It's always good to talk to you. Even when I know you're just trying to make me feel better. Elfgifu and her gods . . . what would your god say to do? I don't think ours came with us. I don't think there are gods any more."

We listened to the wind and the watchman muttering in his sleep.

Next day I was summoned to the hall and found Gunnar by the fire with a scrap of parchment in his hand. "From the Aetheling. The messenger's in the kitchen for some ale. What does it say?"

I scanned the Latin: no urgent news but Icel thought his thegns might be interested in late events in the Midlands. I didn't show Gunnar how much it meant to me. "The Midlands are now without a lord."

"Old Maelgwyn's dead?"

"Of natural causes, so it says."

"You couldn't kill him any other way," said Gunnar. "Tough old hound was seven years the elder of Britain itself."

"Pray God receive his Christian soul." I crossed myself.

"And one less Brit to contend with."

"As you did with such difficulty at Badon," I reminded him tartly. "He was loyal and valiant. Arthur prized him. He's worth my prayers."

"Yes, yes. What of Constantine?"

From old practice piecing intelligence from fragments, I gleaned the picture. Maelgwyn and his sons dead, no one of the Catuvellauni chiefs had enough power to hold them all together or keep an effective force on Badon. Likely most of them slipped away home, as the combrogi did after Arthur's death. In short, the Midlands were his who could take them now.

"Gott!" Gunnar furrowed worrying fingers through his thick hair. "There it lies, begging for good men to take it, and not a hope."

The story of my life and Arthur's. "Yes. Frustrating."

"What else does Icel write?"

"Just this at the end, quote: 'I have sent messengers to Jutland that those Angles who will swear fealty to me shall be welcomed.'"

"And give them what in return?" Gunnar sat on the lip of the firepit. "No lack of heroes, the ships will come. Brave is cheap, brain comes high. Last year, this year, piddling away their strength raiding the south coasts. Never much of a wound but always bleeding. And for

what? Pride and a little profit and a verse in the song of some sour-voiced skald. Ah, Nerta!"

Unsure of her father's mood, the little girl peeked at him from the door to the kitchen bower. Gunnar held out his arms.

"*Kum, lidt skat.* Come to Papa."

She scampered down the hall toward us.

"If we could forgive quick as children, eh, Gwenda?"

"Christ said something about that. Like many of his sayings, it was quite true and quite impractical."

"Now I've got you, girl!" Nerta squealed with delight as Gunnar swept her up, laughing, into his arms. "Now, now, all better. Eadward won't chase you any more, that was wrong of him. How's my baby today?"

The little gown Gwyneth had made for Nerta's last birthday hung looser now. God made children tough. He had to.

Nerta twisted around in Gunnar's arms to point to the kitchen: something very important. "Grandmother hit Raidda," she said solemnly. "And Mor's very angry."

"Well, Mor can manage. Kiss your papa."

Nerta gave him the gift he needed above all others, crushing her small face against his cheek. He looked over her shoulder at me. "I ought to spend more time with the children. How old are you now, Nerta?"

"Eight and a half."

"So old! Then I think you're big enough to help your father. Would you like that?"

"Ja!"

He set her down, holding her hand. "Then we'll go see that things are right at the smith's and then look in on Eadward at his sword practice—"

The door at the end of the hall burst open again in a tide of angry voices. Elfgifu marched straight down the hall to us, a thin arm vised in her vindictive fist and the rest of Rat dangling from it, Nilse marching behind. Elfgifu flung Rat at her son's feet.

"Here's our fine thief, wise son who is too busy to take notice. *I* caught her stealing."

Less vindictive but as firm, Nilse said, "We cannot pass this over. The Prince's messenger was there. She must be punished."

"Lor, I never," Rat pleaded. "I swear I never. Just lookin

in the pot to see what was left 'n what we could put with it."

"Liar," Elfgifu spat. "Half in her mouth it was. Look, there's the grease still."

Gunnar looked away from Rat with distaste. He didn't want to deal with her today and certainly not his rankling mother. He would have enjoyed being a father for one hour, but the lord was needed. As for Elfgifu, she still burned from her shaming the night before. She couldn't forgive with Nerta's facility.

"Give judgment, son. Remember this slave robbed not only yourself but your children."

Gunnar's disgust was not all for Rat. "Stand up, woman."

"Gwenda, yer'll tell the Lord." She clutched at me, convincing herself by need alone of her innocence. "Tell 'em I never stole."

"Oh, Rat!"

That was all I could say before turning away. I warned her so many times, my friend and a thief to the bone, and thank God judgment wasn't mine. I'd grown rusty at it. But I couldn't help her.

Gunnar pushed Nerta to me. "We'll do it later, Nerta. Papa has work. Gwenda, take her out."

I was glad to be away from that, didn't even look back as we went out the door, too sad for Rat to be frightened for her.

English penalties for theft are brutally severe. It must be so; their world is based on personal ownership. In the justice of that hungry winter, no doubt Rat deserved what she got. I had many times dispensed that justice summarily. Nerta and Eadward went to bed hungry, and yet I didn't want to think on Rat whose weakness and strength so resembled my own. In a world of lords and shackled slaves, she learned survival as I did. Where one fist struck with the sword while the other caressed gallant lies from a harp, that was the bond that made us sisters. We both smelled of that world whose truth we would not perfume.

She was to lose her right hand.

They shackled her in the byre close enough to the smith that she could hear the grinding of Cynred's ax. I

took her some of my supper, little as it was. Livid with fear, she still ate mechanically.

"I won't live it out, that's flat. Weren't I there when they put the iron on yer leg, what with the hiss and the smell of't? What'm I gonner do wivout my hand?" She held it up as if it were already gone. "Whyn't yer speak up for me? What'd I do ent been done before?"

"Goddamn it, wasn't I at you all the time to stop?"

She hunched in her blanket and glared at me over her horehound tea. "Yer was my friend and wouldn't speak up for me. That Gunnar, he favors yer. Gotter tell him it ent right."

"If it weren't for the children—"

"Little barstids are fatter'n me."

"Liar, they're sticks! You never think of anything but your goddamned belly, like a hound that can't be taught."

Rat only sulked in her injured way. "Thought yer was my friend."

"I am. And God only knows the strangeness of that."

"Din I tend yer when yer was sick?" Like the child she was, Rat's thoughts ran in a very small circle when she was frightened, always coming back to the fear of the morrow. We heard the rasp of the grindstone from the smithy.

"It ent the ax, it's the closin, like what they done to you. I won't live it out." She snuffled into her tea. "I'll die'n old bitch'll put me on the fire like kindlin, burn me up. Won't be nuffin left. Yer gotter promise to bury me, Gwenda. How's Lor God gonner find me come Judgment, 'n me nuffin but flinders?"

She flared with sudden fierce rebellion, flinging the cup against the wall. "Christ!" It spent all her small strength. Rat wilted over her knees. "I hope there's better comin, Gwenda. Lor God, I hope, cause it ent here. Sometimes I *wanter* die."

I knew I had to try for her.

I don't know why, but I pleaded to Gunnar. Like the oak that fell on the sparrow stealing its acorns, it was too ponderous a sentence. Her guilt would rattle loose in it. Or simply say I was no longer that much of a Guenevere. Nevertheless I put it to Gunnar in private, drawing shamelessly on his affection for me. I found him in the

deserted byre, gloomily rummaging through the baskets of half-grown wool that his peasants had rendered after slaughtering the animals.

"Gunnar, you and I have given to each other and never asked. Now I ask a boon."

He sifted a handful of the wool. "From my large store of boons."

"Rat is too weak to lose a hand. She's sure she'll die from it, and well she might. Make it something else."

"You think I'm not sick of punishing?"

"I never doubted that, nor that she should be punished. But even she's been needed in the fields these last two years. You'll lose a hand from the spring work. And the time she needs to heal. And she cost you two and a half pounds."

Gunnar sat down on an upturned basket. "These new lords, the bear-sarks. They've never had any love for me, less now. If they see us failing, if they see I can't keep order in my own house . . ." He spread his hands. "Shall I take her eye?"

"Let it be the whip. In the courtyard for all to see. I did as much, tried to escape. She's never done that."

"The lash is not enough. Someone might be hungry enough to steal themselves."

An old ghost stirred in me. "And an example must be made?"

He said it without relish. "That's a good way to put it."

"It's been said before, my Lord." I inspected a handful of the dull brown wool. "Shoddy stuff, barely worth the shearing. Where will the pence come from to restock?"

"Ask Woden. I've burned late candles over that."

"Gunnar, be sensible." I pressed his face to my breasts. "You're one of the few men I've loved with no thought to profit, but why not speak of profit? Rat is the most covetous miser in your house. It pains her to spend a farthing on a meat pie in Wicandaen fair. Give her the whip and a money fine. She'll remember that. Make it meaningful."

In the end Gunnar made it the whip, but it was Elfgifu who counted the pennies. We were all there in the gray cold courtyard when they led Rat out and tied her to a wagon. And I was in the kitchen bower when Elfgifu tore through Rat's possessions. Her money, which would have gone to Gunnar in any case, amounted to three pound/

ten. Elfgifu took it all, throwing the tattered rest of Rat's things into a corner, pouring the coins into a sack.

"What are you lowering at, Gwenda? She's lucky."

"Yes."

"Wouldn't have thought the kotze had this much money. It will buy some of what we need at least."

"Yes. Hlafdian. I will tend Rat myself."

That was nothing to Elfgifu. "You started by wanting to kill her. Now you give her more respect than me."

"I don't respect Rat at all, Hlafdian Elfgifu." I clipped off the words with edged distaste. "You I respect. Her I call friend."

She smirked grimly. "Well understood, little Brit. None of your kind have ever known dark from light. Murder and weep in the same breath. I'm close to seventy, but I'll put you both on the fire and walk away. Go on, see to the rodent."

In trying to save Rat, I'd sealed her end. I didn't know her deep through after all, never realized how frail was her hold on life and by what she measured it.

"Took it all," she whimpered on her pallet in the darkened hall as I bent over her, fingering hyssop poultice into the mess of her scrawny back. "All I had, Gwenda."

"Better than your hand."

But it wasn't. The loss broke Rat. The money, the stupid three pound/ten. No reasoning with her that she'd always have a bed and clothing and something to eat. That hard silver was security to her, all of balm and joy, probably all of real faith she'd ever known in a handful of coins so worn you couldn't tell one Caesar from another. She never spent them. They were safety against the ever-lurking Not Enough, the fear that drove her to tuck away bits of bread in her pallet even when she wasn't hungry. No doubt she lay awake many a night, counting the numbers of her safety like a catechism.

"Well," I tried lamely to console her, "they'll use it for all of us. You'll get some use of it one way or the other."

Much as it tortured her back, Rat twisted around to me in the gloom. Her battered, chinless face was dignified with its terminal truth. "What for, Gwenda?"

She took a chill almost immediately and never left her bed afterward except to be moved to Edytha's bower. The

cough deepened, became painful to hear as well as to her, then a frightful hoarseness, then a wasting fever. I did what I could, chopped and carried extra wood and coals for her fire. Inconsistently, Nilse brought her that extra food for which she'd been punished, but Rat couldn't eat much. I can't say whether she decided that night not to live any more or simply found it too difficult or pointless.

She had our toughness, Elfgifu, but you and I were given a variety, even a poetry of reasons for life. Rat was given facts. She thrived by them until they were taken away. Don't mouth such words as hope or ambition to Rat, they are irrelevant.

I tended to Rat myself, cleaned her, fed her when she could eat, tiny mouthfuls of soup with Gwyneth holding her up to receive it. I sat by her bed and tried to sustain her with huge promises.

"Look here, sweet. I've got a bit put by from Wican-daen, this and that. If you'll try to get well, I'll cut the lot with you, Rat. Old miser, that ought to get you out of bed."

She patted my hand with a bony claw that grew colder each day. "Don't yer fret. Old bitch ent had the best of me yet."

"She won't last till proper spring," Gwyneth was sure. Long before that we all knew Rat would be gone before first thaw.

Toward the end of March she became feverishly obsessed with her last rights. We'd long since eaten the last horses, no one could journey on foot so far as court for a priest who might not even be there now. Rat made her confession to me—much less damning than mine, my lords, and no business but hers. The distillate sins of her forty years required few more words than that. Tidy, as this world goes. Rat was immensely pleased that I wrote it in Latin and made me read it back to her several times. Not a point missed. That would go better for her, she thought. If a naïve Christian, she was tenfold the Catholic of me; the letter of the ritual was all to her. I had to promise to wash her before burial and watch at her wake. She didn't expect more, though I gave it. My Merlin, my sister, the incongruous symbol of my own stubborn survival. Perhaps that's why she mattered so much.

Kindness is always delayed too long and usually paid to the wrong place. So with me; I bustled about and hovered over Rat with useless attentions that should have gone to Arthur or any one of a dozen lives lacerated along my way. Rat basked in it, puffed and primped when I did her hair or bathed her with sweet unguents, and never knew the pathetic fraud of it all.

But she lingered from the habit of survival. The organism went on twitching without purpose. On the last day I lay beside her so long with her head on my arm that I felt cruelly cramped.

"Gwenda!"

"What? What is it?"

Her cold hand groped for mine. "Hold me, Gwenda? I'm goin. I'm slippin off'n they'll get me."

"Who?"

"Devils."

Her terror was very real, real as mine when I thought it was my time and all the worse because Rat *knew* what was waiting for her behind the dark and the thunder. She needed all the comforts of the Church now, and there was only me. Not enough. She tried to fight, to rally against that falling night, but she hadn't the strength. Her eyes glazed with terror. She was too weak to cry now, only gaped and struggled. I screamed silently at God to open his hand and let her live or take her quickly. No luck either way. Rat clung as tenaciously to the end of life as she had to the rest of it.

"What'm I gonner do till yer get to a priest? Might be months. Might not be any help 'tall. They're gonner get me first afore Lor God even knows I'm gone."

I thought of all the soothing lies I'd fed her in ten years, like dealing with Thor to turn his hammer aside. She always believed. What white lie now would make the going a little easier? The answer was something of a surprise: the truth. But then I'd always saved that for emergencies.

"No demons will have you. Not my Raidda. Mark me: in Eburacum there's a chapel built with my own money. Brigid chapel it's called."

"Yer ent from there. Yer said Hull all these years."

A conspiratorial glance at the door. "I didn't dare tell truth. Understand? Rat, I'm trusting you with my most

dangerous secrets now. If you get well—and well you might—where would I be and you knowing all?"

"Oh . . ." Rat was more curious than dying just then. "What, what?"

"Your promise not to tell."

"Swear on Cross, Gwenda."

"Eburacum."

"Coo!"

"I built Brigid chapel. Every day of the week Father Donal says mass and lights candles to Mary and Brigid for my family as they will for me."

Rat managed a sputtering cackle of vindication. "Din I have the right of you straight off? Always knew yer were more'n yer let on."

"No, I couldn't cozen you, could I? On my hope of heaven, they'll pray for you too. Every day."

God's Eyes, I meant it. My friend might have lived with nothing but she would not die frightened if I could help it. "My girl, you'll be home snug and smug before the demons have bare wind you're off from here. I promise it, Rat."

Father Donal, the chapel rector, would say I was presuming on my patronage, but it worked because Rat was a child and believed in the literal. The novenas and candles were promised, and it would go hard for me if the smallest part were left out. Even now she tried me to make sure I wasn't lying to her.

". . . In kindness like, but still a lie, and there I am wivout so much's a candle or one croakin monk."

"Believe me, Rat."

"Wisht I could, but yer been the fox afore, Gwenda. Don't lie now. *Can't yer see how scared I am?*"

"Oh, Rat, what must I do for you?"

"Tell me truth's all. Ent like I was off to Wicandaen fair'n home again."

Just truth. To hell with it. I gave her the last gift in my power, sent for Gwyneth who came with that cloying sweetness one saves for deathbeds.

"And how is't, Raidda? We hoped you'd join us in the hall tonight."

"Ow, sod off. What yer need her for, Gwenda?"

"You asked for truth, that's all I've left. You know Gwyneth heard my confession when I thought to die."

Gwyneth darted me an apprehensive glance. "I did."

"A confession is truth spoken to God, Rat. And in my own name. Gwyneth, for this moment I release you of that much. Speak the name I gave to God. I want my friend to know it."

Gwyneth twisted her hands together and mumbled it. "Guenevere, Queen of Britain."

"And of your own witness, did I lie?"

Gwyneth jerked her head from side to side. "I saw the Queen when she was young, Rat. It is she and none other."

Gwyneth was still uncomfortable with the subject, not at all sure Rat wouldn't bray it to someone else and cause trouble. I motioned her to the door. "Pray your silence still. God keep you."

"Rhodri and I will pray for you, Raidda."

"We'll hold you to that," I said as she slipped out the door. "Do you believe now, Rat?"

"Lor God!" Very little light left in her eyes but it was transcendent. She might have died in fear of hell and tinged with doubts about my honesty. She loved Gwenda, but Guenevere was capitals carved in enduring stone. Her candles and prayers were assured, the door to paradise flung wide, angels beckoning, ledgers balanced at last. But she still found some small room for injury.

"And yer kept that from yer best friend all these years."

"Well, now I've put it right. The chapel will last. Each prayer for me will be followed with one for you."

She managed a weak snicker. "Yer must've been frighted as me."

"Putting by for a bad day, as you always did."

"Hold me up, Gwenda?"

"There, you have to cough?"

"No . . . gotter laugh, 'n it hurts."

I supported her frail shoulders while the spasm of weak laughter took her, no more than a spattering rasp. "Five pound the bleedin pair of us. Old Bridden was sold on the cheap that year, wunnit? Let me lie down . . . coo, wouldn't old bitch love to know that? Thought she'd call a holiday when she pinched my silver. Never trusted 'em not to. So I din never keep it all in one place. Told yer I'd be straight wiv yer, Gwenda. Come here, close."

I bent over her dry lips.

"In the byre," she croaked, "empty stall wiv the white oak post in back."

It was an effort, but Rat made it, struggled to tell me. Under the white oak post was the rest of her savings, laid by for a day like this when the English might steal the rest. Oh, Rat never trusted a one of them, not Gunnar nor any man that went by the name. She did them good all those years at Wicandaen fair. Got them drunk, got them ready as she certainly knew how, and then didn't she rob the bleeders blind? Easy enough, they were just men, only thinking of the one thing. Any road, it was all mine for being her one true friend since Cilla. Seeing as I was once rutting lady of the lot, maybe I could use it to get back and set things right, now I knew how the world really was. And I was to give a whole shilling to Brigid chapel in her name—but *only* if they toed the mark and prayed regular and weren't mean about the candles. Rat wanted her money's worth.

"Full measure," I promised, tucking the covers around her throat.

"Stay by me? Yer won't go off now?"

"I'll be here."

"Remember them candles now. And tell Mary Virgin who they're for, mind."

"And a shilling to the priests." I stroked her wasted cheek. She took a deep, ragged breath. "Could sleep good now. A nice nap."

When her labored breathing was more regular, I tried to doze a little myself. There would be the washing and shrouding to come. . . .

"Gwenda?" Her voice, a bare whisper, brought me back from the brink of sleep. "Yer hear me?"

"Aye, love."

"Them priests at Brigid? Sod a shillin." Even at the end, Rat's prim sense of values clamored against extravagance. Her thin mouth contorted with its perpetual disgust. "Not for them."

"What shall it be then?"

I thought her breath had began to labor toward the end, but Rat was laughing again. "Ha'pny, Gwenda. Not a farthin more." I felt the tiny, dry pressure of her cold lips on my cheek. "That's all they ever give me, innit? Cunting barstids."

She went in her sleep and at peace. That was only right, but still I hope it will count for me that I helped her to it. Even heaven comes higher than ha'pny, but Rat never lacked for prayers in Brigid chapel.

Rat died in the late evening. Gwyneth and I washed the body, dressed Rat in her holiday gown, shrouded her in linen. Rhodri came to watch with us. Our English masters were not familiar with the custom of the wake, but they gave us candles for our vigil and we made a wake with ale. Gwyneth keened for Rat, I sang as much of the requiem as I remembered, and the three of us waxed as melancholy as our small ration of ale would allow. To Rhodri it was not much of a wake by respectable British standards. Uisge should flow like water at such times.

"And to think you used it on an Englishwoman," he mourned. "Ale won't do it. A wake needs tears and madness."

We watched until the last candle burned low and we had to sleep ourselves against the hard work of the morrow. I went to bed and slept almost dead as Rat.

Early next morning, when I brought their porridge to Gunnar and Nilse in the hall, I inquired about Elfgifu. "Will she be in for breakfast?"

"Mother ate in the kitchen. She had work," Nilse told me.

"I'd be grateful for an hour's time to bury Rat at the edge of my garden."

Gunnar frowned up from his bowl. "Bury? That's where Mother is now, seeing to the pyre."

"*She's going to burn Rat?*"

Nilse shrugged. "Don't we always?"

"Not to Christians. Not to Rat. I promised her."

"It's honorable enough for a lord; it will do for Rat." Gunnar wouldn't hear any more about it. "I've ridden over Mother's wishes and given you much rein, Gwenda. I won't balk her in a thing like this. Now you have work of your own to do."

I stared at them, beginning to seethe. "No."

"What?"

"I said no, Hlaford Gunnar Eanboldson. Rat's not

going to burn. Think you else, you'd best have your whip to hand, because you will need it."

I bolted out the door, across the courtyard and through the open gate. Hurrying as fast as my bad leg would permit, I saw no smoke beyond the walls, but they weren't far from it. Elfgifu stood by the pyre, Cynred beside her just lighting his torch. Rhodri was there, no doubt ordered to carry the body with him and not at all happy about it. A frugal pyre, the seasoned logs eked out with brush, just enough and no more than was needed to consume the small shrouded body that rested on it.

"Put down that torch, Cynred."

They all turned, surprised. Of my own kind and beliefs, Rhodri read very well my purpose as I descended on them.

"Down, I say. I'm going to bury her."

Elfgifu blocked my way, cold and bristling. I was opposing her again openly as I'd done silently for ten years. "You don't have the land to bury her, fool."

I didn't bother to disguise the contempt. "My garden. Mine by law. She'll help grow vegetables, Hlafdian. You'll have use of her even in death. One imagines you'd like that."

As I made to move by her, she grabbed my shoulder and pushed me back. "Cynred, light the fire."

"Rhodri! Take that torch and step on it! I command you."

Rhodri obeyed from a lifetime of habit, not to betray me. He relieved the bewildered blacksmith of the torch and stamped it out as Cynred gaped.

"What means all this, Rhodri?"

"It means matter between the ladies and none of ours," Rhodri cautioned tactfully.

Elfgifu pulled a stout faggot from the pyre and closed on me. Not Rat that mattered now but that I'd openly challenged her authority with that part of me that would never bend. "Burning is an honorable way, little Brit. Don't earn yourself a beating."

"Honorable! To be burned like garbage on a midden heap and her soul wandering forever? I saw you pawing through her things, Elfgifu: it was indecent, right as you were. But you won't spit on her now. Rhodri, come help."

I stretched over the pyre to pull at the body. The stick

came down on my back with numbing force. I crumpled under it, then coiled. Elfgifu waited for me to step back, give it up. The stick poised.

"Why not the midden heap, Gwenda? Isn't that where your kind put my children?"

"Don't strike me again, Elfgifu."

"Get away from there." She raised the stick.

I held in check the mayhem the blow had lighted in me, put it all in my eyes and voice. "Once you were stronger than me. Now you're just bigger. I've learned much from you, Elfgifu. It's your turn. If your children went on that heap, so did my own life. In a way you will never understand. The world owes us nothing, either of us. And if you strike again, we'll both regret it."

It was not all cruelty that made her strike again. I saw the years and the loss in her eyes as well as the iron thing that made Elfgifu what she was. And Gunnar leaning against the gate, quite aware we could settle this ourselves.

"You *were* one of them!" The stick whistled down. I caught it easily, twisted it out of her grip and broke it. "Damn you!" She came at me, fist raised. I caught her wrist. The blow did not even rock my arm. We poised there, Elfgifu speechless at my resistance, but she couldn't loosen my grip on her right arm. I turned her wrist inexorably, pushing her off balance. She stumbled to gain a purchase with her feet and swung her left fist at me. She was strong yet. I saw sudden lights as Elfgifu clubbed at my face, but kept on twisting. Again and again she battered at me, wherever she could reach—less and less as I forced her further off balance. I tasted blood in my mouth, felt the bruises on my face, but kept twisting until Elfgifu was forced to her knees, then onto her back.

"You have grown old," I said, "but you have never grown up. I will bury my friend."

"Gwenda, you'll break her arm!" Cynred moved to part me from her, but Rhodri stepped in front of him, easy but firm. "Don't, mun. This was a long time wanting."

Even down and helpless, Elfgifu defied me. "Break it, slave. If you can't I'll whip you to death."

I don't know what would have happened then had not

the other hand come down and torn me loose from Elfgifu. Gunnar jerked his mother to her feet and shoved her away.

"Not a word, either of you." Gunnar swept his arm in a backhanded slap that caught me on the cheek and knocked me against the pyre. "The slave has been punished, Mother. Go to the hall."

"She—I'll kill her—"

"She never struck you, just stopped you. *Go.*" With the same fierce energy, Gunnar lifted Rat's body from the pyre and barked at Rhodri. "You! You believe in this burying nonsense. Get the tools. And you shut up, Gwenda. You're as thick as Mother. Get the mattocks, Rhodri."

Like a man Gunnar took it out on the hard ground of the kitchen garden, swinging the mattock against the earth as if it had insulted him, stopping only to let Rhodri scoop out the loose dirt. When the grave was deep enough, they lowered Rat, then pushed and scooped the earth over her, marking it with a stake. Rhodri and I knelt while I said what prayers I could think of. Gunnar waited us out with tight patience. What little religion he practiced didn't seem right without a fire.

"Are you finished?"

"Aye, and we thank you, Hlaford." Rhodri bobbed his head. "Letting her have proper rest as you have."

When Rhodri went back to the forge, Gunnar sat on the ground near the new grave, tossing a lump of earth from one hand to the other. "Was it so important, Gwenda?"

"She was. We understood each other. She loved me."

"I love you, and I'll certainly never understand you."

"That's the cornerstone of faith, Gunnar. I would not change it."

He brushed lightly at my bruised cheek. "Does it hurt?"

"No. I'd take three more of the same for half a good meal. My God, what is it holding me up? When my mother-in-law was my age, they were carrying her in a litter."

Gunnar helped me stand. "You're strong as Mother now. We gave you that, Elfgifu no less than me." I fol-

lowed the line of his gaze to the bare fields. "Almost time to plow. We need a new brace of oxen. Ewes . . . a ram." He flung the clod away, weary with the immensity of all we needed to start over. "Get one, there can't be the other. Scarce an animal left anywhere after last winter."

"We've the one ox, old Borba."

"Hoof-rotted. Should have cooked him last year. I can't tax my people what they don't have. Eadward, who should be off to court this year, will have to work in the fields again. Even Nerta. On less food. A miracle is needed." Gunnar struck his hands together. "We will do a miracle."

That night when I finished serving in the hall, I went to the byre and dug into the packed earth around the white oak post. Rat had buried it deep, but out of the rotting hide sack I poured a cornucopia. Miser she was, probably carrying more than a pound with her when she sold herself. She once showed me how to conceal money, not delicate but effective, and she'd added to it over the years from the men, theft, any way she could, grudging every minim spent. I counted more than two pounds, most of it in bronze half pennies, a number of minims, sesterces and some Gaulish coins not seen west of Londinium for years.

I pocketed a pound, bunched the rest in my fist and walked through the dry wind to the hall where the family still savored the last of their ale before bed.

"Lord Gunnar."

The coins jingled out of my hand onto the board before them. "You asked for a miracle or a brace of oxen. Buy them and the rest of what we need."

Gunnar poked at the coins like manna, exactly what they were. "What is this?"

"From Rat, sir. Since you'd not free me in any case, the money's not that much use to me if I'm starving. But she gave it to you, no one else could." I held Elfgifu's eyes. "Pray you all remember that. And buy what we need."

Rat wouldn't like it, but nothing else would serve. The offering moved Elfgifu profoundly because she couldn't understand it. I was putting a few early flowers on Rat's grave next day when I heard the sound of a footstep behind me: Elfgifu, her cloak and veil fluttering in the

wind. As she spoke, there was none of the habitual contempt.

"Why did you do that, Gwenda? The money?"

"We can't eat silver."

"You could have hidden it. You did not. Why?"

For the first time in ten years, she'd addressed me with the intimate *du*. Perhaps, even to her hard and unforgiving lights, I'd earned the right at last. She knelt to help me as I patted a little earth over the flower stems to hold them in place. "Not deep enough." Her large red hands bit into the earth, scooping a better purchase for the flowers.

"Why will I never understand the like of you? You make no sense at all."

I tried to articulate for a foreigner what I'd never had to put in words before, the Brit beneath the Roman. "With us it's always been not so much honor, certainly not business, but what is fitting. And what's fitting is not always of this world, Hlafdian, or even of common sense as you know it." I touched her arm. "But you and I need fight no more. Old women should forget certain things."

She patted the earth more carefully about the plants. "You're right. But it is hard."

"And not for me? Don't I remember the night you brought us here, the collar already chafing my neck and . . . oh, Rat. Rat! It was the three of us, you, me and Rat. And for all she's under the ground, she may have saved the pack of us. *Ach-y-fi*, but I'd adore getting drunk tonight; just a little so I could weep or a good deal to roar at the gods before I fell down mumbling."

"Mad, all of you. Kill for a penny, spit on a pound."

"And cry for night in the middle of sunlight. That's why we're marvelous Christians and deplorable politicians. Come, you'll get chill on your knees. Why don't I make us a touch of tea?"

No order really needed to be given to assemble for the spring plowing. Gunnar's men knew the soil as well as he; already some had stopped by the hall to inquire, though with less enthusiasm than in previous years. When the day came, they gathered more out of duty than purpose. Men, women and children, all were thinned out and undernourished. They clumped together listening to

Gunnar in dull silence. His land must be plowed first. That he'd paupered himself feeding them his sheep was not forgotten, but what of now and next week? In past years they'd come leading their yoked oxen. None were in the field now except old Borba. Gunnar asked no questions. They had nothing else to eat. The last of their turnips and barley went first, then whatever roots they could find. Finally the pig, the few chickens, then the oxen. You don't reason with hunger.

"I've sent Beorn to Wicandaen," Gunnar told them, "and wherever fresh teams may be had. Until then, we will work with Borba. To the forest."

All of us were in the fields now—Elfgifu and Nilse with their skirts tucked up into their waist strings, Ase unloading buckets from the wagon, young Eadward fourteen now and just beginning to lengthen in the bone toward his father's frame but long used to working his heart out under patient Beorn and here in the fields.

We noted one farmer missing from the first gathering. "He has a fever," the wife told Gunnar. "Hlaford knows he would not shirk, but he can't rise from his bed."

The earth was terribly dry, the small clods crumbled too easily in the hand. A Brit peasant would have said it was too early. This year anything else would have been too late. Fires would have to be kindled all over the fields. For two days I swung an ax with young Eadward, cutting the wood for the fires to thaw the earth before plowing. The smoke rose up to blacken the sky as all the lords of the Iclingas prepared with us.

Gunnar was everywhere, directing his people, playing the optimist. Better times were surely just ahead. We even managed to joke a bit over the thin soup and hard bread that would be our only meal that day. Our laughter died when we looked to our one pathetic old ox and saw the fields and how much was to be done.

We dredged muddy water from the brook, now mere pools seeping away into the bed. The farmers set aside a little for drinking, but the rest went into the soil. On the third day, two more farmers failed to appear.

"Where *are* they? We're too damned few now."

"They have the fever, Hlaford."

"And the flux, sir. Their bowels move all the time."

Whatever, the fever went through our people like

plague, opening their bowels, robbing their strength, doubling them over with sudden cramps as they worked. It may have been the brackish water. Certain alchemists have maintained that evil humors can taint the purest water now and then, especially if it stands. That may have been why Gunnar and I escaped the fever. Neither of us ever liked water, contenting ourselves with an occasional swallow of ale. And we were usually at a distance from the bucket. If it was the water, that's why the folk of Gunnarsburh were the last to succumb, habitually drinking more ale than water. But it took them; first Elfgifu and Gytha could not rise from their beds, then Nilse, Ase, finally hale young Eadward doubled over next to me as we worked and stumbled for the edge of the woods. Cynred and Rhodri staggered along for a time before they took to their beds. I tended Elfgifu in her chills and fever as she rambled darkly of the workings of Loki. Stricken Gwyneth saw it as witness to Scripture: the world was indeed ending, we'd see. And Gunnar fretted over Beorn—"He should be back now"—while I tended Ase and tried to comfort her in the knight's absence.

"Perhaps he has the fever, Ase. It's taken Witgar's people. Maybe it's in Wicandaen as well."

There came a morning with the first real hint of warm spring when there were only the two of us in the hall at daybreak over porridge and ale. Gwyneth and Rhodri lay helpless on their pallets in a corner. The hall was quiet and dark, a little chill without the fire. I folded down over my arms; only morning and a whole day to go before rest again. Days unnumbered beyond that.

"How many are there for today?"

"Us," said Gunnar.

"You're joking."

"Getting light outside. Let's to it."

"The two of us alone? What of the new lords; won't they help?"

"You think I haven't asked?" Gunnar sounded bored with the question. "Bad off as we are. They laughed at me. 'Gunnar is a leech at the breast of *gesithcund*. Gunnar is a traitor to his kind.'"

"You gave those bastards their land!"

"And helped the commons cut the fat living out from

under them. They said no more could be expected from a man not warrior-born, no matter who his father was."

I swallowed the last of my ale and stared into the bottom of the cup. "God, I'm tired of that argument. Suddenly and profoundly sick of it."

"They enjoyed refusing me and waving their moth-eaten ancestors in my face. But the one thing they won't see is you and me giving in."

"No." I tried honestly to summon the determination. "Not yet."

Filling my pouch with ale and my pockets with bread in the kitchen, I felt Gunnar's arms go around me from behind. His hands cupped my breasts, pressing me to him.

"You're a lovely man with no sense of occasion."

"I just wanted to hold you a little."

We stood motionless, his bearded cheek against mine. "A man's lucky to find one good woman in a lifetime," he said. "I've found two."

"You've taught me so much, Gunnar."

"I've learned from you."

"I always resented love in my strange way, but not with you. If I have to drop down dead in that rutting field, I couldn't do it in better company."

Gunnar raised my chin to smile at me. "That's my wish. I just wanted you to know."

When he went to fetch Borba from his stall, the silence of ailing, failing Gunnarsburh closed around me. I tended to Gwyneth and Rhodri, weak as they were. Nilse had enough strength to worry over Nerta lying next to her, shuddering with chills.

"Hold her head up, Gwenda. Make her drink the ale. How will it go today? How many are you?"

"Just Gunnar and myself, sweet. Can I get you something?"

Her head moved weakly on the pillow. "No . . . this will pass. We've all had it before, just never this bad. We must save the food then for Gunnar and you."

"We'll start the plowing today. If Borba can last. Poor old beast, I look to him to fall so we can cook him."

"So have I." Nilse closed her eyes, tired just from her few words. "See to Mother before you go."

Elfgifu made herself ration the ale I brought her; only

a small swallow. She felt the defeat around her, saw the hopelessness in me sitting on the edge of her bed.

"We have been low before, Gwenda."

But never so low as this, I read her silence, *never so close to the edge.* All of her driving will wrapped itself tight around Elfgifu now at the end and clamped her mouth down like a siege.

"Just you and my son? Hear me: if Borba has to feed us, see the children eat first. And some little part should go on the altar. We must not forget the gods. With their meager gifts to us this year, the offering need not be large." The grim smile creased her strong mouth. "If it comes to that, you must do magic."

I wondered if she wasn't wandering-fey as myself in my sickness. Elfgifu seemed serious. She struggled to sit up; I propped the pillow behind her head. Almost seventy now but still vital, she worshiped hard gods all her hard life and lived by principles rigid as the sword she gave and took in betrothal. Only dark magic could defeat her kind; now in her extremity she would invoke even that.

"You Welsh have sorcery we don't know about. I know the spell you've put on my son. Don't deny it, I'm not a fool to babble everything I see. You have magic. And your men, they used magic, had to. Why did they not give up at Eburacum and Badon when they'd given in for a generation before that? Magic, that's all it could be. If Gunnar fails, if he can't go on, you must summon that magic: devils, gods, spirits of the dead, anything to keep him going, *anything*. So he won't give up now. He's only a man. Men break so easily. There's a demon in you, I saw it that first night I brought you here. But sentimental, too. That's the weak Welsh of you. That's why we'll win in the end. I have driven my son. I have kept the old gods and the old ways because we needed a *spine*, Gwenda. You are strong. You are my equal, I've seen that. So I beg you, what magic you have, use it now for my son."

As we led lumbering Borba out the gate to the field, there was not even a watchman in the tower. We kept hoping as the sun rose higher on a fair day that others would appear from the cottages, but knowing they wouldn't. The fever held all of Gunnarsburh in its hot,

dry hand. No sign of life. No sound except us and the birds.

"Perhaps some will come later."

"Perhaps." Gunnar kicked at the hard ground. "It will be work for Borba to pull through this."

"I can work ahead of the plow and break the ground first. That may help."

"Yes."

We didn't say what we thought, ignored the hopelessness like stubborn children, that it might somehow turn into hope. We took just enough ale to wet our throats, then Gunnar grasped the plow handles, I picked up the mattock and we began.

By midday the sun was warm, the weather mockingly perfect. I worked ahead of the plow, breaking the clods before Borba hauled the plow through them. The hoe didn't help much. The ground would have been hard for a prime team. Borba strained and stumbled, lurched forward and stopped as the plow stuck, switching his tail in dull misery at the flies swarming about his haunches.

We spoke little, saving our breath for work. Only toward dusk did we look back at the little done and the mountain waiting. Poor Borba was blessed for not knowing the impossibility of it all. His hoofs were rot-eaten stumps, his best years long gone. While I dropped down in the furrow to rest, Gunnar went to the ox and put his sunburned arms around the thick, bowed neck.

The next day was even warmer, the sky monotonously clear. Already the little we'd plowed was drying in the sun. We waited a little by Borba, pretending to stay for whatever workers might appear, but really to delay for a few minutes longer grappling with the undone mountain. Then Gunnar passed me the ale, drank himself, and we began again.

"There'll be the others to help when the fever runs its course," Gunnar said. "Perhaps even tomorrow."

Not tomorrow or even the day after. Fever is one thing, hunger another. One can work all day on a little food once inured to it, but there must be something steadily. You can't drain strength without replenishment. That we did was from doing it for years, but now it was a diminishing return. We tired more quickly as the plow inched along the furrows. We spoke hardly at all, the sun limned

our shadow behind us, under us, lengthened it ahead of us. We did not rise as quickly from rest; we crawled up, then pushed ourselves up. Finally, as the shadows merged into dusk, we drained the last of the ale and unhitched Borba from the plow. As I started to lead him away, the ox bawled in a plaintive timbre and hung back. Gunnar inspected the worn rear hoofs.

"Split. Poor old thing." He patted Borba's fly-bitten neck. "When you stall him tonight, give him plenty of grain, all he wants."

"There's not much left."

"Then give him all of it," he said impatiently. "Empty the bin. Why not?"

I felt as fatalistic. "Why not indeed? He's finished."

"So feed him well tonight. Tomorrow he goes in the pot."

I couldn't mourn much for Borba; at least for a day or two we'd eat a little better. We lurched on toward the stockade with the crippled ox hobbling behind. There was a question I didn't want to ask, though it had to be voiced. "And the plowing? There's not an ox left in two days' walk."

"I can pull it."

"No, Gunnar."

"I'll *pull* it. You guide it. We have to, for Gott's sake."

"Which god?" I snarled out of my own hunger and exhaustion. "None of them will help us."

"Who cares? Woden, Christ, Freya, let them fight for heaven-room, I don't care any more. But this is Gunnarsburh."

Not the mundane earth, but Gunnarsburh. He hooked three fingers in my slave collar and pulled me to him, hard. "And I wear its yoke as you wear mine. I'll work us until we drop, and then I'll—"

He didn't know what then, neither did I. A miracle, some of the magic Elfgifu entreated. And God knows from where.

"We'll wet the ground and break it with the hoes for a good space," he planned. "Then I'll pull the plow. I've heard your tribes in the western mountains do it that way."

"That's true. And not much more than a shoulder-bone for a plow."

"We can do it, Gwenda."

"I suppose . . ."

Next day no one in Gunnarsburh should have been up, but Gwyneth and Rhodri managed to totter about. Between them they managed to butcher the ox.

"Poor old brute," Rhodri mourned. "Were we not so in need, I would've cried over him."

Gunnar and I were in the field as the sun broke over the eastern trees, chewing our hard bread and sharing an even smaller ration of ale. For an hour or so we trudged from the shriveled brook to the fields, dribbling water along the furrows and breaking the moistened ground with hoes. We had to scoop out the brook bed to fill the buckets. Gunnar sniffed at the water.

"Stinks. I wouldn't drink it if I loved the stuff."

When we'd broken as much as we could plow before noon, Gunnar put on his loose linen blouse and twisted his way into the plow harness. I grasped the plow handles.

"Gwenda, you know what 'lord' means in English?"

"Bread-giver. The first word I learned from you."

Gunnar's fists knotted about the harness, tightening it to his shoulders. "Then let's make some bread."

He threw his weight against the lines. The plow bucked and lurched forward, then caught. I strained with him, angling the plow to free it. Gunnar strained again; the lines went taut. The plow began to move.

I don't know how we struggled through that torturing day. Gunnar's shoulders went raw under his shirt, then bled through the linen. The callus on my hands cracked and left a blood trace on the handles. At dusk Gunnar called a halt. It was too dark to see any more. I slumped over the plow. Gunnar disengaged himself from the harness, stood weaving for a moment, then dropped down on the earth. So we stayed for a long time.

"An ox has a miserable life," Gunnar breathed. "Let's get some water. Wash."

It seemed a marvelous idea. My skin was tight and sticky with sweat, but I couldn't move just then. "In a moment."

"Yes."

In a moment or an hour, Gunnar got up one joint at a time and together we wove like drunks across the field to

the brook, the bucket banging against my wobbly legs. We undressed like sleepy children with no thought to modesty and washed each other's clammy skin with slow, stiff movements. We'd not made love since that night years ago here in the fields before Port came, and certainly neither of us had it in mind now. As I patted the water over his bleeding shoulders, the most erotic thing I could manage was a light kiss to brush the raw-rubbed flesh while thinking *at least there's meat tonight*. I slipped my arms around Gunnar; neither of us moved or spoke; we hadn't the energy. All that was needed for tomorrow when somehow we had to do it all again and the next day and the next and time out of mind before anyone could help us.

When we could, we dressed and stumbled home.

They'd cooked the whole ox since it wouldn't keep. I nodded over my portion, not able to eat it all, that tired and my belly shrunken from tiny meals. Gwyneth put it aside for me, then crept back to her bed as the fever took her again.

The next day rose warm and cloudless as the one before and those to come—all of them, damn them, there'd never be rain again.

"All right," Gunnar cursed the clear skies. "Don't rain. Don't rain ever again, you bitch."

I'd brought linen from Nilse's store and wrapped his shoulders the best I could. What was left I bound round my raw hands. We filled our buckets and began again, breaking the earth and watering it. Then it was time for the plow.

Gunnar took a deep breath and let it out slowly before he picked up the harness and twisted his way into it. I closed my aching hands around the plow handles. Then Gunnar's weight strained forward to break out the blade. Slowly, ever so slowly, the furrow lengthened behind us.

We went on hour after hour as the sun climbed, hovered at zenith and began the long fall down the western sky. In the giddiness of my fatigue I fancied Arthur balancing on the plow, laughing at me. The plow handles went slippery with blood oozing from under the linen bandages, darkening the sweat on Gunnar's shirt. He dared not stop now; his whole being was screwed tight to

the forward motion, dragging the plow one more foot, one more foot, another after that.

When we worked toward Gunnarsburh, I looked to see smoke, any sign of life to know the world was not really shrunk to the two of us and the dry earth, but there was nothing.

The plow caught. Gunnar lurched against it with a sound of pain. I bit down on the cry as the handles pressed into my laid-open hands. The blade wouldn't move.

"Wait."

I went on my knees to claw the large stone from the earth. "All right, it's clear."

But Gunnar was down, slumped over to one side.

"Gunnar?"

He didn't move. I stumbled forward to him. He barely raised his head to me, dull-eyed. "Let me. My hands are hurting on the plow as it is."

"You can't pull it, Gwenda."

"Can you?" His shoulders might have been scraped with the jagged edge of a knife.

"No."

"Wrap your hands. I'll try."

"If I can't—"

"I'll try, damn it."

Without another word Gunnar moved away to the plow. I looped the harness over my own shoulders, took up the slack and heaved. The plow didn't move. I gathered myself again, praying: God, Goddess, Epona, Brigid, one of you, all of you, all-one of you, sit in my shoulders and legs. Christ, priests, angels, monks, earn your keep this day and let—me—*do*—it—

The plow lurched and stuck. I dug my toes in, bent double and pulled. With Gunnar pushing hard on the handles, the miserable plow broke free and began to move through the dry earth. By the time we'd come to the end of the furrow, my hands were cramped on the harness and my shoulders already felt the leather biting into them. So much effort, so little gained, and even further to go next time and the next.

"You're right. An ox has no life worthy of the name."

I threw myself against the weight of the plow, felt Gunnar's strength push it free, and we went on like the other

animals. On and on through the dry afternoon, unable to stop once a furrow was started for fear I couldn't begin again. My shoulders ached, then chafed but I pushed on through the half-done field, not thinking of the rest to be done, not praying now, not thinking at all. There was nothing but the jolting ground in front of me, the next step forward, the next gulp of air in my lungs already burning with dust and strain.

One moment my legs were pushing under me, then I was down, blinking at dancing lights as the rough earth scraped my face. The next memory was opening my eyes to Gunnar swabbing my face with a bit of linen. My lips moved thickly.

"Hopeless, man. We've got to wait for the others. Beorn when he comes back."

"If he comes back. Anything could've happened to him now."

"Yes. Poor Ase."

Gunnar twisted about to look over the field. "Half finished. This one at least."

"Doesn't matter now."

"Get up."

"I can't."

"You said you'd try."

"I did. I did try, damn you—"

"Take the reins."

While I struggled up to stretch and relieve the cramp in my back, Gunnar went to the bucket to soak the stiffened linen. He called me to help him rewind it about his shoulders.

"Gunnar, you can't."

He jerked his head toward the plow, then fitted the harness to his shoulders, wincing as the leather tightened over his lacerated flesh. "Take the reins."

"You can't."

"Will tomorrow be any easier?" he sobbed out of his rawed throat. "You want to die here, woman? We could. You want to know how close we are to it?" Fierce, not to be denied by me or the gods, he whipped his arm toward the plow handles. "Take the reins!"

I don't know how we did it, through the hot sun of the day into the long twilight and dusk. The sweat streamed down between my breasts and legs, then dried sticky as

the heat went out of the day. The world was an illusion;
there was only Gunnar and I, the harness and the plow.
Licking at the caked stickiness around my lips, my eye
might wander to the sky that jolted this way and that, no
longer blue but white and dry as sand. We didn't speak at
all, not even at the end of the furrows when we came
together to turn the plow and set it for the next. I didn't
want to look at Gunnar then as he poured water over the
linen to keep the blood from caking stiff. The material
was dark-soaked now as we started into still another
row. The plow ground to a halt after a few feet. Gunnar
staggered in the harness and hurled himself against it
with all his remaining strength. The plow wouldn't
move. His legs simply went out from under him. Gunnar
went down on his knees and didn't rise.

I hung over the plow handles as if impaled on them,
then heard his dry sob.

"Bitch."

I stumbled forward to sink down beside him on the
earth, sloshing the ale pouch. Almost empty. I gave him
the last of it. Gunnar ducked his head that I wouldn't see
his tears. He couldn't rise, couldn't begin to rise. The sun
was down now and all the shadows merged and thickening toward night over the field.

"Freya, the bitch," Gunnar rasped. "Her. Freya, the
only one of them I ever really believed in. I've done everything but open my veins and pour my blood into her."
He slammed a weak fist against the earth. "You want
that too, you greedy bitch? You got the best of all of us.
We never forgot you."

Dusk and silence deepened around us. Neither of us
moved. Gunnarsburh seemed miles away. I knew we'd
never do it; now Gunnar knew. Like all his kind, defeat
was never the logical result of cause but a puzzle he'd
break himself to unravel. It weighted his exhaustion with
a hurt I longed to salve. All of his dreams and Elfgifu's
ground to a halt here in this dry field, the future shrank
to this, to the two of us beaten on the half-worked earth.
Reason and will had tried and proved not enough.

Reason had strained to the end of its tether. What I did
then was not logical or even very sane. Those clear lights
had guttered and gone out, leaving only the childish
hope of miracles. I remembered Elfgifu's plea: I must do

magic. Magic of the oldest and most potent sort. The last magic left me.

Gunnar didn't move when I rose stiffly and took the bucket to the brook. Undressing with the clumsiness of exhaustion, I stood naked in the dark and poured half the bucket over me, then dipped at the rest to wash as best I could, rinsing my mouth with a double handful. I loosed the thong and let the uncut hair fall over my shoulders and back. While the bucket filled again, I stood erect in the darkness, bare to night and Hecate, the sun's heat throbbing in my skin against the cool dark, and raised my hands in prayer as I'd done so long ago in Eburacum before each of my lovers came for their own reasons.

But this prayer and magic was for Gunnar.

Goddess, have mercy on him. He has never forgotten you. Though he called you by another name, he has been faithful. He has burned offerings to other gods, but you are the one he stroked as a lover, you are the wife who curves into the hollow of his soul. So many times you've filled me, given me your shape and glory when it mattered far less. Fill me now that we may make this magic together. It's all I have to give him. We've already lost; that's our humanity. We will go on somehow, that's our glory. Come into me now.

So I stood erect and bare as the sky-clad daughters of Hecate summoned her to fill them, until the quivering of tired muscles ceased and I was composed. Until I felt the Goddess enter me, fill me with the relaxation, until I was both in one, our combined power like coiled rope. Then I carried the filled bucket back to Gunnar.

I helped him pull the shirt off his sticky back. His hand stroked my naked leg in weary affection, and I felt his bearded lips brush against the puckered scar on my thigh.

"Where are your clothes?"

"Epona doesn't need them." I unwound the stiff linen from his shoulders, wincing at the cruel lacerations. "Be silent, man. She brings you her gifts, the first that men such as you ever asked and were freely given. Sacred gifts are received in holy silence."

From exhaustion or wisdom, Gunnar said nothing as I washed his face and kissed each eyelid. "Blessed be thine eyes that shall seek wisdom."

And his strong mouth. "Blessed be thy mouth that shall speak the truth of the Goddess."

Washing slowly down his body, ever so gentle on the torn flesh of his shoulders, to his furred chest to kiss each nipple with the blessing. At my bidding he stood up while I stripped the loose trousers from him and unwound the breechclout, ladling the water from the bucket to wash the grime of defeat from his flesh, fondling his penis as the most sacred organ, washing it ritually before kissing it.

"Blessed by thy organ of generation, for without it we would not be."

Stroking his thighs, my voice lulling, I felt the quickening in Gunnar. Not much; he was too tired to respond rapidly, too far gone to harden for me just now, but I went on washing until I spilled the last of the consecrated water over his feet and kissed them.

"And blessed be thy feet which have brought thee hither." I raised my hands to him. "Lie down, man. Don't speak. We've only made holy that which is still to be done. Lie down, lie here by me."

Gunnar folded down beside me. It was not lust now, no part of lust. Of all the men who ever came to me, Gunnar was—besides Arthur—the most innate believer, accepting in reverent silence. He held me as all men have held the woman-goddess-mother since time began, frightened of her and being frightened, needing to deny, to dominate, to escape, but returning always in spite of that to the need and trust, to the joining of womb and seed.

I ran my tongue over his dry lips, fingers grooving through the shaggy mane of his hair. "Gunnar, do you believe?"

His belief surged in the way he stroked me. Because now, in the warm night of a dry spring there was the heat of our bodies and the feel of the sun in our skins. His soft penis pressed against my leg, still unable with the weariness in him, but Gunnar needed and believed without words, the way it must be.

"Listen," I whispered, my lips very close to his, kisses for punctuation, the true caress of the Goddess. "Soon it will be Bel-tein, the time of the sacred fire, the dropping of lambs and foals, the time when my people did this magic in the furrows of the field, for what happens to the

spirit occurs in the flesh, and it has been so since my people first rafted their cattle and goatskin tents across the water from Gaul to Britain. At the Bel-tein fire, the women ask the Goddess to enter them. They stretch on their backs in the fields, become the field and the furrow, the man the plow and the seed. You have sacrificed to me, sweet man." I drew his mouth to mine in a long, languorous kiss. "Now touch me. Reach inside me. Plant the seed. Make the barley."

"Gwenda, I can't. I love you and I want to, but I can't."

"You can." I slid my tongue down across his throat and chest, across his hunger-flat belly to his groin, kissing the softer skin on the inside of his thighs and the tender flesh of his testicles. "It is not only a loving now, not Gwenda but the Goddess. I am your woman. I am all women, all woman, but still only half. Give me your seed."

Poor desperate, believing man. I felt him start to harden under my caressing lips. Nilse never did this for him, never even knew of it, but the mouth is to kiss, to taste, to take and give pleasure. The mouth is the first orifice the child uses by instinct. Whatever the frightened little half-men say, the mouth is of the Goddess. I licked at the length and engorging head of Gunnar's penis until he writhed with a desire his body could barely answer. Twice he swelled in my mouth only to go flaccid with the exhaustion that pulled him toward sleep. The third time when I felt the weak pulse that told me he was about to finish, I broke it off against the protest of his thighs, straddled him and eased him into my own readiness, clasping and unclasping the length of his penis until Gunnar was deep-sheathed in me. I could barely see his face in the dark, I bent close over him, brushing my nipples across the hair of his chest, stiffening them toward my own pleasure.

"You are the Goddess," he whispered.

"Let the magic work."

The pleasure grew slowly for both of us, our senses heightened with fatigue. I felt Gunnar firm inside me now as I moved gently on him and his mouth found my nipples. His body was drunk with exhaustion. I felt him nearing his own finish much sooner than he wanted to. He was almost ready, and still, by the arts my mother taught me, I held him off, held him back, soothing with

my kisses the raw, torn skin of his shoulders. My own movements were imperceptibly longer, deeper, lifting and sinking again and again, a little faster—

Gunnar groaned. His hard fingers gripped cruelly at my waist, and when I cried out at the pressure, he let go. His thighs shuddered under me, then he forced me down hard as he arched up to meet me. Gunnar made a sound between a gasp and a sob, gripping and ungripping my body from thighs to shoulders. I pushed myself down hard on him, squeezing tight.

"Yes," he breathed. "Don't leave me yet. Let me stay inside you."

His spasm passed; that he wanted me still started the hot pendulum for me. The tingling warmth spread outward from my deep belly as I thrust down on him—out, out, warming along my limbs in a growing sweet agony. My back arched, the cry deep and primal in my throat, the first wave exploding outward from my belly, then wave after shattering wave took me in a grip crueler than Gunnar's and hurled me for a vaulting instant through the stars, head lashing back and forth, and only at the end of this whip-madness did I feel the dull reality of his iron collar at the back of my neck.

It chilled me, brought me back to the dry crust of unmagicked reality. I bent low over the man. His eyes were closed. He might have seen my true likeness then, the goddess of me, spent as I was. From pure exhaustion I melted away from Gunnar and slipped down onto the earth. He didn't move or open his eyes.

"That is your people's magic?"

"Yes."

"Perhaps it is." He thought about it. "We were like sky and earth coming together."

"In believing is the magic."

We lay quiet together for a long time, our exhaustion mellowed by the loving, that part of us at least fed.

"When you think that the whole flower is curled in the seed," Gunnar dreamed, "the whole oak snugged away in an acorn. You know, for one instant I saw the stars close enough to touch. Closer than that, part of me. Are they really so far or just that we never reach for them?"

Stars or not, he touched me saying it. Then, like a man, he blunted poetry with the practical. "Gott, I'm hungry."

He didn't understand my dolorous laughter. We retrieved our sweat-stiffened clothes and crept home, leaning on each other.

Next morning I helped pale Gwyneth see to our ladies and the children who were now well enough to be up again. Gunnar and I breakfasted on strong tea and frugal slices of meat. It was still dark in the hall when Eadward and Nerta came in, the girl preening in the new garment I'd put on her, Eadward all arms, legs and big feet now, awkward between boy and man, his voice breaking when he hailed his father.

Gunnar swept Nerta up in his arms, but he took Eadward's hand as one man to another. Small distance, but a distance none the less. From now on, that handclasp said, love between father and son would be cloaked in reserve. Something might be lost, a thing Gunnar might still lavish on Nerta, but so it must be.

"Well, Eadward. The fever's left you."

Eadward straddled the bench by his father's side. "I can come work with you today."

"You're still pale, son. We're pulling the plow ourselves."

Instant challenge to very new manhood: "If Gwenda can do it, so can I."

"Let him come," I urged. "If the fever's passed, then perhaps there'll be others from the cottages as well."

"And me!" Nerta pulled her father's beard until he stopped her. "Let me go too."

"All right." Gunner let her drink from his tea. "We'll all go. You can help with the watering. But you must stop if you feel weak."

"I feel strong," Eadward protested. "Beorn's worked me hard. I'll put a penny my sword arm's almost as good as yours, Father."

"That's well. You're fourteen. A man. Someday your shield will hang on the wall where mine is. You'll be thegn, perhaps even an earl."

"An earl, no less of a man," I echoed.

"And the young aetheling will be your sister's son, your own nephew. So it's no disgrace for such a highly connected lord to know his holding from the ground up, and your geburs and cottagers will follow all the readier when they see that Thegn Eadward Gunnarson knows

the seed as well as the sword. The sword is only now and then, son. The seed goes on always. And nothing you ask of them"—Gunnar's hand strayed to his bandaged shoulder—"that you won't first demand of yourself. That's what makes a man that men will follow. Do you know why?"

"No, Father."

Gunnar put a tender arm about his son's bony shoulders. "Because that way each man sees in his lord the best of himself and the best of what he can be. In a way the lord is hung up like his shield, a reminder of that best. So! Gwenda, take some ale and bread to the fields. We'll be along. No—wait, children." He stayed them as they moved to follow me. "Please wait."

There was a note of wistfulness in Gunnar as he invited them to stay. "We have a little while before we must go out. Stay with your father."

Nerta clambered back onto the bench under Gunnar's arm, Eadward under the other. I poured the ale for them and Eadward toasted his father.

"Hoch, min far."

"Hoch, Gunnarson."

What he said at table haunted my mind as I trudged across the courtyard to the gate. A good lord is followed because each man sees in him the best of themselves and the best of what they could be. Yes . . .

That was it, *that* was the magic Arthur had that I so envied and never defined. All of them—Bedivere, Gareth, Gawain—saw that quality in Arthur whose eyes were for his vision alone, who reached out to grasp it without pausing to consider if any of the others could even see it; who drove himself harder and further than any man who called him lord. This is what men will follow. I had the determination, but Arthur had the ease of it, the magic that made his yoke a light one for men to bear.

How simple a thing to elude me so long. Or perhaps because it was so simple.

Another cloudless day. By midsummer the ground would be parched and the brook a dry crack in the earth. We couldn't think of that, we'd never get anything done. Perhaps today with the children helping and perhaps some of the cottagers . . .

Even as I thought it the first men emerged from the

forest. My heart swelled for a moment: there, even now some of them were coming back to work. . . .

But they were not cottagers. More and more of them poured out of the wood from the Wicandaen road, moving toward the pale post, helmeted men with spears and shields. As they merged into a force of dozens, then a hundred and more, I hurried back inside to bar the gate and scramble up into the watchtower to pull frantically on the bell rope, shattering the morning with my alarm.

"Up! Out! Men at the pale. Gunnar, Cynred, Rhodri, out!"

Cynred came to the door of the smithy, then Gunnar shot out of the hall, sword in hand, Eadward loping behind, colt after stallion. Gunnar reached the tower at a dead run and leaped at the ladder, throwing the order to his son—

"Arm the men. See to your mother and sister."

The boy spun about in quick obedience as Gunnar leaped onto the platform.

"I thought they were our people at first."

We heard the horn sound from the pale.

"Friends, you think?"

Gunnar said it flatly. "If they're not, there's not much we can do about it."

The horn sounded again.

"Close to two hundred." My stomach began to flutter. What a way to die, without a chance. "They don't look English, Gunnar."

"No, I'd say not." Gunnar took down the tower horn and blew an answering blast. "We might as well. They'll come on anyway."

I watched the strangers surge forward. "The pickings are lean today if they've come for plunder."

"Come, let's meet them on the wall."

When the host came within hailing distance, the entire ravaged population of Gunnarsburh was waiting on the wall. Every woman, even old Gytha, had risen from her bed. Gunnar stood flanked by his gaunt mother and pale wife, Nerta by me, Eadward clutching his sword too hard, Rhodri and Cynred with spears and bows. A poor showing, but that was the lot of us.

"They will not take me in my bed," Nilse vowed lethally. "I will die here by my Lord."

"Jackals," Elfgifu spat with a disgust deep as my own. "They've heard we're finished and they come to pick the carcass. By Loki, I wish we had just one foxglove bell to wear for them."

"Just let me take one," Rhodri prayed as Gwyneth nestled in close to him.

"And one or two for the lost Lindissi," she said. Then a furtive glance at me. "And holy Arthur."

The wind was from the east behind the strangers. Ase stiffened suddenly, went alert, ear cocked to one side. "Listen!"

Gunnar caught it too. "Cattle."

"And sheep," Elfgifu confirmed. "Hear them?"

I did not. "Ghosts, then. Nothing on four feet that hasn't been eaten."

When the first dirty-white sheep dribbled from the forest, Elfgifu said, "Will you never learn to believe me, little Brit?"

The newcomers appeared to be led by a husky young man whose dull yellow braids thrust out from under a ruined leather helmet. He paced without hesitation to the wall just below us. A moment of tense shuffling silence among the strangers, then the young leader drew his sword and jammed it into the earth. At this signal, all other weapons were grounded.

"We would speak with the Hlaford," he said in his Jutish accent.

"You are," Gunnar responded laconically. "Gunnar Eanboldson, thegn to Icel. Who are you?"

"Teutons, Lord."

"And yourself. Thegn or boat-chief?"

The youth removed his helmet. "I led the ships, but we have no lord." A few of his men laughed sourly. Gunnar pointed with his sword.

"If you come for plunder, you're a bit late. But I call your attention to the decorations on our wall. They were once Varingas. Now they're leather."

"We have heard of Gunnar Eanboldson. My name is Wickstan and we are no pirates," the young man replied with some edge, that his intentions were so mistaken. "We have no land. The Geats have seen to that. We were well-governed men in Jutland." He took something from his belt, impaled it on a spear and lifted it to Gunnar: a

wrinkled scrap of parchment. Gunnar pretended to peruse it, then passed it to me.

"A moment, Wickstan. We are a civilized court here. My clerk will overread this writing."

I breathed one delicious breath of air, happy that it wouldn't be among my last. "It's from Icel."

So it was: his invitation to landless Jutes of honor to swear fealty to him and live among Iclingas.

"We hear in Jutland that Icel is a prince strong enough to bend even bear-sarks to the law," Wickstan said.

"That is so. That is . . ." Gunnar fingered the message, looking from wife to mother to children. It seemed to me the same comprehension lit all of us. *God, Goddess, thank you.*

"Now," said Gunnar. He spun around to grin down at young Wickstan. "If you come as friends, then welcome."

"And I regret that we have nothing to feast you with," Nilse offered.

"But we have!" Wickstan laughed expansively as the tension dissolved. He wheeled his bare arm toward the distant sheep still milling in profusion from the forest. As we watched, a man broke clear of the trees leading a brace of oxen. "Even your own shepherd."

And then the staid Ase belied all the years I'd known her. Weak with fever, her back still snapped straight as Rhodri's spear as she lifted her arms to the provident gods. "Beorn! Look, Gunnar Eanboldson, where comes your gebur-knight. Hoch, Beorn! Hail the risen Baldur-hero. *Beorn!*"

"Our women and more men wait at your place called Wicandaen," Wickstan told us, spreading his arms in the ceremonial request for hospitality. "Are we welcome in your house, Thegn Gunnar?"

Gunnar's expression crumpled with fatigue, hunger and relief all melding into a wide, beatific grin. He passed a hand over it all as if to wipe away yesterdays for tomorrow; or perhaps not all of yesterday. Gunnar caught my eye; he said it aloud but the truth was between us. "Yes. Magic enough. Cynred, Rhodri, open the gates."

The Teutons marched in good order through our gate to wait behind Wickstan, who handed his sword to Gunnar in peace only to receive it again in trust. The Teuton

fyrd men peered about at our silent, empty courtyard. Probably some of them considered how easily it could be taken for themselves; others no doubt wondered if they'd fled one desolation for another.

Blanched with fever, Elfgifu leaned on her son's arm, trying to stand straight in front of these new men. "Look," she rasped in a parched voice. "How *fat* they are."

"Yes. Now, Mother."

"Now," said Elfgifu. "The Midlands. We can do it."

"Now or never," Nilse agreed.

"Now." And Elfgifu tottered away to her altar to commune with her gods.

Ase might have echoed them, but she was long out the gate and flying across the field, skirts hitched up like a girl and no thought to redundant dignity as Beorn recognized her and broke into a run himself, scattering sheep to the winds, and it was gorgeous to see them collide and whirl in clumsy joy, even more to see the sheep—so many of them!—and the blessed lambs wobbling along by their mothers, already roasted and succulent in my starved imagination.

Now if ever. They had the fresh blood, good fighting men, sturdy women and a horde of healthy children. They could take the Midlands if the will was there.

TO ICEL, AETHELING—
With these Teutons come to swear their loyalty, I send my own hopes. Prince, our resources are diminished beyond recovery and my thoughts are bent to the future. We are far gone in drought and the future moves to where the Midlands stand empty. Now is the time. We have always been a people to venture, from the fall of dice to the turn of a man's life to the crossing of the sea. We must gamble now for the Midlands. Such a time will not come for us again.

The ideas were Gunnar's, the lucid figures of speech mine, the last trenchant vow Elfgifu's.

We carry our ways and our gods with us.

So they were starting out again, starting over. See the thing logical, worth the gamble, quickly decided, done. The whole nation of the Iclingas—prince, lords, farmer-knights, geburs, cottagers, tradesmen, laet-slaves—were starting over once more to win or lose on one throw. Others would take what they left. Their future lay in the west.

Starting over. The remaining days at Gunnarsburh were aswirl with preparation, comings and goings, packings and messengers back and forth. One of the last things Gunnar did in the week before we left was to manumit Rhodri and Gwyneth to freedom. No sudden altruism based his motives but good English sense. In a new place where land would be more plentiful than people to work it, Gunnar knew it paid to raise slaves to the status of cottagers. For Rhodri and Gwyneth it was manna but little change. They'd still be of the household, kitchen and forge as before, but for having their own to go home to. They could barely conceive of life away from the house of Eanboldson, but part of their yield would henceforth be their indisputable own.

"Glory to God!" Rhodri exalted, rubbing at the old callus on his neck. "Think of it, a whole quarter-hide of our own. I wish I was young again. And what of you, Gwenda?"

Indeed, what of me? Their freedom, the reality of it, made me ache suddenly for my own, brought back in a poignant surge names and faces that had to be dusted off with an effort of memory. Emrys and Gareth and Rhian. Bors and Regan. She'd be close to thirty now if she lived. Though the yearning took me suddenly as it did that day over my flowers when I tried to escape, I knew there'd been a life and a learning at Gunnarsburh, but it was done. I *felt* it end in me as the first Teuton wagons rolled through our gates. I wanted to go—not home, but to the rest of me, the me still becoming. Like Gunnar breaking the soil in his fingers, the time had simply come.

But Gunnar hadn't freed me or even hinted at it. Then one evening he sent for me and bade me walk out in the fields with him. We strolled together across the furrows we'd never finish or sow. Gunnar picked up a clod from time to time and tossed it idly away.

"Well, my Lord. You had some purpose in sending for

me other than to dog your shadow and admire the manly sight of you."

"I know you've wondered why I didn't free you with the others."

"I did think on it, yes."

"They'll never leave. But you—you know how much I'd want you to stay. If I freed you—"

I would go.

"Would you stay as my scribe? You'd be a cottager, perhaps with a servant of your own. Would you stay then?"

I would go. "No, Gunnar."

"Why not?" He halted in his thoughtful rambling and stared at me. "Why not, Gwenda? You've been like a second wife and a friend to me. Where will you go?"

"I don't know. Home."

Gunnar flung his arm toward the west, exasperated. "Stubborn woman, whatever you were, it's no more. It's chaos out there. The Welsh are dying, Gwenda. No real king, no more Rome, no more Arthur or any of it. The combrogi will make no more magic, but who is to say your own sorcery didn't save us? Stay and live. I'd free you in a minute then."

"A comfortable clerk to an English lord while Nilse hangs up British skins? No, my heart wouldn't be in it." *I would go not for want of loving you, but because I hear my own music and must follow it. Because, like you, I was born to choose my own life, not merely accept it.*

"Is that it? That we'd be fighting your people? Hell, your own lords were never that nice in who they killed."

"It doesn't matter what I was, that's dead. And you've been good to me."

"But what? You and I have had a treasure. A marriage. Trust, understanding. But what, Gwenda?"

I pointed across the field. "Just there it was that I came to you as the Goddess and loved you when there was no other sane remedy for anything. There, look."

"I'll never forget," Gunnar said. "It saved a part of my life."

"And even in the joy of loving you, dear man, I felt your iron collar around my neck. Oh, Gunnar, I'd love to lie to you and myself and say I'd be happy spinning out my days as the pampered scribe of an honored lord. A com-

fortable dowager nonentity. No. If you open the cage, this bird will fly."

Manlike, he wouldn't accept what he didn't want to hear. "But why?"

"Because I have the wings for it like you. You'd not love me else."

"There's no order, no law, no safety unless things are owned."

"I wasn't born to this collar, my love. If you want me to stay, you'll have to leave it on me. I'll never forget you, any of you. But as I did that night loving you and tall enough to touch the stars with the Goddess and you deep in me, I'd always feel this iron around my neck. I'm not ungrateful; this collar has taught me more freedom than I ever knew before, but it still has a ring to chain me. You're a beautiful part of my life, but not the end of it."

"And what is?"

"I don't know, Gunnar."

"Oh, you damned stubborn—woman!" Gunnar kicked at the earth in his frustration. "Won't you ever face reality?"

He was so stymied by it, I had to laugh. "Won't you? The money Rat hid I could have kept for myself. I gave it to you out of love, not because I belonged to you. You have to decide whether you love me more than you own me. There are facts for you."

"Facts? Facts?" Gunnar stamped away from me to whirl around when he found an answer, arms a windmill of exasperation. "I thought I offered you gifts. Advancement. Rhodri and Gwyneth took it as such. Well. Well. I won't stand here arguing if you don't want them. I've better things to do and so have you."

He strode away toward the stockade, halting again as his English-logical mind refused to leave it. One male finger pointed and shook itself at me. "Your husband must have been a very patient man. By the gods, he needed it, and that's all I have to say."

Nevertheless, two days later I was summoned to the smithy to find Gunnar and Cynred waiting by the anvil.

"Aye, Lord?"

Gunnar jerked a thumb at the anvil; when I hesitated, he drew me down to it. "Go on, Cynred. Break the bolt."

Cynred raised the hammer and brought it down on the

bolt. He needed several strokes, but the bolt was ten years rusted shut. When it parted at last, Gunnar raised me up, stretched the collar open and removed it. He handed me the old lead seal that Frith stamped for my sale.

"What does this say, exactly?"

After all the years I'd forgotten myself. "Let me see: Gwenda, Parisi woman with the scar. One pound/ten."

Gunnar smiled ruefully. "Well then, Gwenda with the scar, I manumit you to your own freedom, keeping this seal against your inheritance which is mine."

"And good fortune to you," said Cynred.

My neck felt naked without the old weight.

"Leave us a moment, Cynred."

When the smith left us alone, Gunnar toyed with the hammer, clinking it on the anvil. "Well, I thought on it."

"A lovely gift. Thank you, my Lord."

All I could see was the top of his head bent over the anvil, not his face. "I asked myself, did I love you as much as I owned you." He dropped the hammer ringing on the anvil. "And I do. You will still go?"

"Yes."

"I'll never understand that."

"You owned me. You knew I'd go if you opened your hand, and yet you did. That's understanding enough."

"To . . . to let you choose," he said with difficulty. "Must you?"

"As much as you."

Gunnar searched me for reasons. "Why? Where?"

"There are some old friends who'll remember me. Small things, but I've a small life now, so they're important."

And then Gunnar let go the last of me and accepted it. "Do you have enough money, skat?"

"Quite enough. A few pounds."

"I'll give you more before you go. As much as I can spare."

"I don't need—"

"Take it. Don't be proud. Don't you know what I'm saying?"

"Yes." I moved into his arms. His beard was rough and lovely against my cheek. "I'll never forget you," he said.

"Woman, I loved you somehow. I gave you the only thing I could."

His words were always simple, he never needed many of them. And he suspected, perhaps not in comfort, that love was more an open hand than a closed fist.

"Don't expect too much of Eadward just yet."

"No. I'd like him to be a boy longer than I had time for."

"And Nerta. Children are tough as radish. A bath and a kiss now and then, they'll do famously. They can even do without the bath, but the kiss is needed."

I tried to avoid the loss in his eyes, but I couldn't. "This is goodbye, then."

"Yes. We'll see each other for days yet. But now is goodbye."

"I'll always love you, man. Without rhyme or reason but that you're the damned shining sort I've always had to love the few times I've found you. Not always well enough, but with you—yes. A work of art."

Starting over, burrowing deeper into Britain to take firmer root this time, to make an end to mere beginnings. Some of them would die, but not the dream. The halls would rear up behind the stockades, Woden nestle cheek by jowl with Christ. The Catuvellauni cursing Icel's folk would learn to do it in English.

Starting out. The stir within and without the wide-propped gates of the stockade buzzed with purposeful orders—men shouting, cattle bawling and milling about, the high whine of Rhodri's grindstone as spears, swords and tools were sharpened for the last time before the stone was unseated and packed in a wagon. Nothing was left behind that could possibly serve. Even the seasoned timbers of the stockade, as many as could be loaded, were levered out of the ground for defense along the way.

Gunnar was everywhere, seeing to everything as the wagons groaned through the gate to swell their party and be loaded. Nilse marched through it all with Ase and me in her nervous wake, packing each piece of her life with tight-lipped reverence, from the wooden platters to her Cyprian perfume bottle. The uprooting shortened her temper but she reined it tight and only once spanked Nerta for being a noisy bother.

In a fever of excitement, Elfgifu got in everyone's way, sputtering and cursing with no real anger, making sure there was room in her wagon for the worn icon of Woden that hulked over her altar.

And of course the damned Teuton children underfoot everywhere, swinging on the gate, the wagons, stampeding the sheep, climbing on or falling off everything in sight until Eadward planted himself before them to bark in his breaking voice: "You brats behave! Stop getting in the way. What are you laughing at, girl? This isn't play. We should leave you all behind. Gott, you'd drive a man insane."

Rhodri and Gwyneth had a wagon and tools to themselves now. Not much to put in it as yet, but ambition was their new toy. "Thirty new acres," Rhodri dreamed. "A plow and an ox and maybe two next year. Doesn't it *dazzle*, sweeting? Born so poor I had to borrow a shadow, and here I am an owner of land."

"Prince Rhodri, no less." Gwyneth thrust her latest bundle into his arms. "Stow these in the wagon. Och, Gwenda, though—it does make a soul wonder."

"What's that?"

"Where will the like of you go, now that . . . all that's dead and gone?"

"Why, straight to Arthur, who's risen," Rhodri reminded her.

"Yes," I said, and let it go at that.

And at last, the day.

They would journey together to Witgar's holding, join his wagons and then Icel's, trickles becoming a stream becoming a westward rolling river. The Teutons parceled out by Icel traveled with us; the big placid women, most of them pregnant and a child or two trudging behind; the men like Wickstan, not yet used to practical English ways, grave and formal in their old-fashioned gear and bronze-winged helmets. The last folk to come were those from Wicandaen, the common folk in their own wagons or afoot, their whole world in the bundles on their shoulders. Alfred came with them, no doubt sure from birth that this would happen, sure to the jot how much of it he made himself, his eloquence packed up tidy as his bolts of cloth.

"Hael, Gwenda!"

"Hael, law-maker. Whatever will you do with nothing to rail against?"

"Nothing? Ho-ho, listen: those new bear-sark lords, they've got a taste of property now, and they'll be bellowing themselves blue in the gemot for their rights. Well, let 'em roar, Gwenda. Greedy bastards can't argue and rob me at the same time, can they?"

The wagons creaked out of the stockade to join the lengthening train outside. Three, four hundred people and a storm of cattle and sheep, a cacophony of penned-up chickens flurrying on the carts.

"Nerta, see to the old coops, there may be eggs we missed."

The peasant men, the spearmen of the English fyrd, guzzling the last ale with their new Teuton brothers, Ase wringing her hands, swearing she'd forgotten something after a dozen trips to make sure—

"And I'll think of it three days from now. Ach, Gwenda, I wish my children had lived to see this. Well—the fates said no. We will go alone. If they meant to take me and not the children, they would have."

Again, the English for you: all is fate, fate writes all. And all will go into darkness at the end of the world, but for a little while there's light and they will make the most of it.

Then Gunnar trotted away from one of a hundred last details to catch up the astonished Nilse, whirl her about, lift her high in a very un-English bonfire of exuberance— magnificent. He might have been British.

"Put me *down*, husband. Your men are watching. What is it?"

"To the wagons with Nerta. We're ready to start."

"Oh . . ." Nilse looked about with that brimming mix of excitement and sadness that comes with finding the new but already missing the old. "Where is Nerta? Where *is* that girl, Gwenda?"

"Just off to the byre for the eggs. I'll fetch her out."

I was in the open doorway of the byre when the watchtower sounded the horn to assemble. At the blast, the busy people moved faster to complete a dozen things, but Elfgifu stopped dead still. Then, slowly, as if waking out of sleep, the old woman turned her head this way and that—that movement alone, a statue amid scurry. Then

her hands lifted in a kind of uncertain supplication and fell again as she straightened her shoulders and moved to her altar where a few deformed chicks that would have died anyway waited in a small wicker crate.

Elfgifu lit the altar fire and then, as the flames licked up, faced the weather-worn icon of her stern old god.

Whenever I'd heard snatches of her at prayer through the years, it was always the same; not like praying but telling, sometimes imploring. And now as I listened, I knew why. The altar and the sacrifice, these might be for Woden, but her words were for someone closer.

"My Lord, it is happening. And he is leading them, Eanbold. Oh . . . I have chafed him much that he wasn't you, and he shamed me when he burned your shield. But that was only because he is a man and gets discouraged, I should have seen that. But he has done it all. *He* has led them in war and in the fields and the writing of good laws. And now he leads us home. Your son, Eanbold. Where we belong. We will not be burned out again. The crows have long flown over, combrogi magic is old. You barely knew him . . . he wasn't even walking then. But be proud, husband. Cry out in Valhalla that Gunnar the son of Eanbold will feast with his father there."

Almost as an afterthought, Elfgifu made a sign before her eyes and set the wicker cage on the fire. "All-Father Woden, you go with us. Take this offering. Send me a sign that my debt is paid."

"Hlafdian?"

She rubbed a hand over reddened eyes. "Yes, it's time. Help me carry the god to my wagon. Your last duty to me."

"And a last gift." I took a faggot from the fire and ground it out on the altar. "Among my people, a sacred fire is always lit from a piece of the last. Take this and let it be part of your first altar fire in the new place."

Elfgifu turned the stick in her hands. "You must know I am very proud today."

"Of course, Hlafdian."

"I am long unused to joy, Gwenda. So long I thought it was all lost, all for nothing. But now we'll go back to stay." She thrust out her strong red hands to lean against the altar. "I've not done badly. One grandson to be thegn

like his father, another will be prince. That is worthy of Eanbold's wife."

"Here, take my kerchief, your nose is a sight. I'd be less than a good Brit if I thought it was going to be easy for you."

"Brits. You're strange people. Give out where you should hold fast, stone-stubborn when you ought to quit. I didn't think you'd last a year, you or Rat."

"Oh, poor Rat. I must leave her some flowers. She always loved them."

"And sentimental." Elfgifu's snort had no contempt in it. "Your weakness, all of you. Those men around Arthur were all the same. That last day in the Midlands, after all that death, they couldn't manage two more. They found a horse for me, even food to take in a sack." Her flintiness softened as she remembered the Welsh inconsistency that spared her to do it all over again. "The great Gareth mac Diurmuid, the devil on a horse that even Cerdic feared—why he was a *mite* of a man, Gwenda, no bigger than you. He and the Lancelot might pass for honorable in my balance, even kindly. They mashed up pears and goat's milk for Gunnar. I'll never know why they didn't kill me, but not a man would. Even Arthur made only a show of being angry with them.

"It was Arthur himself who put me on the horse. Did you ever see him, Gwenda? Comely enough, but an odd color to his eyes. They didn't go with the rest of him. He lifted the child to me and said, 'Woman, tell your kind this is British land.'"

"Mother!" Nilse hailed from the gate, wrapping a fresh veil about her head. "Come, it's time to start."

"Go on, I'll be there—oh, won't I be there, Gwenda! She worries I'm too old for this." Elfgifu actually grinned with defiant mischief. "Children born this side of the water, they don't know what strong *is*. Put them all on the pyre, I will. I lasted Arthur and most of his Gott-damned combrogi, didn't I? And you know what answer I made to the great Pendragon? I said *no*." Her callused palm struck against the altar wood. "Not Brit, I said, not a foot of it. We grew the barley. That made it ours. But Arthur was thick as you and would never see the sense of that."

"Grandmother, come!" Now it was Nerta hopping up

and down by the gate as the last people lifted their packs and moved out the gate. "We're going*goinggoing*."

"Yes, child." Elfgifu waved her on. "She'll grow strong, that girl. We'll find an earl at least for her, you wait. Always marry upward, it's good business. Well." Elfgifu took a last swipe at her nose and handed me my kerchief. To my astonishment, she bent awkwardly to kiss me, something of a valedictory. "You're free, little Brit. Enough of this, come help me lift the god. And don't drop him, he's old."

I saw Gunnar, distant at the head of the column, stand up and scoop his arm in a great, wheeling circle. The wagons began to move, and I knelt by Rat's grave in the kitchen garden. I said a few of the prayers that came to hurried mind, then one to Mary Virgin to intercede for my friend, crossed myself and patted the flowers into the low mound.

"I'm off to Brigid chapel, Rat. I wish it were the two of us. I could do worse for friends hereafter, but there'll be candles enough to light all Eburacum. Rest you gentle."

I rode west with the Iclingas only a day, then parted when we met a procession of Augustinian monks afoot on a journey to Eburacum. After my farewells to the family, I slipped a folded parchment to Gunnar.

"Keep this safe with my seal."

"Why, what is it?"

"Haven't you told me and told me from here to Samhain that you're my legal heir? Well, here's my will."

Gunnar thrust it in his tunic. "I'll read it close then."

"When you learn to read. Farewell, good master."

Then I ruffled Eadward's hair and kissed Nerta and Nilse, and stood aside for history to pass me by. My last sight of them was from the top of a hill as the monks plodded on before me: the endless wagons, the harried dogs nipping at tardy sheep, the children skipping behind the wagons, the lines and lines of spearmen—and by God, Elfgifu in the lead, ahead of them all, her stride unrelenting as her destiny.

VIII

The Horses Grow Old

ompensations: if there was no hope of regaining my crown, there was no desire for it either. Like my old kirtles, the notion no longer fit. The kennel won't change, as Bedivere said, only the dogs, and why should any of them fight for the others? Britain had a spate of strong dogs; what they needed was a strong people. No, I'd go to Eburacum, keep my promise to Rat, perhaps say farewell to Emrys, pray once more at Arthur's tomb, and then—

And then?

My ten monks were from Londinium where, they said, the Saxons of high and low estate were singularly uninterested in any gods, ours or their own. The monks were on their way to Eburacum and beyond where there might be more need for holiness, and told me what news they'd heard from the west. Constantine's alliance with Aurelius Conant had evaporated in squabbling and then open war. There were no more real principalities or lords, only war bands living off the carcass of the country. Some rode for Constantine, some for Emrys Pendragon, and all plundered for themselves if the truth be told. The west and the Midlands were anarchy, and only Cair Legis still flew the Pendragon.

"And the people? Your flocks, good brothers, the lambs of God? Who's shearing them now, everyone?"

My monks thought that a bold comment from a

woman. They were not of the radical persuasion—that, they muttered sourly, smacked of the troublesome northern monk, Coel. This was the sort of thing he was always on about, departing from his ordainment and contemplative order and stirring the common folk to dissension.

We walked by day and slept where chance found us at night. There were plenty of deserted byres and houses. You would have thought the whole country empty at times, but once north of Humber I was among my own Parisi. The vista wasn't cheery. Even in our most negligent days, my country had never been so desolate. Trev after trev we passed, deserted or burned out, fields gone to seed. Now and then at a distance I might spy a peasant and his wife grubbing over their small patch and sidling off when we came too close. As we neared Eburacum on the paved Roman road, more and more people passed us, dragging handcarts or bent under the load of their few possessions. These were not farmers but city folk, and we stopped to share some bread and water with them in the hot afternoon. They'd all been evicted, dispossessed, tax paupered by the praefect of the city.

"Him, Constantine, that calls himself King. He's taxing the blisters on a poor man's foot," one frail old man said eloquently. "And what he leaves, the bloody praefect snatches up."

His Parisi accent fell like music on my ears after so long. "Can ye nae pay't, don't they take all and thrust you out the gate. Where bound, woman?"

"Something of a pilgrimage."

"No matter. Wherever ye go, it's the same. They'll all rob you. Hide your money. Bury it."

This in a country where once a maiden could walk with her virtue and a sack of gold from Castle Dore to the Wall of Hadrian and arrive with both inviolate.

The city of my ancestors was now no more than an armed camp. Constantine's banners flew everywhere, but there was nothing royal about the littered streets, only garbage and slovenly soldiers. Some I recognized as Cornish by the flower chaplets wrapped about their helmets. A few had the stamp of knights, but most were a coarse lot, unshaven, foul-mouthed, fighting in the middle of the street, drinking or relieving themselves where

and when they pleased. We'd been stopped at the south gate by guards and, after perfunctory questioning, hurried along to the palace to be registered and questioned as strangers. We passed the well where Emrys and I once laughed out our desperation while his horse debated whether to rise again. Then up the steps from which I once greeted the decurions of the city on what was my last return as queen. Now they pushed me and the worried monks up the steps into the very halls I'd fled ten years before.

My first whiff of the interior air made me yearn for the street again. It was no more than a filthy barracks now. Pools of urine fouled the corridors, spilled liquor, rushes moldy and unchanged and hardly a man in sight that Gareth, Bedivere or Arthur would have tolerated among combrogi. Anything of value—furniture, hangings, bronze fixtures—had been stripped away, replaced by rough camp furniture and racks of spears.

The old forum smelled like a stable. In one corner a man, probably a relief guard, snored knottily on a pallet. Near the bare dais a bearded officer grumbled over dispatches written on wax tablets. Fairly squared off, more efficient in his bearing than the others I'd seen, he dispensed quickly with the monks after noting their names, business and destination. He was even cordial, taxing them only a pittance.

"We give the Church no problems. Just have to know who's coming from where. Lot of spies about. You may go, brothers. Not you, woman. Stay."

The guard from the gate pushed me to the table. He quickly emptied my waist-purse onto the table in front of the officer. "That's all she's got."

The captain dabbled among the silver pence. "Search her."

The guard fumbled carelessly about my body; no doubt he would have been more thorough were I younger. He found nothing else, thanks to Rat who taught me to conceal my real purse between the thighs. "That's the lot, sir."

"What are you?"

"Gwenda. A freedwoman."

"This money is Saxon."

Fresh news to the dull guard. "Saxon, no less?"

"I was a slave among them ten years. They freed me. And that's my money."

"Ours now." The captain jingled a handful of the pence. "War tax. Don't feel put upon. Everyone pays it."

"Where's the war?"

He chuckled. "Where isn't it? Why are you in Eburacum?"

"I am Parisi. It's been many years, but I did hear the Holy Grail was brought here by your bishop."

"Grail?" He looked at the guard in mild disbelief. "The Grail's in Witrin where it's always been. Do you know where Witrin is?"

"I've been to there, sir."

"Oh?" He squinted thoughtfully at me. "And who's the Abbot?"

"When I was taken and sold—"

"Taken?" The guard seemed curious at this.

"Yes, yes," my interrogator cut him off. "Traders. Be still and listen. There's a lesson for you in this. Who's the Abbot of Witrin, woman?"

"It was Brochan."

He swept his eyes over me, up and down, not yet convinced. "And his patron?"

"Princess Eleyne of Astolat—when I was there."

"And still, the little ray of sunlight." The captain pushed back his stool and came round the table to inspect my neck. "She's what she says, a Brit freedwoman. But you shards on the gate look sharp at what you pass through. See the callus on her feet? Saxon women have more callus on their feet than their shoes have leather. They never ride horses. And this headdress: they won't go without one. It's immodest to show their hair in public. Shy little violets they are: blush at your kind of language, but they'll gut a man like a fish for dinner. This biddy could've been one of them walking right into Eburacum."

"M-maybe she is," the guard stammered.

"Maybe she is." The captain turned to me casually. "A proper Brit, freed but loyal to her masters. Where's the court of the Sudhymbre Saxons now?"

"Nowhere," I told him. "All the English are moving west."

He gave a final nod of satisfaction. "Damned right they

are, and the King's looking sharp to them, too. And you"—to the chastened guard who'd just begun to relax again—"remember the cut of these clothes and the headdress. Right, you can go."

I breathed easier, glad to be leaving the place. It stank like a latrine. Hard to believe I was born a few paces from this sty. I first set eyes on Arthur just where the littered table stood now.

"Woman, wait. What did you call the Saxons?"

"English, sir."

"English?" The captain's head swerved to his guard for any kind of enlightenment and received none. "English? Never heard of them."

A few streets of boarded-up shops from the desolated palace, Brigid chapel was hardly changed, though it wanted a good sweeping. The mosaic panel of the chi-rho over the altar was flanked by marbles of Mary and Saint Brigid in shallow apses. Brigid had been a goddess before the Church appropriated her. We commissioned Annennius to sculpt her, one of the last really good men in marble. Brigid had made the transition without turning a hair.

While not strictly orthodox, there were good mosaics of Cador and my mother as patrons of the Church, and a mural on a terra-cotta panel of their munificent daughter—decades younger and slimmer in Roman dress and hair style—making a donative to Father Donal to build this chapel while Bishop Patricius blessed the undertaking. Speak of artistic license: I was still playing on Cador's knee when Patricius returned from Ireland with a number of converts and their barbarian children. Donal was one of them, no older than myself. Patricius died within the year, but why spoil a lovely picture?

I genuflected to the altar and crossed myself from the font, waiting for the young priest to notice me.

"What do you want, woman? The poor box is empty. We have nothing to give."

"Then here, I'll sweeten it for you. I should like to see Father Donal if he's still here. Tell him it's an old friend."

The priest paused to light several candles before replying. "Father Donal is at supper in the refectory."

"Good. You may tell him his friend is hungry as well."

The priest gave me a closer inspection, knitting du-

bious black brows. "I've never seen you. Are you not a foreigner?"

"Of Eburacum, but I daresay you were not even ordained when I left. He will want to see me."

Still doubtful, he finished his altar chores and disappeared through a side door. I was studying the mural with philosophic amusement when I heard Donal's bustling step behind me.

"Well? Yes? And what is it?"

"Donal, you old immigrant. This picture flattered us both even then."

He'd gone stout with the years and more florid than I remembered. His red hair, once a flaming pride, was now a thin, snowy wreath about his ears. Kindly Donal was, but not blessed with a large patience for small matters. "Who are you, woman?"

As I removed the English veil, I saw the impatience hesitate, recognize, deny itself and affirm again.

"Lady Guenevere!"

"Donal of Slemish. Look at us up there. Was I ever that young or you that sanctimonious? That was the year Cador dangled me as a royal bride in front of the Picts and I started to blush in the confessional."

Donal glanced about to see if the young priest was within earshot. "The whole of Britain's thought you dead for ten years."

"And Constantine?"

"Aye, that one too. I won't speak his name in my chapel."

"Let's not shatter his illusions just yet. Weren't you at supper? I haven't eaten since early this morning."

"Come, come." He guided me toward the refectory entrance. "But put on that . . . whatever it is. No one will recognize you in that. And few without it, I'll hazard."

In the simple refectory, Donal placed before me a bowl of barley and leeks, stewed in last week's soup, and a large onion. He was appalled at the way I attacked the food. My table manners had gone quite English, which is to say they'd gone.

"You eat an onion as I'd eat an apple."

"Best way," said I between ravenous bites. "Turnips too. Have you one around?"

"Uh . . . no, but there's more barley."

"Good, good. Lord, I'm famished."

When I'd laid waste to his table, I pushed aside the bowl with a sigh of contentment. Over Donal's blessedly offered uisge, I told him of the last ten years and then demanded of my country.

"What's happened to my people? No, first tell me of Lady Rhian. You must remember her, Gareth's wife? She came here often for mass. And Regan. She was about to give birth. What of her?"

Donal didn't remember Regan at all, not even the name. "Of Rhian I can be surer. Constantine took the city, but didn't sack it. No women were harmed save a few peasants. That always happens."

"Yes, doesn't it?"

"Lady Rhian was paroled to Cair Legis."

"There's luck. I'm off that way as soon as I can."

Donal poured himself more uisge and savored it before answering. "You think Legis is any better than this?"

"Arthur's nephew holds it."

"And how, Lady? No city, no place in Britain is any different than this. There is no Britain, just rags. The only thing that abides is what cannot be vanquished. God's domain. The country's gone back to what it was before Ambrosius. A patchwork. No order, every lord for himself. The people need protection. They become clients of any lord that will shelter them. He takes most of what they have. You think Emrys is any better?"

"I don't know. But right now I need your holy office."

He put aside his uisge. "Oh, Lord, and I've been saying ten years of requiem masses for you. Is it confession you want, then?"

"I suppose yes, though my sins have been spare of late. Just adultery."

I'd been too long away from the Church. Donal was surprised into candor. "My God, again?"

"In a good cause, Father."

"It always was."

"The way of it—"

Instantly Donal turned away, shading his eyes. "God's love, you've gone slack, Guenevere. If this is a confession, give me time to turn my back and pretend I don't know who's dropping it in my ear."

"Later for that, Father. Please let me have a stylus and tablet."

When the priest brought them, I wrote the prescription to be appended to the standing offices of the chapel. "I bid you to this as patroness."

Raidda of Londinium, a most devout daughter of the Church, was to be prayed for every day immediately following the prayers for my family. On my own death, to follow those invocations on my behalf. Extra candles were to be purchased and kept lit for her as for my parents and Peredur. For this (forgive me, Rat) five extra shillings in English silver would be my donation to Brigid chapel.

"Not that you need it. We endowed this chapel with enough to see us all to Judgment. Now you may turn your back, Father. I need my purse."

When Donal obliged my modesty, I hitched up the homespun skirt and fumbled between my thighs for the hidden purse. The arrow-scar twinged slightly.

"Going to rain."

"No, we've not had a drop in weeks."

"Longer in the east. Here." I spread the silver coins in front of him together with the folded scrap of parchment. "This was her last confession. I promised to bring it to you for hearing and absolution."

Donal unfolded it. "Who was this woman?"

"Read."

He read, folded it again and laid it aside. He might have said a number of things. Bless Donal, he didn't. "It will be done."

"Today."

"Within the hour."

"Not much for forty years, is it? She stole when she was hungry and sold herself to men. What she knew of kindness she showed to me. I will not have her forgotten of God. Would I had so little to answer myself. As long as this chapel stands for mine, pray for her. Please see it done."

The old priest studied me across the table. "You are much changed, Guenevere."

"And very tired, Father. May I sleep here tonight? It's going to rain. Not divination, just my bad leg tells me."

In the chapel I heard Donal through the first of the masses for Rat, prayed for my own family, then lit candles to Mary and Brigid and set a new one in an unused niche to complete my promise.

Holy Mary, take care of Rat. A bit late and a bit west, she might have been you.

At sunset Father Donal and I watched from the chapel door as a pathetic procession dragged its way toward the west gate of the city.

"More evictions." Donal shook his head pityingly. "The taxes are crushing them, and aren't they off to Legis where there's the same waiting?"

They reminded me in a forlorn way of the Iclingas exodus, but with less hope and purpose. "It's a funeral, the whole country. Pray for me, Father Donal."

"That's my office, Lady."

"No, I mean pray my ignorance be forgiven. God's Eyes, I had such a chance, I had all of Britain. And I tried; in my own way, by all I'd been taught, I tried. Now, when I want to help them so much I'm helpless myself."

"I cannot even now quite think of you as helpless, Guenevere."

We watched with profound sadness as the dreary procession trickled by. "Look at the children, Donal. Not a shoe in the lot. God bless them, Emrys must do better than this. Oh, yes, the Kingdom of God endures, but the Kingdom is not *here*, Donal. I've been a long time in the cold, and it's not enough. Goddamn it, it's not enough for *them*."

As my leg promised, heaven opened that night and turned the city into mud. I heard mass next day, lit another candle for Rat and made my confession to Donal, colorful as he expected. There were few shops still open in the stagnant city, but I managed a decent hand-me-down wool cloak and a new pair of shoes. The dispirited shopkeeper was astonished to see good silver on his board once more. His cash box contained nothing but a few minims and a sesterce or two.

When I walked through the west gate, I raised my head to the parapet. Just here Rhian and I stood to see Gareth and the combrogi come limping in from Legis. The two guards on watch gave me little note as I passed through the open gate and started on the long road to Legis.

Dispossessed people on the road to Legis: the ruin of
my city only mirrored the shambles of my country, one
part fleeing to another for succor that might or might
not be there. We were strung out for ten miles, tinkers,
potters, shoemakers, fullers, children for whom it was all
a lark until they began to get tired and footsore. I
mucked along with this group or that, listening to their
fly-drone complaints and hopes. The Pendragon was a
benevolent lord, they heard; things would be better in
Legis. But they had no Alfred, no notion of an Alfred to
conceive of what and how, nor a Gunnar to link peasant
and prince in any understanding of the need.

Aye, they needed that before all else.

I fell in with Huw and his wife, Lowri, by casual incident. Their cart mired on a stretch of road where the
paving blocks had been ripped up long ago for other
building, and the gravel bed eroded and full of mud now.
While Lowri and their young daughter Mabli hauled on
the shafts, Huw and I strained behind—"Together
now!"—and heaved the laden cart free, pushing until we
reached hard pavement again.

Discouraged at their fortune but still looking for a future, Huw and Lowri were about Gunnar's age. He'd
been an agrimensor like his father, a surveyor of land for
builders.

"Not much of that any more," Huw said.

"And what do you do now?" I asked as we hauled the
cart along.

"Whatever. Carpentry, that sort."

"My Huwcyn can turn his hand to anything," Lowri
stated with pride. "Mabli, stay close, don't run off! Och,
look at her. Ten years old, can't tell her a thing."

"You're familiar, Lowri. Not all that much, but I think
I've seen you before."

Like most of the imposing world, Lowri needed very
little encouragement to launch into her life story. Their
son ran off last year to join some roving band or other;
they'd only Mabli now, and their main hope was employment at Legis. The town was smaller than Eburacum but
not so moribund as not to need a good carpenter, and
Lowri herself was highly skilled—a cook, no less, once

employed at the palace. In Peredur's time that was, rest his soul as finder of the Grail.

"He died young, but he was never well, never. Gentle but absentminded, looked right through you, the half of his food always came back to the kitchen. Toward the end you could see the blood dabbled on his napkin. And then there was his sister. Now *her*—they said she was too proud, hot-tempered. A little bird of a woman, that thin and worried, always more to do than time to do it, and God love me, I'd starve on what she ate, and in those days I'd a neat figure myself. I saw her myself the day she rode in with the King's nephew a prisoner and the poor rag end of the combrogi trailing behind. The Cornishman'd been trying to kill her the summer out, and there was a great red scar across her pretty face. It was all too much, she couldn't carry it. Nae gentle as her brother, but nae always sharp unless you crossed her. Oh-ho, *then* you heard that little bird to the city walls. Mabli! Mind, don't stray off. Stay close, girl."

It rained again toward evening of the first day out from Eburacum, the rain a soft background to the grinding of our wheels and the dull ache of dampness in my leg that made me limp sometimes. When the rain ended in the long twilight, we were just east of a high hill with a crowd of folk busy at the top around a growing fire.

Little Mabli sang out: "Look, da! Building May-fire."

"And I'd forgot with all the troubles. Tonight's Bel-tein," Huw said. "Country folk up there."

"Can I go see the fire, can I, da?"

"Not a fit place for little maidens," Lowri warned delicately.

"What's that mean?"

"To hell with that," Huw said with relish. "Won't there be music and dancing, and how long since you and I jumped through Bel-tein fire together, lass?"

"Och, we're old now."

"Never!"

"Still . . . a great while since we danced together." Her hand strayed across his husky back, lingering. "A great while, Huwcyn . . . sing dogwood, alder, wild cornel . . ."

Oh, years since I heard my own people sing. I thrilled to it now, wallowed in it as a drunkard taking to wine after long abstinence. Lowri sang the first line alone, high and sweet. Before it was done, Mabli was skipping beside her, adding her child-pipe to the carol.

> Sing dogwood, alder, wild cornel,
> The cuckoo's nest is ne'er his own

Now Huw added a different, deeper line of harmony—

> The clover spreads his sweet red bell
> And we'll a-maying go-o-o,
> And we'll a-maying go.

By the second verse everyone within earshot on the road, man, woman or child, was part of the carol. Oh, if carol had a color it would be scarlet ribbon flung against bright green, blue sky or white stars . . . not enough? Well, you have to hear it—the deep bass of the older men, the vibrant tenor of the youths, the warm lines of the women over it—

> Sing rowan, beech and mulberry,
> The nest is full but cuckoo's flown,
> And we'll be bedded, you and me

—And the bright, pure voices of the children over it all, turning the top to delicate silver like sun touching clouds.

> When we a-maying go-o-o
> When we a-maying go.

No one teaches this peculiar gift of melody, but until you've heard my own people sing, let no man speak of music. The Brigantes atop the hill caught the song on the air and some of them leaped high and waved to us. Now, with the song rising up from all of us, Mabli drifted away to join the other sweet-voiced children skipping in time down the center of the road. The music was wine enough; warm with it, we didn't hear the growing rumble behind us.

Aye, there's a lass to marry me
When she runs through the Bel-*tein* fire,
And we'll be childed one-two-*three*!
When we a-maying go-o-o

A delightful unexpected upward twist of the higher voices, women and girls, the gilded capstone to it all:

When we a-maying—GO!

As the carol ended we heard the voices behind us— shouting now, rising with that edge of fear that prickles the hair on the neck. Men cursing, the sudden high scream of a woman, only partly the name of a child or husband, the shrill fear of children. Behind us, people and carts scattered like scalded chickens to left and right of the road before a line of plunging horsemen. One of them carried the king's banner and none slowed at all for the people on the road. I saw one old man go down under the hoofs.

"Mabli!" Lowri twisted about, eyes bright with fear as Huw and I hauled the cart clear of the road. "Mabli?"

She couldn't see the child; that frightened her more than anything else. The children were a knot clogging the men and women ahead of us, still chattering and oblivious. Huw whipped his head this way and that to find her. "Mabli! *Get off the road!*"

I saw her first as the horsemen surged closer, nearly on top of us, still chattering along with the other children. Now even they heard the coming thunder as I ran toward them—"There, Huw, get her"—pushing them right and left out of the horses' path. Huw was quicker, snatching up Mabli and leaping aside, one arm hooked through mine to pull me to safety. The riders passed so close I felt the wind-stir of them on my back and the paving stones shake under me. Frightened, Mabli began to cry in her father's arms while I took out my relief in scolding.

"You little donkey, you might have been killed. There, Lowri, she's right as bread and as dumb. She's all right." I kept saying it over and over as Lowri snatched the child from Huw's breast to her own, all love and maternal anger.

"I told you and *told* you—"

"Bloody patrol from Eburacum," Huw said in clenched hatred. "Gwenda, if it weren't for your sharp eyes . . ."

"And your nimble legs, man. Mine aren't that swift any more."

"There's someone hurt back there. Bastards. Wouldn't even turn aside for children."

"No. Not even for children." The memory mocked me. "God damn them."

"Is it hurt you are, Gwenda?"

"No, Huw." Just an old hawk come home to roost. "God damn them all to hell."

"And home again. And you, girl—" Firmly, Huw plucked Mabli from her mother's clutch and spanked her bottom a few sound whacks, more in relief of his fear than punishment. "You mind! You keep close to Gwenda, not a foot away or you'll get better than this."

We were still near the hill at dusk when the Brigante country folk lit the twin fires at the summit. Many of us climbed the slope to sing and dance with them. I noticed that a good many of them had bundles, homeless as ourselves. They were shy of us at first. Hill folk are backward as Picts in some ways, but then they saw we'd brought city wine and uisge to share and what food we had, and they offered us of their own oatcake and that pungent concoction of pork seasoned with rosemary and sage, cooked in the stomach of a sheep. Arthur always swore by it, though the concept nauseated me until Gwyneth cooked it once at Gunnarsburh.

I perched with Huw and his family on one of the turf ramparts erected for the ancient holiday, passing the uisge between us, tapping my feet as the dancers circled the fire. No place for a priest, this. The young dancers grew drunk, wild and wilder until, two by two, they slipped away into the shadows. The fires were replenished from the separate stacks of nine sacred woods, then Huw and Lowri with a mischievous wink of conspiracy left wide-eyed Mabli with me and joined in the circling dance about the blaze. In the half-light, flickering at the edge of the celebration, couples locked in each other's arms, rolling about in the old invocation to fertility in field and womb. Young men who'd yet to find a girl

to couple with were leaping high, straight through the flames to emerge unscathed on the other sides to squeals of feminine admiration or horror when their clothes caught fire and had to be beaten out, whereupon the proud, smoking youth would snort and rear like a stallion and plunge across the flame again.

Content, mellow with uisge, I hugged Mabli close and sang with the others, watching Huw cut his rusty capers with Lowri.

"Ay, Gwenda—watch!" Hand in hand they rushed through the narrow space between the fires and back again to tumble, sweating and ecstatic at my feet.

"Gwenda, go in the fire."

"Oh, no . . ."

"Na, na, in the fire with you," Huw insisted, unwinding my English veil. "Give us a year of good luck. We don't half need it."

"Into the fire, you who helped save my child," Lowri demanded, pulling the bone stays from my hair and shaking out the mass of it. "God, such hair, a white river of it. Go, give us a blessing from Epona."

"Look at the like of us," Huw chortled. "Good Christians calling on Epona."

"Brigid was at the fire ere the chapel, husband. Epona'll be sainted too, mark. Dance, Gwenda. Call us a blessing. If Christ's forgotten us, the old gods won't."

With my hair unbound I stepped out of my shoes, tucked up my skirts and joined the circling dance once around the fire, then danced into the searing heat between the two pyres. In the hard light, flushed with heat and drink, I raised my arms to the stars.

"Brigid, Goddess of Brigantia: hear your people and give them good harvest and flocks this year. Let the seed find welcome in the soil."

The heat stung my skin. People stopped dancing. They stared solemnly at me.

"Epona, Goddess of the Parisi, horse-goddess, mated with the house of Cador, smile upon your people. Give life to the seed. Give children to the young ewes and the new wives. *Ia! Evohe!* Brigid and Epona, see our fires and the testament of our strength and joy. Smile upon us."

And so I stood rigid, my face tingling with the heat of the fires, hands up and supplicating—

"It *is* her."

The ring of dancers surged closer, then Lowri broke through with Huw after her, to pull me away from the fires. "Bring torches here."

Then I was ringed with new light borne by the Brigante men—fierce men of the hills, some of them with old tribal scars cut across their cheeks. They thrust the torches into the ground as Lowri knelt to me and then rose to touch with the greatest reverence the old white scar on my brown face.

"Hear me! Was I not on the steps when Gwenhwyfar ferch-Cador returned to her people? This scar was red and new then, but it is she and no other. She has returned."

"Queen no longer, Lowri. Just Guenevere."

"It was many a time that I brought your dinner to Imogen's hands. And the voice. I remember your voice, my Queen. The years have done much to you, but that's not changed. This is the Queen, daughter of Epona," Lowri attested to the crowd. "The flesh of the Goddess."

But it was my Brigantes who remembered me most as goddess incarnate, the old folk whom the cross only lightly shadowed. They were a folk of signs and portents, and perhaps it was not so much the miracle of me as their need for one then that made them kneel and believe. But Mabli, who knew more than any of us about love and joy, wiggled through the knot of men and women straight to be swept up in my arms, pressing her small, moist mouth to my cheek.

"Ay, Gwenda, are you going to bless us? Do some magic."

Bless them? That was all I could do. I faced them with Mabli in my arms as the others hovered with their own needing children, swallowing back my own helplessness.

"Let the children come closer. All of you, come close. Let me bless you."

Next morning there were offerings of food by Huw's wagon and the shy, curious children to gawk at me. I couldn't find my veil, nor would anyone even look for it:

the incarnation of Epona should not hide the wealth of her hair.

So, from a ragged train of refugees, somehow we'd become a pilgrimage without a point save that they insisted I lead them toward Legis. The line on the road grew longer behind me through the day.

"Brigantes from the Bel-tein fire," Huw told me.

"Why are they following us?"

"They follow you, Lady. They've nothing to go home to, most of them."

"Keep your eye peeled on the road behind us," I said. "I want no more people hurt."

In the evening by the fires set from wagon to wagon, I went among them because they expected it. At each place a share of food was left for me whether I ate or not, although I must take a sip of wine or mead and bless the children. My God, they were all children. They knew in a child's vague way that miracles would come of my return, and hung on my every word as I sat cross-legged by their fires. There was usually a child on each knee and sometimes another draped around my neck playing with my hair while I told them the old stories that were as much legend to them as to the Iclingas—history, as it were, with its shoes off.

". . . And then King Arthur saw the giants about to attack—"

"Were they really giants?" asked one pragmatic little boy.

"Well, in their bleak and blighted homeland they were called bear-sarks, some of them big as two good Brits one standing on the other's shoulders."

"*Dyw*, that's big."

And a bigger lie, but didn't it make a grand story? From fire to fire, children to be storied before they slept, and loving it myself, to be honest.

". . . And so, with the magic and invisible Merlin whispering in his ear, Arthur mounted the hill of the choosing. And there were with him the best lords of the combrogi. Gareth of the Thousand Eyes and Kay, Arthur's wise brother. There was Trystan the bard whose harp knew the thousand sacred verses, and even Prince Geraint—aye, he that stopped Cerdic at Llongborth and fell in doing it. Each of them had on his lance the head of

a Cornishman who tried to keep Arthur from the crown. As Arthur stretched out his hand to take the sword from the stones, all the people on the plain knelt in a great *shout* of choosing. Not a man, woman, boy or girl, pig or chicken in the land of Britain that didn't know they'd found a King. So, with the ancient Roman sword on his saddle, on rode our new King to Eburacum."

"Why Eburacum?" demanded my pragmatist.

"Why, to marry me, goose. And that's tomorrow's tale. To bed with you."

Later, when the children had bickered, punched and wrestled each other to sleep, I spoke to the men and women who gathered around me, but in a different vein. Where they would leave a reverent space around me, I bade them sit close where I could touch them, where they could see in my eyes the truth I told them.

"You speak of lords as an evil, and yet you are so ready to follow me again. What can even the best lord do with such as you who wait to be led, who wait to be pushed here and there like leaves underfoot? I have spent ten years as a slave and yet I was freer thus than any of you. I was among lords who worked the ground with their own people. See here on my shoulders the marks where I pulled the plow myself, my lord guiding it. These are such people as have not been seen before in Britain. Each man has his own by law and no man's above that law. When we reach Legis, you must seek out the decurions of the city and make yourselves known to them that they can take your needs to Prince Emrys. You must ask to sit in their councils that the problems of the city are known to you."

But there were no more decurions, I was told. They were a thing of the past. The younger folk remembered them only dimly as something of the Romans, and who cared for that any more?

Walking ahead of the rest, I was first to see the crowd at the junction of the spur road to Bancor and Viroconium. As customary in the west, the crossroad was marked with a large stone cross mounted on a wide block. From this eminence a man in the dun robe of a monk was exhorting the crowd.

"Most like Brother Coel," Huw guessed. "Praefect put him out of Eburacum for speaking against the King."

"Then he's worth listening to."

Reforming monks were an embarrassment to the Church and now and then to myself as Queen. In the two hundred years since Christ became the official deity of Rome, his Church had grown to power and wealth by aligning itself with both along the way. This entails a good deal of tact and a short memory. Firmly entrenched now, it must make them blush in their opulence to hear a fiery young man remind them of their simple first principles as expounded on the shores of Galilee. Rather like having one's old love letters read out in public.

The crowd around the cross were mostly country folk, some of them refugees like us. I pushed through them to get a closer look at this Coel: dark as a Brigante and with the burr of their hills in his tongue to edge the truth he spat at his listeners. Once neatly tonsured, the crisp hair was growing in again in tight black curls. The energy of him seemed more of purpose than constitution, not unhealthy but ascetic, not a man of inherent fire as I measured him, but kindled to it from without, by a world that disgusted him.

"Why do they speak of Christ in this sorry land when Christ is forgotten?" Coel challenged his hearers. "Oh, he's here, he's all over Britain every day. Why do you think I left the cloister where I prayed and fixed my eyes and heart upon Jesu since my fifteenth year? Because I couldn't kneel and pray to Him while He called me from outside my gate and Himself still bleeding.

"The Church fathers, the bishops, look you what they raise up as King over us. Why, the latrines of Pilate and Herod were cleaner places. Where are the people for whom He shared out the loaves and fishes? Do not they deserve some part in the feast now? There was a time for greatness and a man to fit that time. I watched at his bedside while he died and saw the sun set over Britain when he did. And now if Jesu walks this land, it's not inside a cloister or the hall of a lord or the nave of any cathedral, but here with you! And you! And you!"

Coel jabbed his finger at one and another of us, voicing the sedition that got him ousted from my city. It would have been rather commonplace in Wicandaen where

men like Alfred and Brand argued change over every cup
of ale.

"It was written long ago in Rome—and by a Briton,
I'm proud to say—that God's a fair executor. Who has He
disinherited from His sweet air or water, the warmth of
His sun, the produce of His seed? None of us. Where did
He say that one man may have more than another? Nowhere. These fat bishops with oil in their hair and jewels
on their fingers, these latter-day and sorry lords who
know only how to take with nothing given in return:
would they deign to sit with the poor as Jesu did and
share dry bread and unseasoned fish? Not likely with
what they've waiting at home. God will not reach
through the fog of this back-broken island until *all* the
wealth of His sweet earth is parceled evenly. That simple
it is. When there are no more rich, as the good Briton
wrote, there will be no more poor. Old woman, why do
you laugh? Are you not one of the poor like the rest of
us?"

"Poor as the rest," I assured him. "But you exhort the
wrong congregation."

Lowri tugged me forward. "Speak to the people, Lady.
Speak to them as you do to us around the fire."

"Do that," Huw urged as others around us took up the
plea, sibilant at first, then louder like an incoming tide.

"Gwenhwyfar . . . let Gwenhwyfar stand with the holy
monk."

"Let God and the old gods stand together."

Little Mabli darted to the cross, bobbed a curtsy to
Coel and hopped up beside him to shrill to the crowd.
"See, see! This is Gwenhwyfar, the daughter of the God-
dess. Oh, see!"

"The wife of Arthur," Lowri raised her voice.

"Guenevere?" Brother Coel came down from the block,
suffused with a radiance I did not yet understand.
"Guenevere the Queen?"

"No, don't kneel. This is a time to stand up, Brother
Coel. All of you, come close about the cross."

I heard my name go through them like a wind as Coel
and I mounted the stone block together. "Is't she . . . is't
Guenevere? Nae, cannot be, she's dead. But it is."

"Brother Coel is right. The heart of Britain has always
been in such monks as he, not the priest or bishop; in the

cloister, not the Romish Church. But he preaches to the converted. Which of us here doesn't believe poverty is real or unjust? My God, even I've been that hungry in my time. Queen I was, but I tell you now that if anyone here has a loaf and a fish to share, I'll not cavil to sit with him. Yes, I was wife to Arthur, but I've been a slave—see here on my neck the mark of the collar—and I tell you there's a better way. I've seen it."

"Ah, God, look at them," Coel glowed. "Would I had the silver of your tongue, Lady."

"Among the Saxons whom you despise was I a slave for ten years. And yet not a one of them who'd stand for what you suffer. Who will free you? You will. Who will help you? None but men like this Coel with the heart to feel and the eyes to see. But first you must wake and rise. The Britain you knew is gone, children, but you've grown as used to a collar in your so-called freedom as I did as a slave. Crying against the lords who tax you, you're too slothful to see that first help must come from yourselves. 'Gird up thy loins like a man,' God said to Job. 'Thy right hand can save thee.' Well, what in bloody hell do you people think that means?"

Speak of full circle. I broke off in a wry grin at the personal joke. Good God, ten years ago I would have me arrested on the spot for voicing such thoughts and ponder the culprit as something incomprehensible.

"Guenevere, return," I heard from the crowd in my silence. "Rule over us."

"Ferch-Cador, rule over us. Take back the crown."

"There, you see? You rise from one knee only to bend the other. Not me, my people. I've had enough of ruling, even now when I've learned how. And I'm old. Help you? Yes, while I'm here and able, and that's not long. And men like Coel will help you. But when are you going to help your*selves*?"

Heads were turning to the west where a line of mounted men appeared over the crest of a hill on the road from Cair Legis.

"More lords," Huw muttered. "More trouble for us."

"Why do you set them to the impossible?" Coel beseeched me. "What can they do but hope?"

"And what have you done, Coel-fach, but tell them they're sick with a plague of lords? They know that.

What they don't know, have never known, is that if they expect to find physic, they've got to get off their own arse."

He seemed to relish the bluntness, grinning with a kind of reminiscence. "You speak plain as Arthur did."

As the galloping column drew closer, I pushed through my own people to meet them, men looking worried, mothers warning children close. I recognized a golden cup on the shield of the leading rider: a Grail knight, and that's all I saw before he was past me and the rest after him, scattering men, women and children over the road and heath before his circling riders began to herd them back together with spare, neat excursions of their mounts. The bearded, scar-faced Grail knight stood up in the stirrups and bellowed his orders.

"Stay where you are! Don't run, you can't get away. By order of Prince Emrys, since you cross his land, you are to be taxed. One-half sestertius from each head of a family before you enter his city."

"Taxed?" Huw threw up his hands. "Great Lord, why are we here? Weren't we taxed out of our own city?"

The knight ignored him. "Line them up. No one will be hurt. Women and children to one side, men in a line. Look sharp, now."

But I'd recognized certain marks about these shabby knights: the fluid, easy manner in which they controlled obedient horses, the manner in which their mail was packed behind the saddle, even a face here and there. I dodged in and out of the wheeling horses, trying to get their attention. "Leave these folk alone. You! I know you, you were combrogi once. And you rode with Lord Penrwd. Leave them alone! Have combrogi fallen to banditry?"

They paid me no attention at all. I barely whisked two children out of harm's way, blistering after the heedless riders: "The shame of God on you! Coel, come. Where's he who leads this pack?"

"There." Seething with the wrath of angels, Coel strode to the scar-faced knight, with me not half a pace behind, and seized the horse's bridle. "Are you knight or thief? There's nothing here your kind haven't taken already. God's hand on you if you rob them further."

The knight removed his helmet to mop his sweaty face

and untrimmed beard. "You'd be that monk we heard of. They come to be clients, don't they? Protection costs; stand aside."

"We will not, sir." I recognized the shield and the face now, changed as it was. "Has the pride of Britain become its shame? Don't you know your Queen, Ifan? You carried my sword once. Don't raise it against my own."

He spared me a quick, impatient scrutiny. "Daft old woman—"

"*I bid you stand, Lord Ifan*. Yes, you recognize the voice if nothing else. And this scar. You were at Glevum when I bled with it, and Lord Gwenlys dead at our feet."

Ifan hesitated, looked closer at me. "Holy God." In a trice he was off the horse, calling. "Wait! Wait! Bors, come quickly."

"It is the Queen," Coel affirmed with audible pride.

"Bors! Lady, it was given out—"

"Don't harm my folk, Ifan. I'll pay their tax in good silver. My nephew will be content."

"Where in all these years have you—?"

But then I was turned firmly about to look up into the face of my own Bors—heavier, rougher, harder for the years gone by but my dear Bors still. Neither of us was very coherent.

"Is it you, mum? Where—they said you were killed."

"What of Regan, lad? Did she get through? Oh, call off your men, these folk haven't a minim among them. Damn it, boy, what of my Regan?"

As my name coursed through the horsemen, they forgot the peasants and rode in closer. I recognized, in their patched leathern trousers and tunics, older men who'd ridden with Arthur and Geraint. "My Lords, you know me—Arthur's wife and this monk his friend. Give us kindness if nothing else. Is Regan safe?"

"Safe, mum. She was paroled."

"And the child?"

"The bairn . . ." His eyes clouded, still confused at what he was seeing.

"Son, son, they dragged me out that night, Bedivere and the rest. I wouldn't have left her else."

"There were none to attend her." His bitterness was old and dry as my own. "The babe didn't live. But we have other children now. God is kind."

"And you won through!" I punched gleefully at his chest. "Don't I remember the night I sent you out."

"Cut 'em to kindling we did." Ifan grinned. "We were still on the road when we heard of Eburacum and knew we were alone."

Brief, illusory, but I felt the old pride thrill my blood. "Lift me up, up!"

"To horse, Lady?"

"To your shoulders, lummox."

Elevated by Bors and Ifan, I raised my hands high to knights and peasants. "Look, all of you. *Here* is the heart of Britain as it could beat. Lord, monk and people together. Put your wagons in line. On to the city."

"On to Legis!"

Bors shouted: "A horse for the Queen."

"No, put me down. No horse for me. Brother Coel and I will walk with them. But stay with me, Bors, tell me of Regan. Is she well? Oh, Bors . . . how has it been?"

Coel sang out to the people tugging at their wagons. "Follow Guenevere!"

As the long snake of us began to move, someone in the rear took up the song and not alone by the second line.

> Sing dogwood, alder, wild cornel
> The cuckoo's nest is ne'er his own,
> The clover spreads his sweet red bell
> When we a-maying go-o-o—

"Sing, Bors! They're wanting a good tenor."

> When we a-maying GO!

The pocked, stained walls of Legis displayed its will to survive, though its spiritless population appeared as transient and purposeless as those who trooped behind me through the gates. Emrys' house, the old forum in the center of the town, was ravaged as the rest—unwashed floors, whole patches of tile torn up, all in the same disrepair as my own palace and as much of a barracks. Like Eburacum, an armed camp with a fringe of beggars.

News of my coming sped with Ifan to Emrys before me. A welcome of sorts, assembled in haste and considerable shock, was waiting me in the unswept triclinium.

My heart hurt to see the knot of them gathered under the dingy murals reproachful as myself in their reminder of empire. See my people as I did then, Bors and I standing in the center of their dining couches as Bors announced with muted pride:

"Lady Guenevere, the Queen that was."

Look at them and reflect that there's nothing more embarrassing to mourners than the resurrection of the mourned. Gareth and Rhian—old now, much older in wear than myself. And Bedivere, snagged like myself on the spur of events, he'd still not found that place of peace he so wanted. I wondered if Myfanwy was with him.

And my dear Regan who once bubbled and skipped at my side, near thirty now, her face harder in its set. She'd such a dazzling smile. Her teeth were broken now where the Silures had handled her with less than gentleness. Not bitter but, like Bors, no longer expecting much of this world.

My nephew Emrys, the risen Arthur. No . . . there was no longer much resemblance. I saw the measuring in his glance before any welcome: What did this change? What would it cost him? Where was his advantage? The hand resting on the low table before his couch was minus a finger, and gray showed in his beard.

And another grim hawk come home to peck at my culpable liver: Blodwen next to her son, vindictive as might be expected. She wouldn't miss this for the crown and a high seat in paradise. Doubtless she'd have me on my knees were she still in command, but no one commanded that son of hers now. I'd helped him to that.

They all seemed more worn than robust. The men's swords were unbuckled but set close to the tables as in barracks, the floor's rushes strewn with leavings. Perhaps the most telling point was their raiment. Although Blodwen derived visible amusement from my ragged homespun, the faded and patched condition of her once-fine kirtle straining over the fat of age, and that of Regan, now carefully mended and let out in the back for her added weight, the cracked leather of Emrys' tunic, all told on them more truly than my hand-me-downs. And yet they clung to the faded finery of a past they couldn't restore and wouldn't relinquish. They reminded me of myself once, painting my face with too much cosmetic

against the first signs of age. The dishes from which they'd eaten before my arrival were of silver and bronze, but dented and greenish about the edges with the tarnish of encroaching neglect.

One man was a stranger to me, easily the best-groomed man in the chamber, presented to me later as ambassador from the court of Constantinople. In contrast to the others, it was startling to see him lolling on his couch in immaculate white with a cloth-of-gold Byzantine collar, jeweled hands dipping morsels in *liquamen* and nibbling in the fastidious manner of a bygone era.

My first impression of Lucullus Aurelianus, like Arthur's, was contradictory. A strong, competent man who chose the role of the fop and played it to perfection, every line of virility carefully curved into the effete but not quite able to hide its force. The expression under carefully plucked brows was bored, supercilious, but watchful. The son of Ambrosius, he might have been emperor in Arthur's place but proclaimed pleasure to be his sole religion. Yet he wielded a sword at Badon, however reluctantly, and he and Gareth were the only two men in the triclinium who rose in courtesy when I entered.

"Well, Nephew."

"Dear Aunt, most welcome."

"And Bedivere. Is this the place you found to watch the world go by?"

Still lean he was, the rusted copper hair now white as mine. "Na, lass. I've left off the looking for it."

"Regan! *Sut mae'r mab*, my darling. Gareth, Rhian, bless you. All of you. I can't tell you how good it is to see you."

"And me, Guenevere?" Blodwen didn't hide her smirk. "You bless me too?"

"And crave your pardon for many wrongs."

"Um." She considered that over her drink, chuckling with a private joke. "We hear you've been slave among the Saxons." Her bleary gaze was still indirect, the face bloated with years of heavy drinking. "One finds one's destined level, don't they?"

"Apparently, Blodwen."

"Did you tax them, Bors?" Emrys queried. "Sorry, Aunt, but it must be. You can see conditions."

I dropped the purse in front of him. "For each family head in good silver weight. You wish to count it?"

Emrys only jounced it once on his palm and passed it to an unkempt servitor behind him. "It is the times."

"Yes, the times. But I am very glad to see you, Nephew." I could hold back the poignant question no longer. "What in hell has happened to my people?"

"*Her* people," Blodwen echoed sardonically.

"What you see." Bedivere shrugged. "We tax them to make some kind of order. To live ourselves. So we can fight. I could have told you this ten years ago."

"Yes. Regan, come kiss me. I've thought of you so often, and we both deserve that much. It's all too sad."

The lightness was gone from Regan's step. Each of us was a ghost to the other, known and unknown, and the sadness of our knowledge couldn't be masked.

"I'm close to a thousand years old, Regan, and you're getting on yourself." The age of her would mean nothing if I could have seen something like hope in her eyes. There was none. And the reassurance of her was very self-contained.

"It's all right, mum. I lost the child and I was frightened without Bors or you, but it's past. And I have other children. One of them is named for you."

"Marvelous! Let me see her soon. Rhian, come to me. And you, Gareth. Would it endanger your modesty to know what the English call you? Devil on a horse, no less."

And yet even the devil grew old; the hand I pressed was now swollen with arthritis, and Rhian was well past the hard vigor of her middle age.

"You look well," was her blunt assessment. "You've got heavier."

"I was a bit of a wraith before. Oh, it is so good to be with you all again."

A sad lie. The tatter of them, the worn end of what was, made me hurt. The pristine Lucullus was almost a reproof when he bent over my hand.

"I had not the pleasure of meeting you on my last visit, Lady."

"Arthur and I weren't speaking that month. But he called Lucullus Aurelianus a friend."

"The late King called me a number of things." Lucullus smiled easily. "But friend at the last."

"Isn't this all cakes and milk," Blodwen brayed. "Have you forgotten, son, how she put us on our knees, put you to shame and left me to defend our city?"

"It would have been lost anyway, Mother."

"Not so proud now, is she?"

"Be still!" Emrys silenced her more savagely than the reproof warranted. I saw the reason as he rose to come around the table. He reached for a cane and moved with difficulty, not old but gnarled with war and some of his mother's bitterness and dissipation. "Aunt Guenevere was my teacher. If anyone saved me, she did. I learned too late. We're all too bloody late."

"Emrys, the monk who came with me, the other people—what provision can be made for them?"

"Out of what? Fields that haven't been worked for want of peasants? Empty granaries?" Emrys winced as he pegged toward me.

"You're in pain, Nephew. Please sit."

"It is nothing. A gift from the Cornish not yet healed. Later for the monk; he's a small nettle I won't brush from my coat if he's discreet. It's the realities that concern us now."

"Yes, they followed me through your gates. A handful of beggars at a prince's door can be sprinkled with pennies and forgotten, but a country full of them is a reality of some magnitude."

"Don't be obtuse, Aunt. You see what we've come to. I am the legitimate continuance of your rule in Britain. I doubt even you could have done more. And I have sons."

"I am glad to hear it."

"And I will pass what I can to them."

Blodwen began, "Those folk out there—"

"Mother, *I* am prince here," Emrys quashed her efficiently.

"So you are, royal son, but don't miss the point. That rabble out there have made her thrice valuable to us."

"Quite so. Fill your cup and let me rule." Emrys caned his tortuous way to the open casement. "The Church had no real choice in crowning Constantine. He would have murdered every bishop in Britain otherwise as quickly

as he did Maelgwyn's sons. Those people out there follow you because they think they have nothing else."

"A reasonable assumption." Only Lucullus smiled at that.

"But if you made public your choice of me as successor."

"You never did," Blodwen reminded me pointedly.

"I didn't expect to leave the throne so suddenly."

"You were the great one for letters of state, but you never put that in writing."

"I was a bit rushed, Blodwen. Your son was just learning at my knee the rudiments of rule. What is it you want then? My redundant abdication? You can have it with ribbons."

"That's not enough, Aunt. I have sons."

"And Constantine has none?"

"None," Blodwen snorted. "And none likely, the sodomite. The only women in his house are his cooks. He couples with one of his knights."

I sensed an uncomfortable silence. Then Blodwen, with some deference, inclined her head to Lucullus. "The Ambassador's pardon. I except his grace."

"Not at all." Lucullus waved it away with exquisite good grace. "Not at all, Lady. Like most of my habits, the custom was fashionable for a time. I never followed it with Constantine's ruinous conviction. Please don't inhibit candor on my account."

I reminded my nephew of a long-standing truth. "There's never been a rule or even a custom of filial succession in Britain."

"Britain will go as we sway it." The hardness in Emrys' truth was undisguised. "Think, decide and do, Aunt. You taught me that. If you've had a brutal ten years, so have I. Worse. I won't live to your age. I want a clear choice for myself and my sons. That crowd that came warbling through the gates with you will follow anything that leads. Lead them to me, Aunt. That's all I want. Fair and logical."

"If there were just more of us," Gareth said. "We've never really lost against Constantine."

"Or really won," Bedivere reflected.

"Gareth is right, Aunt. Once I move against Con-

stantine, not just to raid but to retake Camelot and the west for good, Eleyne will break her treaty."

That was news to me. "What treaty?"

They told me then, completed my education. Within a year of my rout, Eleyne made pact not to oppose Constantine in any way. That left Dyfneint alone, a neutral principality, and freed Constantine's siege troops to mobility. It also explained why I missed Galahalt from the present company.

Emrys pressed his point. "This could be a new age. Proclaim me as your choice, as Ambrosius did Arthur, and we'll have Astolat in our camp."

"Eleyne's always been loyal, but at the risk of her country?"

"True. Well." Emrys hesitated, clearing his throat. "I was thinking more of Lancelot."

"I see. You had more talent than I knew."

"You were a fine teacher. Guenevere dead, Lancelot couldn't care less who ruled. Guenevere returned is a different matter."

"Yes, a great deal of talent. Has it occurred to my eager heirs that an old woman might like to sit down?"

Instantly Bors steered me to the couch Lucullus vacated for me. The ambassador poured me wine and Regan presented it.

"I welcome you home, mum. Not a night I closed my eyes without praying for you."

"Or I you, Regan."

"You never knew who your true friends were, never," Blodwen admonished in a voice full of spleen. "You could have settled on Emrys ten years ago, but because I asked, you took us for traitors."

"That was a mistake."

"You made too many mistakes!"

"So I did. I also made a prince out of your son, and a prince he is, of my own cut. Without me he'd be dead in Glevum with—oh God! I forgot. Flavia. Emrys, is she still alive? Is she here?"

"No, Aunt. She died at home."

Blodwen's satisfaction was indecent. "She didn't last out the siege."

"A servant found her," Emrys said. "She was lying in bed with the wine cup in her hand. It was her favorite,

the last of the set Augustulus sent her." I heard the genuine regret. For a moment when Emrys sat beside me and took my hand, we were close again as that early morning long ago at the well in Eburacum. "Her going was easy, I think. She put something in the wine."

Yes, she would. Flavia Marcella, that thoroughly Roman woman, would leave the game with her dignity intact. She offered me that cup once, knowing one or both of us would need it.

"You must burn a little incense to your grandmother, Emrys. She had impeccable taste." I held out my cup to the chamber at large, for all I was to them now—old friend, discomforting ghost or political godsend. "Well, children, here I am."

And welcome home, Mother.

Strange limbo summer in Legis. If no royal joy, at least keen royal interest in my resurrection, and miracles expected high and low. A flurry of covert letters went by swift ship from Emrys to Eleyne: Guenevere is returned and what price treaties? Letters back from Astolat: Guenevere is right welcome home. The very stones of Witrin sing out, where she is invited to sojourn or anywhere within holy Astolat—

Providing, as Emrys made clear, I published him as my choice to succeed. "It's just, Aunt. You did proclaim Constantine a usurper."

Dryly comic summer as the convened bishops of the west wrestled over their position and future safety in the matter, frowned on the radical taint of my sentiments and delayed the proclamation with cavils of their own.

"This truant monk Coel must recant the heresy of his speeches."

Strange, ominous summer, a slow passage of time to the quick beat of hoofs as Emrys dashed about, scraping the bottom of the bucket for one more try at destiny, abetted by an Astolat straining at the leash to aid insurrection.

The Dyfneint cavalry, led by my husband, even he called the Lancelot, and by my blessed and only son, Galahalt, are pledged to Emrys and Guenevere.

"Damned woman never could say her mind without flags and trumpets."

"She's with us," Emrys was satisfied, "but adds her reservations about Coel. She suggests you urge him to discretion."

"She wants him to belt up, is that it?"

"She and the bishops. The man is totally unrealistic, Aunt. Share our wealth? As if we had it! Now you suggest they share in power and by a process which, if *I* can't understand it, Eleyne will call screaming heresy. And you and I, dear Guenevere, need all the allies we can muster."

Summer of respite for Emrys. Constantine was in the Midlands, countering a new threat. Post riders brought us a foggy but clearing picture of the king's forces and those of Icel fumbling for each other's throats like hostile dogs in the dark along the wooded banks of River Trent. Day by day the riders came as they did to me at Eburacum. Constantine is in contact with them . . . is not . . . is again. They feint and fade before him . . . no decisive action yet. Emrys finds one observation mightily puzzling.

"What's this about plowing? They say the Saxons are laying out fields. Not even won the land yet and the buggers are plowing it?"

"It's late in the season. They want to get something into the ground. Speaking of that, Nephew, could you spare me a good blacksmith?"

Distracted by a thousand things to do, pained by his unhealed leg, Emrys could spare that much—and a piece of charcoal from the smith's forge, a worn bit of palimpsest to draw on while the Dobunni smith scratched his head over my creation.

"That's a hard curve to put in the blade, Lady."

"The curve is the crux. Look on it as a challenge, lad."

Emrys granted me a house near the city walls where I promptly ensconced Coel, Huw and Lowri as my little family. There were plenty of empty houses in Legis when we arrived, now filling up as the indigent population swelled from week to week, some of them taxed out of Eburacum, all of them drawn by, hanging on, the name of Guenevere. Constantine must surely have heard of me

by now. How it must gentle his sleep on Trent to know he'd my death to do all over.

Rainless summer—not the drought of the east but parched enough. Trusting, the hungry people of Legis followed me out the gates to the neglected fields. Britons ever, they knew to deck the horns of the oxen with flowers, but stared at the new plow the blacksmith lifted from the cart.

"I told you to help yourselves. And this is a start." I harnessed the oxen to the new plow. "Brother Coel will pray for rain, and Epona will do what she can. Now see what this new plow does."

Most of them had never seen an iron plow and none an English blade that turned the sod neatly aside as it broke and furrowed it. Brother Coel walked beside the flower-decked oxen, chanting:

"O Arglywdd, who divided the waters from the land, who let the earth bring forth the herb yielding seed—as it was in the beginning, let the waters bring forth abundantly of thy gifts in the name of Christ Jesu."

"Amen!" I cried. "The rain will come at God's will, but no one said you can't bucket water from the wells. Come, let's water this earth."

It disturbed even radical Coel to invoke one deity while I made the old sacrifices to another.

"Coel, did not my husband open his heart to you at the end? And was Arthur above calling on any god to hand? Come, bring the doves, and remember what a heretic Jesu was in his own time. You men! Who'll be the first to learn this plow?"

Mabli took pride in sweeping my house immaculate, but I was rarely home between dawn and dark. More used to the open air, walls and roof cramped me now but I took pleasure in planning a dinner for my old friends. Bors and Regan were to come, and Gareth and Rhian.

"And tell Bedivere he must bring Myfanwy. I've not seen her for that long."

"Myfanwy's dead," Rhian said shortly. "Nor would I speak of it to the Gryffyn."

"When? How?"

"Who knows?" Gareth rubbed his swollen knuckles. "He came back to Cair Legis the summer after we lost you. House burned, servants scattered."

At least four tribes had poured over Dobunni land after the loss of Glevum, ramping back and forth in an orgy of righteous and profitable pillage. Bedivere found his wife's grave. Someone did that much for her.

"But he never speaks of it," Gareth warned. "Not even to me, not even over a cup. Do you not either."

"Bring him anyway. And drink this potion for the arthritis. Vinegar and water. It will ease the swelling."

"Jesus God, it's worse than the ache."

"Drink it every day. The English swear by it. And look you bring Bedivere to dinner."

Strange, sad summer, like an autumn in the heart. My friends came, but there hung over my table a pall of reserve. Huw and Lowri served and then sat down at my thoughtless bidding as they did on any day. They spoke not at all and left as quickly as they finished. I was a little hurt at the diffidence of close friends after I'd so looked forward to sitting with them. "What's the matter with you all? You've hardly spoken."

None volunteered at first; they seemed embarrassed. Then Rhian made a stab at it. "You are so different. We're not used to sitting down with servants any more, and that's the whole of it."

"Oh. I see."

Perhaps I finally did see what Gwyneth meant. *You are not like us.* The confession surprised and then troubled me more and more, indicative as it was. Like her husband, Rhian had been born in a sod hut next to an Irish bog. Bors could claim little better ancestry than Bedivere, for all his honors under Arthur. Regan was the daughter of a minor tribal factotum. But we raised them all to privilege across the otherwise unbridgeable gap from their beginnings, and they'd grown used to it in less than a lifetime. I wondered if the peasants they now spurned out of habit could grow to self-awareness as quickly. My two old knights, Bedivere and Gareth: I remembered over my wine cup how I'd humbled them once as the lowest of the low, raised more by Arthur's fondness than any merit. Such was my own intractable arrogance: how could I blame it in them?

"And you, Bedivere? My unregenerate son of a groom? You once came over me with a girl I pushed in the mud. Would it demean you to break bread with her now?"

He acknowledged the tacit truth of it before he spoke. "Na, it would not. Less trouble for me than it will be for you, Guenevere."

Regan plunged in: "Mum, you know we love you . . ."

"But. Such beginnings always have a but."

"You don't know the problems we have. You don't know the times."

"Regan, the times are being made on River Trent even as we sit here."

"Will you *listen* to me, mum, and not leap down my throat for trying to help you? And you, Brother Coel. Please listen to Bors."

Bors, the adopted son of my heart, tried with difficulty. "You confuse everyone with these strange teachings. The Prince is not against you, but what's he to think when you incite the peasants to form these—what call you them?"

"Folk meetings."

"For what purpose, mum? Government, property, they know nothing of these things."

Sadly true. My exhortations usually produced no more than a wish that I return to the throne. They understood nothing.

"Blodwen's at Emrys day and night to have the succession writ and signed and you out of Legis."

"Yes, Godspeed and begone. So?"

"And Brother Coel must not call the lords thieves because we manage the best we can," Bors concluded.

"You're being watched," Bedivere informed Coel. "Emrys doesn't like it at all."

"And there it is," Gareth mourned. "What are we expected to do then, when we must fight with no regular revenue, no anything and the country a ruin around us?"

"Do we not have a right to live?" Rhian demanded. "Have not we earned that in hard years and harder service? Praise God I'm alive to say it, Guenevere, but you were not the lightest hand on the rein, and more men died in Arthur's service than had our good luck to survive. But look at the world as it *is*. And let us live what time we've left."

Bedivere squinted at me. "You always played devious games. There's those wondering what you want. The crown?"

"God, no."

"But you still want to muck in royal business."

"Has your philosophy turned with your fortunes, Lord Bedivere?"

He understood my meaning, years past the sting of it. "Guenevere, if I believed in anything any more I'd put it in a box and light candles to it. But against Constantine, we're *something*, woman. We tax the people to live and fight."

"And the kennel won't change, just the dogs."

"*Aye, so it won't!* What would you have us do?" The burst of feeling twisted him away from me in his chair, one hand over his mouth and the frustration he felt. "What would you have? I should have died with Artos. Nothing's been whole or made sense since."

Coel raised his head to Bedivere. "That's blasphemy."

"What?" Bedivere turned in to the little monk who'd barely spoken through supper but followed the conversation with slow-seething disgust.

"Blasphemy to wish yourself dead when God gives you more time to choose your life."

"You? You were there when I brought him in dying. You're too old for that sort of innocence. You were a proper little monk then, praying was your business as it is now. Why in hell are you off your knees and on to us, screaming for our blood? We kept your kind safe, we still do. Must we do it with nothing in our bellies or on our backs?"

Full circle. Even Bedivere, saddest of all. Coel put down his fruit knife and folded his hands in front of the plate. "Why am I off my knees? Because when you brought the King to our cloister, my knees were the only part of me that bent, my Lord. My vows were a sham and so was I. I dreamed of being an abbot then; not only that but confessor and confidant to the Queen herself. Not an unforgivable dream for a boy who never even knew his own mother. I craved definition. Influence. I'd stand in the streets of Eburacum and cheer with the rest when you rode past, Lady. Who knows, perhaps I was in love with the glamour of you."

"Coel, I'm charmed. You never told me."

"Thank God for that." He smiled. "I was insufferable. And when your husband came to his last sickbed in our

cloister, the little holiness I had was pushed aside by the swelling of my pride. Now, I thought, I am at the elbow of the mighty and I will be changed forever.

"I wrote letters for the King, wrote his thoughts, and I *was* changed because . . . I learned from him. He had a direct and very pungent turn of speech. Time after time I'd suggest that his words were too plain for posterity, too common for a King already a legend, and even re-draft them in a more elevated manner. But my words didn't fit his thoughts. The King always said, no, leave it plain. And he was right, Lord Bedivere."

By his manner and enthusiasm, I'd thought Brother Coel younger than he was, but he'd lived and above all, he'd thought on life more than prayed over it.

"After he died I couldn't put him out of mind, not even to pray. I said, what is it about this man? He's too simple, too casual, too unkingly for a king, doesn't give a pig's squeal for his own dignity. Yet he was not simple but profound, and the dignity never left him. And when I read over what I'd tried to put in his mouth as sentiment proper to a king, the words were stale. Empty. Dead beside his own that still glowed with life. And life is God, is it not? From that day the cloister grew too small, too cramped for me. You see . . . you, I, all of us believe in God. We hope in God. But that man *knew* him and had seen his face. As I saw it in Arthur."

Gareth crossed himself. "Amen."

"No, Lord Gareth." Coel shook his head with a slight smile. "Not an amen, not a gesture, that's easy. A life! His life. His meaning. I know how he felt about the people, for he came out of them. Their mark was all over him. And *that's* why I'm out among them, Lord Bedivere. Stirring them up, making them think. Putting some of his plain anger and plain common sense into them. Because Arthur would. He'd be out there too and more dangerous than me. He knew life, that man, and never forgot what it showed him. Well, his world is falling apart, but so long as I've a tongue in my head I'm going to be out there mending and complaining."

Coel rose and bowed to us. "My Lords. Lady, will you excuse me? I promised to talk to some people. New folk, just arrived."

The table was silent for a space after Coel left. Then

Bedivere roused himself. "Little boyo has a way of putting things, doesn't he?"

"Well." Gareth was obviously touched as the rest of us. "I hope he comes to no harm. Through himself or anyone else."

"Amen to that," I said. "Lowri? Come fill the cups. Let's finish the wine, my friends."

"None for me." Bedivere got up from the table and inclined his head to me. "I'll be off. Thank you and good night."

"Off so soon and the wine not gone?" Gareth chided him.

"I thought to catch up Brother Coel. Just to talk with him. Good night."

Coel was arrested that night, taken in the middle of an address to new refugees at the city gates. Lowri was turning down my bed when Huw panted home with the news.

"Where have they taken him, Huw?"

"To the Prince and not that gently. Are you going there, Lady? I'll attend you."

"No, stay here." No need to put Huw and his own in danger. My stomach told me they'd be coming for me soon in any case.

"Why is this man under arrest!" I demanded of Emrys and his bloated mother.

"Quite simply, he's become an embarrassment," Emrys said. "As you have. Mucking about with plows and nonsense about folk meetings."

"You're ostentatious, like all reformers," Blodwen declared with audible relish. "Being one of the people takes accustoming. I was born to it. As you and Flavia reminded me so often."

"But I'm glad you came, Aunt. It saved me a summons."

The hour was late. Only two lamps burned in the dingy triclinium. Emrys and his mother rested on couches in front of a low table that held the cold remains of their supper and Blodwen's ubiquitous pitcher of uisge. Coel stood before them with a stony guard behind him. To one side, Lucullus Aurelianus reclined on his couch, delicately savoring his wine. Now Emrys rose to sit on the

edge of his couch, toying in the rushes with the tip of his cane.

"Brother Coel, many lords would simply dispose of you and pay the price of churchly outrage. Yours would be small. I don't hate you; I can even sympathize with the poor, being one of them." Emrys pointed his cane about the room. "You call this opulence? My country is one step from anarchy, monk. You have no sense of reality."

"Like the Queen," Coel retorted, "I'm becoming wearied of that word."

"The Bishop of Cair Legis and his advisers have suggested for you a pilgrimage to Ynnis Witrin. A spiritual journey that you recall your vows of contemplation."

"How can I meditate in God's house while someone's setting fire to the gate? I knew your uncle; this is not the Britain he tried to build."

Emrys agreed wearily. "No, it's not Arthur's dream. It is the reality. Meanwhile you can strive to convince Abbot Brochan of your views. I want you gone in three days."

"With as many of your flock as you can draw away with you," Blodwen slurred over her drink. "They crowd our streets to no purpose."

"As for you, Aunt Guenevere." Emrys paid me the courtesy to rise; I saw the effort it cost. "Lucullus has safe conduct from myself as well as Constantine. He asked that you might travel with him."

"Say rather hoped," Lucullus amended with his liquid grace. "The honor would be mine. My embassy takes me east in any case. I entreat you join me, Lady."

I didn't quite understand it all. "And where shall I journey, if it matters?"

"To Witrin with Coel." Blodwen plucked a folded letter from between the dishes. "Astolat invites you. Eleyne, Lancelot, the psalm-singing pack of them. They love you still. Very good fortune, my dear."

"Thank you—dear. Well, Coel? Pilgrimage or exile, what shall we call it?"

"Call it the times." Emrys took a larger parchment from the table and briefly perused it. "Your formal letter of succession, Aunt. Somewhat delayed; the bishop

wanted Coel silenced, but he'll settle for him tucked under Brochan's wing."

The document was a simple and straightforward statement of my will that Emrys succeed me, which decided no more than Ambrosius naming Arthur, but with several important churchmen already subscribing. The letter stipulated no other concessions from me, nor was I naïve enough to ponder the result if I didn't sign. The choice was academic now. Emrys at his best could do little more than Constantine at his worst. Both physicians used the same ineffective physic on a dying body.

"So I am ostentatious? Do you have any idea what I was trying to do? Those people out there were always led, taxed, told what to do and then told to get out of the way. These meetings would give them something, a vested interest in their own lives, not just squatting there as a hindrance to your government, but part of it."

Blodwen grunted. "Impossible."

"No. I've seen genius come out of such meetings among the English. They're as ambitious as you were when you married Kay Pendragon, and just as acquisitive. They're out to hold their own and add to it. And the lords don't give any more than they have to, but at least there's a meeting of *minds* in it, a sense of permanence and belonging that goes right down to the plow. You won't see them dragging from one place to another, hoping someone like you will be kind, creeping away when you're not—"

"I don't understand this any more than the peasants who crowd around you to touch the Goddess." No, Emrys wouldn't. His mother knew the early poverty, but Emrys grew up with the servants easy to hand and habit. Not a tyrant, but with his own definition of government as I shaped it for him. He held out the stylus to me. "They haven't the ghost of a notion what you urge them to. What can I do for them until I have the power? That's the reality, Aunt—as you taught it to me."

"All I taught you was how to survive. I taught you power and how to hold it."

"As you had to."

"Very true. And so all you learned was my ignorance, my own prejudices, my mistakes and what I called cleverness. Power was the game. But wrap that power in

a mortal body, call it king or queen or god as we have done for a thousand years, and every few decades you need a new king, a new god, a new icon. It's only going to last when the roots go deeper than your ability to make war. The house supports the roof. We have been a roof trying to hold up the house, so long as it kept its place and behaved. Here." I dipped the stylus and put my name to the proclamation. "Long live the King."

Blodwen sat back with some relief. "We thought you'd be more difficult."

"Why? Emrys says he can do nothing with the peasants until he has power. I know he can do very little of permanence without them. What's it matter what I sign? You'll grab this, Constantine that, back and forth. And neither of you will win or any like you."

"You lessen yourself." Emrys inspected the signature and rolled up the proclamation. "You were a Queen to remember. A woman of will. You wouldn't give up to Constantine; neither will I. You had a contempt for peasants that once rankled even me. If you recant your teachings, I will not. They worked. You trusted none. Neither will I."

Leaning on his cane, Emrys bent painfully to kiss me. "My blessing to you, Aunt. Lucullus, take good care of her."

Walking home through the dark lanes of Legis toward our house with Lucullus and myself, Brother Coel philosophized on our exile. "I've always wanted to see Witrin and the Grail. But, Lord, I thought I'd have to put her right when she called you ostentatious. I suppose the moneylenders in the temple said as much of Christ."

"A point of view," Lucullus observed with his usual subtlety. "The Queen does wear homespun with a certain flair."

"I don't have the vanity for fashion any more—or the figure, come to that. Where do you stand in all this, Lucullus?"

The Roman could turn even a shrug into elegance. "On the side as usual. My mission is to observe, smooth the way for new trade. Find where Constantinople can open new lines of negotiation and amity."

"In other words, see what's left and who's worth dealing with?"

Lucullus shot me a sidelong glance of amusement, enjoying the candor. "Quite so, Lady."

"Then you plan to meet with Prince Icel."

"Do you know him?"

"Yes. I wrote out one of his more significant laws. Drafted by a farmer lord and three very shrewd peasants."

Lucullus studied me with close interest. "You are a fascinating woman, Guenevere. We must talk further."

IX

Rise Up with Saints

t was to be a gift for Constantine's consort."
Lucullus turned the exquisite little dagger
in white fingers. "Who was in fact a rather
massive Cornish knight—named Alun, I believe. Quite inappropriate. It fits a smaller
hand and better taste."

Coel had left us for a time to see to his followers. We sat
together by the side of the road as the fog thickened
around us. Lowri, despairing over the crinkling of my
hair in the damp, volunteered to put it up with little
bone pins of her own.

We were not far from the disused Roman villa where,
on Lucullus' suggestion, the house of Astolat agreed to
meet us. The small villa straddled the junction of the
Viroconium and Cair Legis roads; from there, Lucullus
would turn east on his own business.

"It is magnificent, Lucullus. Thank you."

The dagger might have been made for my own hand.
Three hairs, allegedly from the head of a saint, were
molded in a crystal teardrop at the pommel. The handle
of intertwined silver and gold wire was reinforced beneath with strips of lead to give it extra weight. But the
slim little blade was a work of art. By now a fair judge of
blades, I appreciated the surgeon's edge and needle
point. The sheath was of soft rabbit skin attached to an
open circlet of light whalebone too narrow even for a
child's waist. "How does one wear it?"

"It was designed for women who actually *want* to protect their virtue," Lucullus instructed. "A last attempt to dissuade the single-minded suitor. Lowri, take down her hair in back."

When she undid me, Lucullus fitted the circlet against my scalp and bade Lowri do it up again, concealing the whole apparatus.

"The women of Constantinople style their hair intricately, and they prize the subtle. One very feminine gesture, a hand fluttering to the hair—what more natural?" His own hand described it authentically. "And I can't think of anyone so in need of it as you, Guenevere."

"You are kind. Lowri, go fetch Brother Coel. We should be starting up again. So many of them. I hope there'll be room at the villa."

We watched Lowri slip away along the road before she disappeared into the fog.

"Britain was always less than a joy to visit." Lucullus gazed around at the gray mist. "But meeting you has paid me tenfold. I respected Arthur and went with him to Badon—with less than enthusiasm, to be sure."

"I hear you were dragged to glory."

"Protesting vigorously. I've always been trundled off to significance like a truant schoolboy."

Curious, this Lucullus. It seemed his pleasure to hide his intellect under frivolity and his strength under foppishness, though doubtless it helped him live longer. As an ambassador he could court any man or cause with fluent charm. The jewels weighed down his pale hands, the fine-carded white wool of his cloak and tunic were immaculate—he never wore a tunic more than twice—and edged with eccentric whorls in purple, his comment on the senatorial honors to which he was born as the son of Ambrosius Aurelianus. His notorious taste for ambidextrous love affairs very likely gained him readier access to Constantine.

"We got on swimmingly," Lucullus affirmed. "A safe conduct anywhere and God help him who trod on my littlest toe. A lonely man, Constantine. I was someone he could talk to, frivolous as I am."

"Lucullus, why do you sham like this?"

He blinked indolently. "Lady?"

"This negative passion for playing the fop, the retreat

from everything that smacks of honor or virtue. You don't fool me."

"Perhaps because I find to my surprise that virtue is all I have left."

"Oh, come!"

"And, frankly, a terminal disgust from my early youth at the sewer of the virtuous."

His youth in Rome was well known. Arthur said he was wont to dye his hair. Like so much else, that had passed. It was shot through with gray, but still neatly barbered in the Roman fashion and fixed in little curls about his white forehead. Where once he wouldn't think of traveling without two or three young consorts of either sex, Lucullus now preferred solitude. Of my age, he rode well and kept the supple tone of continual exercise. Fastidiousness alone would not desert him. To see me devouring chunks of turnip or onion off the blade of a knife elicited in Lucullus a keen interest in the landscape to his far side.

Arthur had found him a welter of contradictions—cynical, effete, painted like an aging whore, courageous, unfashionably honest, hedonistic, in love with life as one who'd bed a beautiful but stupid woman: for the charm, not the value. The close-set eyes and long, severe nose might remind you of certain ascetics but for the mouth—frank and sensual. One could not question his competence as a statesman. Before leaving Cair Legis he supped with me alone, charming and trivial until Lowri retired. Then Lucullus plucked a few pimpernel from a bowl on the window ledge and laid them between us on the table.

"For want of a rose."

I understood the Roman convention. Anything said from this point was in confidence. "Tell me about this Icel and his lords. Everything you can."

Lucullus listened attentively, asking casual but precise questions here and there. "All things change, Guenevere. Thirty years ago we were all outraged at these pirates plundering a province of the empire. Now the gamesters give different odds. One must look to the future."

"And none knows that better than Icel. Lucullus, take something with you. A letter to my old master. We were friends."

And here in the remains of Britain, in a thick fog, sat this contradiction with me. "Arthur said you wanted nothing but to make love and grow grapes."

Lucullus appeared a little embarrassed at the recollection. "Like so many of my flippancies, easily said and even believed then. The music of the senses: how I tired of it. The gluttons were coarse, the libertines shallow, the epicures dull. But the stink of the virtuous was nausea. The cruelty that oozed like excess saliva from their righteous little smiles. I reflected that the fallen at least had style."

"Until it all sagged, yes?"

Lucullus rolled up his eyes in surfeited agreement. "Deadly. I sent my pretty little friends back to their own firefly ends and started sleeping alone and much more restfully. One cleric commented that virtue agreed with me, when I was merely bored. It does pall, all of it."

"And the residue? What remains, Lucullus? Tell me. I really want to know."

"What remains." He reflected, seeking his answer in the fog rolling about us. "A different passion, perhaps. A reflective, arm's-length desire to take it all and make some sense of it."

"Yes. So with me."

"That's why you intrigue me, Guenevere." He flashed his charming smile. "I daresay you've schooled yourself through every known folly and appetite and come to the same conclusion." He rose, carefully arranging the white cloak, and offered me his arm. "You enjoy your unspeakable raw turnips more than Constantine his whole flimsy reign. But then you've wearied of that sweet and the turnip is tangible."

"Many things are less important now, even death. Like you, I've been too long at the feast. Still . . ."

The fog muffled the creaking wheels as people moved along the road toward us, yet invisible.

"Do you believe in the prophecy of dreams, Lucullus?"

"In my time."

"I've dreamed of dying too often to take it so."

And yet this fog. Lowri dreamed of fog the night before we left Legis. A man came toward us out of the fog carrying a silver vessel of costly wine. He didn't offer it but

poured it on the ground at my feet. And when Lowri scolded him for the waste, he only said, "It is paid for."

The people wouldn't let us leave Cair Legis without them. Indigents all, they simply packed their bundles, carts and children and streamed out the city gates behind us to Blodwen's gratified applause. The journey fired them before the first step was taken, hybrid as it was. Neither strictly Christian nor solely of the Goddess, Coel and I were the poles that drew them. The Holy Grail, Christian theft of a pagan aspiration, melded our journey into a true pilgrimage. The cautious Bishop of Cair Legis was relieved to see the back of both of us.

So were my friends, sadly. New realities strained the seams of old friendship, but they did purchase horses and food for us. Bors and Regan furnished me with a saddle, Rhian helped me pack and washed my hair, Gareth very humbly asked if he could kiss me goodbye.

"Gareth-fach, many times Arthur wanted to hug you. Come here to me."

Bedivere remained Bedivere, cinching my saddle and offering me a leg up. "You're a damned fool, Guenevere. I'm not for hugging, but I'll pray for you. There's none in Britain who so needs it."

We troubled him, Coel and I. Possibly we heated his congealed despair, made it seethe again.

"Thank you all. I doubt we'll meet again, so take my blessing. Regan, kiss little Gwen for me."

"I will, mum. Fare thee well."

"Coel! People!" I stood in the stirrups and raised my arm to my waiting pilgrims. "On to Witrin and the Grail."

And so the slow procession of us along the fog-shrouded road, three hundred men, women and children, following Coel, who rode or walked with the high cross in his hand to show all we met that this journey was blessed and no man might interfere with us. Then the fog crept in and hung over us. Lowri and Huw kept their cart close to my horse, as much for their protection as mine. Lowri felt the fog to be unnatural.

"It's evil. Smells evil."

Lucullus halted his mount, straining to see through the enshrouding mist. "We should see the villa by now."

I seemed to remember this place. "The villa should be on our . . . left?"

"No, to the right. I think." He wasn't sure. "Without the fog we could see it."

"Let's nose about both ways. Brother Coel! Halt them here. We're going to look about."

Lowri caught at my bridle, beseeching. "Let me go with you."

"And me," Huw insisted. "Mabli, stay with the cart."

"Oh, you silly—"

"By your leave, Lady." Huw was not to be denied. "Lowri's no fool old woman explaining dreams for a penny. She has the sight. If she smells evil in the fog, it is here. You were lost to Britain once. We will come with you."

Lucullus trotted off west of the road while I turned over the broken heath to the east. In moments the wagons grew dim, then ghostly, then disappeared as the fog crawled between us. Huw hallooed back to them from time to time. Muffled in the mist, sound played tricks on us. The answering voices came from nowhere and everywhere.

"A-ho!"

A-ho . . .

I dismounted, led my mare by her bridle, my friends on either side.

"A-ho!"

A-ho . . . The voice seemed so far away, though we weren't far from the road. Lowri caught at my arm. "Wait!"

"What?"

"It's here." She crossed herself, turning about in apprehensive recognition. "The cold heart of it. This is where the wine was poured." We both heard it at the same time, the approaching footsteps. "We must go back, Lady. Quick!"

One person coming alone with a soft, measured tread. And the voice that called my name.

"Guenevere!"

"Lady, please." Lowri tugged at me, frightened, while Huw drew his knife and glared into the fog.

"Guenevere!"

"This is Guenevere. Who calls me?"

Huw pointed with his knife. "Over there he is."

"No, over there."

"Everywhere," Lowri whispered.

"There," said Huw. And Lowri froze.

"It's him, Lady. It is him. As the sight of me saw him."

The small cowled form flowed out of the fog, yet the voice came from another side. "Guenevere?"

Off to the left, coming closer. The small man advanced to within a few paces and halted. "Oy greet yew from moy masters, Lady."

I knew him after a moment: older, but the face and the peasant Cornish argot unmistakable. Galahalt's groom, Sawel.

"Och, man, you gave us a fright. This place is ghostly enough. We're among friends, Huw. Bring the others."

Now the other man came out of the fog, much better known and loved. Lancelot strode toward me, grasped my hands and pressed them to his lips. That much older, heavier, the mute unhappiness a little deeper about his mouth. "Guenevere?"

"Of course, sweet."

"I would . . . not have known you. What's happened to you?"

"Nothing but I'm a thousand years old. You look magnificent as usual." A gallant lie. Lancelot sagged with more than his years, drawn and unhappy.

"When those at Hull said they found your horse and the sword—"

"A good thing, that. But Constantine must know by now."

"Not from us." Lancelot kissed my hands again. "Come to the villa. Eleyne is waiting. You, fellow—" He snapped his fingers at Huw. "See to the horse. Woman, don't crowd the Queen. Have you no respect?"

"These are my friends, Lancelot."

"These?" That mystified him as much as the altered sight of me, but then Lucullus trotted toward us out of the fog and there was no more time for disillusionment just then.

They were a small party, just the family, Sawel and nine knights. Constantine still thought them loyal; they could travel freely. Lancelot greeted Lucullus coolly, no more than an acknowledgment of his presence. They'd

ridden together at Badon and in Gaul. Lancelot respected the competence and detested the man.

Long before her features were discernible, I recognized the woman waiting for us by the villa's broken gate: Eleyne, hands demurely laced in front of her. She barely inclined her head to me.

"Holy Astolat welcomes Guenevere. I trow this fog is like to a symbol. It will fade, the light return and Britain rise in Grace again."

"Dear Eleyne. My people thank you." We embraced formally.

"Your people?"

"The hundreds who follow me to Witrin and the Grail. They've made a holy pilgrimage out of it."

Eleyne scrutinized me as curiously as Lancelot, then Huw and Lowri. "Such as these? We will speak of them. And of this monk who travels with you. We are loyal but not heretic. Husband, I wish the monk and my Lord Ambassador within. The commons will remain outside the gate."

I tried to mediate. "Eleyne, may I—"

"Let it not dismay you." She rode iron-shod over my half-born protest. "We shall give them alms. Come." The Princess of Astolat turned without further invitation and walked through the gate across the overgrown atrium, her boots echoing on the paving stones.

She was fifty now, the flesh sagging about her mouth and chin, but even more implacable, however small her domain. As much icon as ruler, no one was allowed to sit in her presence until she did and Eleyne chose now to stand, flanked by Lancelot and Galahalt in the villa's triclinium, depressing and dingy as that at Legis in its forlorn reminder of better days. Although the occasion hardly warranted, Eleyne made ours a formal audience, Lucullus, Coel and I arrayed before her like petitioners, an impression she bolstered with her distant manner.

Galahalt had fulfilled the early promise of his father's constitution, heavy-boned, tending even more to flesh than Lancelot at the same age. The round boy's face was setting into jowls, the whole mien as superior and unperceptive as on his fifteenth birthday.

"We will rest here tonight," Eleyne announced in a tone that brooked no discussion, "and set out for Dyf-

neint in the morning. Meanwhile, you are all right welcome. Brother Coel, the Bishop of Legis writes to his sorrow and mine that you abandoned your vows to incite rebellion."

"Reform, Lady," the monk modified.

"Much the same. You are an ordained priest, we hear, besides your monastic calling. What prompts you to this heretical error? Was not yours a vow of contemplation and obedience?"

"Eleyne," I reminded her, "the monks of Britain have been preaching social reform for an hundred years."

"Heretics."

"And the late King was in some ways of my mind," Coel asserted.

"To whose memory we are loyal and to whose works we are pledged." Eleyne's answer was couched in more diplomacy than usual, perhaps in deference to Lucullus' envoy. "A strong Britain under one crown and one Christ—whose Grace is your province, monk, not the secular world."

Brother Coel was respectful but a rock himself. "Not so, Lady."

"What!" The cold deepened about Eleyne as she glared at his contradiction.

"As long as Christ himself went among beggars—"

"You will not attempt to school me in Scripture?"

"Do you not know my mother is of the blood of Arimathea?" Galahalt demanded.

"No man who doesn't know that, sir."

"Or should forget it . . . what?" Galahalt inclined his head to Sawel's whisper. The stoop-shouldered little servant waited at his elbow with a goblet on a tray. "Mother, your medicine."

"Eleyne has not been well," Lancelot said.

"Nothing serious, I hope."

Eleyne drained the goblet with absent distaste and simply tossed it at Sawel with a backhanded motion. He caught it with the ease of practice. "No, nothing serious. A general perniciousness. My physicians cannot treat that which cannot be named. But if I have not Geraint's constitution, I match him in resolution. Monk, you and your pilgrims may sojourn at Witrin. Where you may

pray to the benefit of their souls and your own, for the lifting of error as this fog outside."

Her hands were palsied. I'd not noticed it before. She held them together to still the shaking. Far from well: not dissipation like Blodwen's, but a sourness like bad air around her. The skin was blotchy and dull as clay. "But I will suffer no treason or heresy in my realm, Brother Coel. Look to it. You may leave us now." She dismissed him as one might snuff a candle. "Son?"

Galahalt flung a purse to Coel. "You may distribute this among your people. We won't melt down the silver crosses as you bid us do, but we are reminded of charity. Go."

It seemed a superfluous arrogance, but Eleyne beamed on her son. Coel's response was weighted with laconic irony. "I will tell them it is thus. They will be grateful." He bowed and withdrew.

"And you, Lucullus." Eleyne's voice, never musical, had worn in age to a thin, harsh edge like the drone of a weary fly. "There is a room prepared for you."

"Thank you, Princess. I plan to be away quite early."

"But give us leave now, Ambassador," Lancelot requested. "We have some private conference with the Queen. And you must have your own business in mind."

The dislike was barely masked. Unruffled as always, Lucullus made a graceful bow to me. "Majesty." Then, pointedly to Eleyne as one of secondary rank, "Highness." And he flowed out of the chamber, his white cloak fluttering behind him. Eleyne did not miss the distinction in his leave-taking.

Galahalt made a sound of disgust. "Degenerate."

"Don't trouble yourself, dear son. No doubt the degenerate King found him diverting. No more of that. Now, Guenevere, have you signed the succession?"

"Yes."

Lancelot struck his palms together. "Then we're ready, Gwen." He smiled for the first time since we met in the fog. "The men of Dyfneint have chafed under the treaty since—"

"It was necessary, husband," Eleyne interrupted in her peremptory manner. "We survived in order to restore the Pendragon."

"And now we can," Galahalt said. "We can strike back while Constantine's main power is in the Midlands."

"Emrys writes that you are as queer in your opinions now as that monk," Eleyne said. "I can order him to silence. I request it of you as Arthur's widow. The people of Dyfneint know us as an holy and unbroken line from Christ. You would confuse them."

"Gwen will be sensible; she always was." Lancelot was more concerned with imminent matters. "The King will close with these Saxons any day, any hour. Perhaps already. We're safe tonight, but we must be gone by morning. Trent is not that far."

"And my folk outside the gate?"

That concerned Lancelot no more than Eleyne. "At their own speed, but you must be away. You are the key, Gwen. The symbol. You must be safe."

"Quite so." Eleyne's hands, unclenched for the moment, trembled visibly. "We have only the nine knights of our escort."

"Post them at dusk, son," Lancelot instructed. "Spread them well to the mile marker, you know the place. And remember, from this night we're rebels. We can afford no mistakes. We'll inspect them together before light."

Eleyne frowned. "Surely not. I'll not have my husband who needs his rest, nor my heir forced from sleep when a knight will serve to inspect them."

"Wife, we're very close to the King to trust someone else's eyes and ears."

"No. I'll not let you." Eleyne took his arm. "You know how I hate to wake at night and find you gone. I sleep poorly as it is and never when you absent yourself. I can't close my eyes until you're returned. It upsets me. Galahalt, set your guards and choose a knight to inspect them."

"Aye, Mother." Quite clear whom the boy considered authority. No more imagination than when I'd tried to care for him. Galahalt had only the dull fact of his faith. "I am shriven, Father. There's no fear of dying."

"I know that, boy. I *know* that." In the brief flush of irritation, I saw so poignantly the age encroaching on my erstwhile lover. He had an old man's short patience with being crossed. "But there's more to it than holiness. There's efficiency as well. Go see to the men."

Galahalt bowed to his parents and departed, Sawel gliding soundlessly in his wake.

"It is a poor father who chides his son for Christian observance."

"Oh, nothing of the sort, Eleyne. Here, come sit with me." When she settled herself on the couch, Lancelot dropped his aging bulk beside her with a sigh of relief. "Your son prays more than he rides. In the old days Gareth would have run the suet off him soon enough. Gwen, did you know Gareth was my old centurion on the Wall?"

"Yes, I remember."

"Lord, how we rode! The Saxons never saw anything like us. They couldn't believe it."

"They remember you from the Midlands. They call it the Time of the Smoke."

"Oh? Eleyne, you must get in the habit of sitting when you give audiences. Your ankles are swollen."

"I know, my love." She laced her fingers with his, leaning on his thick shoulder.

"I barely remember the Midlands," Lancelot murmured. "There was a woman and child. We let them go."

"Husband, will you take supper?" Eleyne asked.

"I was always glad of that . . . what, my dear?"

"Shall I tell Sawel to lay supper?"

"Oh, yes, yes. Gwen must be famished."

"He always talks of the old days," Eleyne said, still clinging possessively to Lancelot's hand. "They do us no good now. Do they, Guenevere?"

The fog thickened as night fell and the refugees from Cair Legis settled by their wagons. At my behest Eleyne relented and allowed Coel and Huw's family within the gates to sleep in the stable with our horses. The rest did what they could against the encroaching damp that throbbed in my scarred leg since the weather changed. I limped from wagon to wagon, bidding good night, helping here and there to coax a child to bed; then to the stable where Huw was rationing grain to my horse. Mabli slept, blanketed in straw. Lowri had prayed with Coel and now took me aside, still apprehensive.

"I won't close my eyes till we're quit of this place," she vowed.

"Don't be an old woman. This was once a very lovely place in the long peace."

She wasn't convinced. "I feel the ghosts."

"Well, they're Roman then and quite civilized."

"No, not these. Unquiet dead. They want payment like the wine spilled in my dream. They smother me. I can smell them."

"Fog and wet peat. Go to sleep. Brother Coel?" I knelt beside him where he lay with his arms behind his head. "Don't smart too much under Eleyne. I told you she was holier than Rome."

He wrinkled his nose at me. "I'm used to that. And Rome wasn't built in a day."

"That's the style. Abbot Brochan is a match for her. He once told me I was unfit to enter the house of God."

"No!"

"True enough, I suppose. We'd just done for Mark right there in his chapel—Jesus, the blood of those years, it just went on and on. Brochan will be your friend, you little John o' the desert—but do allow the good Abbot his own opinions now and then. Pray for me before you sleep."

The villa was built like Pendragon but smaller, a square with my chamber in the west wing, the family in the east. None of the rooms were very clean. Sawel had swept out my space and put me a candle by the bare, rickety couch. I prayed, rolled up in my cloak fully dressed and sleep came as it always does to the healthy: swiftly and without Lowri's troubling dreams.

Nothing special woke me, simply ten years of rising before the birds. Still dark, but I could smell morning in the air. From the courtyard I heard voices and the soft *clop* of several horses. Some of the guard, I thought; then I recognized the timbre of the voice and called softly from my doorway to the familiar form of him by his horse. "Lancelot?"

"Gwen? You're up early."

"Farmer's habit." I moved across the atrium, rubbing my eyes. "Where do you ride?"

"To inspect the guard with Galahalt."

"Against mother's orders?"

"Eleyne's gotten too used to giving orders without thought." Lancelot clapped a gauntleted hand across his

saddle. "But *I* lead Dyfneint's horse. Son! Ride out, I'll join you."

The mounted figure trotted toward us from the stable. "What muck, this fog. Won't be able to see anything in this. G'morrow, Lady."

"Ride out and wait for me. And don't be careening off on your own, boy. Stay close."

Galahalt clattered away through the gate as his father turned to me, earnest. "I won't leave your safety to anyone else, especially Galahalt. Got as much common sense as Geraint, rest his soul."

"Amen. And that was scant, brave as he was. You are kind to give me sanctuary."

"Kind, Gwen?" he echoed with a tenderness that expected no return now. "Eleyne signed the filthy pact with Constantine, Eleyne will break it, but you are *my* charge. No, don't speak." He rested his gauntleted hand lightly on my shoulder. "That's all past and gone. But . . . you are so changed, Gwen. This new nonsense with the peasants."

"I was a slave ten years, Lancelot."

"You a slave: that was sin."

"No, dear, that was education. The making of me."

"You must curb it in Astolat. Eleyne is very ill. Any resistance upsets her. She gives little place to things she can't understand."

"Lancelot, she looks ghastly. She ought to take the air more, get out, exercise. What do the physicians call her illness?"

"A melancholy of humors. A wasting."

"In short, they don't know. And you? How've you been, my dear?"

"Oh . . . always the same." He shrugged. We both understood. "One accepts. I'll never leave her, Guenevere. Not now."

"Of course not."

He seemed about to say more, then changed his mind. Lancelot set a foot in the stirrup and hauled himself into the saddle. His breath whistled with the effort now. "But welcome to Astolat, Gwen. Old friends should visit often."

"Old friends will."

"Tell Eleyne we'll be back by light." He cantered the

horse toward the gate and vanished. I lingered in the fog-shrouded atrium for a few minutes, glad of the little morning freshness in the air. As I turned back to the portico, a door opened somewhere along it and a querulous command issued forth.

"Who's there? Who's there! Husband?"

"No, it's me." I stepped onto the portico as Eleyne came closer in the gloom.

"Where are my husband and my son?" Even in the dark I caught the unreasonable fear in her voice and the hands that clutched at me. "Where *are* they, woman?"

"They decided to inspect the guard themselves. They'll be back before the sun's up."

"Oh, God . . ."

She was much sicker than I thought. I tried to ease her. "His old combrogi habit of thoroughness. He's always been conscientious about things like this."

"Yes. Yes, he would be that now, wouldn't he?" Eleyne reeled against me. "God help me. It is a judgment."

"Eleyne, you *are* ill, and none of that nonsense about humors. Here, lean on me. Let me get you to your chamber."

Unprotesting, she let me guide her back along the portico, that pettish, droning voice at my ear. "God . . . what have you brought us to, Guenevere?"

"I'm grateful to both of you. Do you want your medicine?"

"Judgment . . ."

"Where's Sawel? He'll fetch your potion." But Sawel was up and alert, a stunted shadow by her door. "Here, get your mistress inside."

Sawel slipped his shoulder under the weight of Eleyne and eased her into the bedchamber and down onto the couch she shared with Lancelot. Reverently he tipped the ready potion to her lips. Gradually her agitation quieted. I sniffed at the goblet.

"What do they give you? Perhaps I can suggest something."

"Would they knew. I could tell them, couldn't I, Guenevere? Sawel, see to the door."

The silent shadow of him slipped to the door and barred it.

"Where are they now? Where are they now?" Eleyne

begged of the dark. Her head lolled toward me on the pillow. "Bring the candle closer so I can see you."

The dampness twinged in my leg as I moved the candle.

"You limp, Guenevere."

"In the wet. My left leg's all scar down to the bone."

"So even you grow old at last."

Something in her tone chilled me. Eleyne's doughy features were contorted with naked hatred. "Even the great whore. She's killed them, Sawel. She deserves this. Keep her silent."

He'd slid behind me, soundless as always. My head snapped back as the folded linen went over my mouth. Sawel knotted it behind as Eleyne rose from the bed, quivering, fixed on me.

"You think I gave an idle command to my husband and son? You've killed them. He went because of you, but then he always did. 'Gwen is coming. We must see to Gwen's safety. Yes, let us have supper, Gwen must be famished.' Always *you*."

Eleyne flailed out and struck me across the face. She had no more strength than Rat, but Sawel twisted me back into a chair by the bare table and drew another close to guard me like the well-trained dog he was, devoid of expression, a blankness I'd once put down to deficiency of mind. He gripped my arm hard to warn against struggling, then looked expectantly to his mistress for her next orders: good dog.

"They are coming, you see," Eleyne fretted in that oversimple manner one uses on a backward child. "I sent for them to end it. Tonight. And because of you, all I love in this world . . . because of you—"

Eleyne fumbled for her goblet of medicine, but it slipped out of her vague grasp and spilled to the floor. "Well enough. It does not matter now." She clasped her twitching hands together, rocking back and forth. "You selfish whore, you lay with every man in Britain. Your very soul is a brothel. Did you need him as well?"

Out of the monotonous voice and jagged thoughts, I began to understand as she dragged me back past Gunnarsburh, past Eburacum and Glevum to years I'd long packed away but Eleyne never moved beyond.

"You thought me a pitiful little lump of prayers and

duty, didn't you? That I couldn't want a man your way. But I saw the man I wanted."

I shifted in the chair; only a slight movement but Sawel stayed me, drawing his dagger, laying it near to hand. "Do not."

"Blessed Sawel." Eleyne stroked his head. "I pray for him every day. He hears everything and nothing. What he dares for my blood and the Grail is absolved even as it's done. Do you hear me, whore? You've killed my husband and son . . . my Lancelot. I gave myself to him so gladly. Better than you. Even there in the bed, I loved him better than you ever could. You would not know such a hunger. I would pray and think of him, hungry before the amen; see to my duties and go to him before they were well finished. For once there was something I loved more than—I heard music in his arms, he—"

Haggard and shaking—the torment released at last. No one had dug the arrow from her wound, and it suppurated thirty years to burst now. She'd worn older than myself with it.

"I went to him even before we were married, so much I wanted him. I would pay the cost of it, but how could there be sin in so much happiness? And in the morning when I kissed his eyes open so I could see my own happiness shine out at me, I saw only kindness and pity." Eleyne gave them the value they held for her. "Kindness and pity. And nothing else since. He'd already looked to Babylon." She scraped at the bottom of her pain to say it: "But he was an honorable man. God in heaven . . . honorable. All because of you, Guenevere. Why? I will hear it from you. Why?"

At her sign, Sawel loosened my gag, still hovering close.

"If she raises her voice, kill her." The whole thing was sick beyond imagining. She'd betrayed us to Constantine, put herself in danger, perhaps thrown away Lancelot's life and those of her knights.

"Why, Guenevere?"

What could I tell her? It was years past, no part of me any more. "Because I was a coward for a time. As far from my right mind as you are now."

"From my wits? No." Her head bent to one side, alert to something below the silence. "Is't them? You hear,

Sawel? They're coming. They'll take this woman and put it right . . . leave us be. Leave us clean at last."

There was no sound from the dark and fog outside. No world at all beyond this dim, dirty room and Eleyne. If I weren't so frightened, I might have pitied her. "Eleyne, it was so long ago. I was a different person. I did you wrong, but it's years dead."

"You despised me."

"I lived in this world, not a holy myth."

"You laughed at me, like that other whore that wedded Mark and bedded Trystan." Eleyne's mouth distorted in a parody of a smile. She giggled uncleanly. "You know where she is now? A nun in Avebury. Praying, the fat old thing. Imagine that on its knees for something holy? Britain needs to be clean again."

The sight of her made me sick. Comprehension grew like nausea in my stomach. "We never got on, but I thought at least you were loyal."

"I was loyal to Arthur. He gave me Lancelot."

But Arthur died and the whore couldn't bring herself to give up the royal bed where God so denied her that she couldn't even make Arthur a child as Eleyne did for Lancelot in joy beyond duty. No, greedy Guenevere still wanted the crown and sent to loyal little Astolat for their support. Loyal friends: Lancelot would not even give audience to Constantine's envoys.

"But I would, because now I had my weapon: your ambition and Constantine's. I gave them public rebuke and private assurances."

"Eleyne . . . I hope I don't understand this."

She leaned across the table, close to me. "*I* understand, Guenevere. While my Galahalt grew in wisdom and grace, what matter for a few years which degenerate wore the crown, whore or sodomite? Both alike, foul alike with the rot that has hidden holy Britain from the sight of God for an hundred years; so blighted that the Grail disappeared from mortal sight and the charge of my blood. As it could again."

"No, mistress." Sawel appealed to her. "It must not. It must stay with us."

"But it could fade, Sawel," Eleyne fretted, "unless Britain is restored to God's own line of succession."

Not only afraid for myself now; as Eleyne wandered in

her febrile way, I began to grasp the sanctified horror of what she'd loosed.

"Christ sat with thieves. I bargained with the damned: Galahalt to succeed Constantine. Letters sealed in secret, sworn on the Grail itself. And that ambitious creature's scant but desperate hope of heaven. What clergy would not back Galahalt? We would restore them to a power equal to the Bishop of Rome."

Her sudden primness chilled me more than the madness that licked about its edges. "But the devil minds his own. You escaped at Witrin. Your men were too quick and the sodomite too tardy. You escaped my own knife in the battle afterward when that fool of a Cornishman came between us and I had to kill him or lose all I wanted for Galahalt."

"God help you, Eleyne."

"You say that? You, the great logician? Of course Constantine besieged Astolat. So I could pact, treaty and leave my husband *safe*."

"Safe . . ."

"Innocent as he was. He would not turn on you. Never on you."

"But you gave me Galahalt."

"For the time," she said. "So I could give you Sawel as well." Eleyne smoothed her hand over his shoulder like a trusted pet. "They will come straight, Sawel? They would not hurt my men?"

"Certes not," he soothed her. "Will be light enow to see soon, mistress. Yew must rest yorself."

He cared for her; she meant all to this animal. If she wanted me dead now, Sawel would do it without a thought, incapable of reflecting on it. *He hears everything and nothing.* Does everything and nothing, absolved of all. As he was ordered.

As he waited to do from the day I took Galahalt while Constantine butchered my folk in Camelot.

As he tried to kill me in Blodwen's villa, rousing me to a violence that savaged more lives than I could count.

As his obedient treachery opened the gates of Eburacum. As he took my Imogen with his own hands and set me on the cold road that ended with Frith and a slave collar. Gwenda with the scar, one pound/ten.

Gradually my trembling ceased. I felt cold and dead,

but focused at last on the core of it all. Eleyne. For her son and her warped dream of a Britain conjured from her unreal visions and fermented wrongs, she'd murdered the reality, sent men to their deaths as servants to a kitchen, torn open cities, sundered lives, turned out hundreds like Huw and Lowri to choke the roads. She never thought of the numbers or put faces or hopes to any of them. That was beneath and beyond Eleyne. She'd flung to hell forever any hope of a Britain to stand in a real world. She was Elfgifu gone rotten—courage, determination, soured longing, insanity like encroaching mildew.

"Woman, do you know what you've done?"

Eleyne knew. "I've saved them all, saved their souls from you. And they will be grateful, even Lancelot when he understands. I—" She faltered, swaying over the table. "Sawel, if your masters are killed—if they are dead . . ."

He rose to steady her. "Lady, you must to bed."

"No, leave off. Hear me. If they are even hurt, you will finish it here. Before the door is unbarred."

"Oy will that, mistress."

"In my sight, Sawel."

"With a good will, Lady," he soothed her. "Now you must go to bed."

"No . . . no, leave me alone. I want more speech with this woman."

Pliant creature, even Imogen trusted Sawel at the last moment of her life, standing in the light at the foot of the scullery steps, the only one of us who saw him. *Aye, well met! Come down and give us a bit of help.*

If I never left this room neither would Sawel. While he tried to coax Eleyne to bed, leaning over the table to her, my fingers strayed over my bound-up hair, slid in, touched the handle of the small knife. Distracted for the moment, Sawel missed the movement. Eleyne did not, but too late. Before he could understand her wail of warning, before his head was half turned to me, the vicious little blade went across his throat with all my plow-hardened arm behind it.

The blood geysered up and out, splattering Eleyne. She retreated with a shriek, clawed at the heavy bar over the door. I caught her and hurled her back across the

chamber to sprawl on the dingy tiles, still screaming. And then I turned with a colder justice on Sawel.

Obedient to the end, he'd tried to help her, but he couldn't help himself. His dagger clattered to the floor and Sawel crumpled after it, trying to hold his throat closed, making a wet sound I remembered very well, convulsing, fighting to breathe against the blood drowning him. Eleyne went on screaming, not even knowing who might help her.

"Guards! Help! Help! Lucullus!"

"There are no guards, Eleyne. They're all on the road."

I hauled her up and dragged the feebly resisting weight of her to the table, snatching up Sawel's knife. "You did it all."

She fought me as well as she could, no match with both arms for one of mine now. *"Lucullus, help me!"* I forced her down over the table and splayed her right hand against it. "You did it all with your own—little—hand." I drove Sawel's dagger through her hand deep into the wood of the table, pinning her. "That's just for me."

Through her high-pitched scream I heard the pounding at the door. "This is Lucullus. What is it? Open the door. Who called?"

"This is Guenevere. Get away from the door, Lucullus."

"Open it! What's happened?" More pounding. "Guenevere, what's happening?"

"They sold me again. It's a trap. The King's men are coming." I leaned my head a moment against the cool hardness of the door. "They won't harm you, but I probably won't leave here alive. Fare you well, Lucullus."

"What . . . ? I hear trumpets on the road. Someone's coming. Guenevere, open the door!"

I heard them now, thin in the fog. "Go, Lucullus. I'm all right. There's something must be done."

The horns again, closer. Footsteps hurrying away down the hall as I turned to Eleyne. Far too weak to free herself from the knife that impaled her hand, she only huddled over the table, goggling at the wound, at me. ". . . Deeper in hell for this, Guenevere."

"You sainted obscenity." I stepped to the twitching Sawel where he lay with his eyes bulging up at me. Barely alive, but enough. Quickly I cut and tore away the

garments, baring his chest. "The English have one punishment for traitors, Sawel. It is rendered by the woman of the house. And Britain was my house."

Meticulously as Nilse or Elfgifu, revulsion dulled by purpose, the first long slash from breastbone to navel. "For Glevum and Camelot. For Gwenlys and Flavia Marcella."

Eleyne slumped over her grotesquely pinioned arm, not too mad to be horrified. "My God . . . help me."

The second incision across, forming a neat *T*. "For Eburacum. For all the good men sold and gone."

There was a muffled commotion from the atrium, voices coming closer, but slowly, with need to hurry now. I was almost finished, swallowing back the last squeamishness.

"And for my Imogen whom I loved." I scooped deep with the small blade, working with both red hands. Finished. Sawel no longer moved. I rose and bore the result of my surgery to Eleyne. She could scream no longer, only a sound between a gasp and a choking moan when I pulled the knife free and put the offering in her bloody hand. The thing still pulsed feebly.

"This is always given to the god. But I'll settle for you, you're a relative."

"Open the door! Ancellius is hurt."

When I unbarred the door it swung in to reveal Lancelot in early morning light, slumped against taller Lucullus. Eleyne saw him too and pushed herself up. "Husband—"

I read it in an instant: chalk-white, the great wound in his middle, hobbling forward only with Lucullus' help. Something he couldn't understand or make sense of . . .

"Gwen, we were . . ."

"Husband!"

His dimming gaze wavered from Eleyne to me for some answer to insanity. "Betrayed . . . they were waiting for us."

He could manage no further. Lucullus lifted him to the bed. I saw how much of the blood discolored his white tunic. Eleyne stumbled to the bed and fell down by Lancelot.

"The King's men are here," Lucullus murmured to me.

He winced at the sight of Sawel and the mess on the table. "What in the name of—?"

Heavy boots thudding along the portico.

"Tell the English it's theirs. Or anyone's now. What's left."

"Husband, where is my son?" Eleyne mewed pathetically. "Where is my Galahalt?"

He couldn't tell her. Lancelot no longer needed to understand any of it.

"Where is my son . . . ?"

She was still asking of the boy as the footsteps stopped at the door, still asking long after any coherence fled from the sounds.

Father and son were laid out together on the bed, nor would Eleyne leave their side. The sobbing ended after a long time. No other word came from her after that but a low, animal keening. Oblivious to Brother Coel kneeling beside her as she was to everything else, even the wound in her hand. The Cornishmen did what they could for her and then left her alone.

They'd troubles of their own, been in a fight and a bad one by the mauled look of them. Half a squadron, all Constantine could spare but enough to hold me till he came, enough to butcher eleven men instead of nine in the fog.

"We didn't want that," my Cornish guard confided distastefully. "The King's mood is black enough with his sweet Alun gone. And, Christ, haven't we all seen enough blood this week?"

So they had, most of it their own. Still brilliant and fumbling by turns, Constantine lost most of his cavalry in the forests along Trent River. My guard was not a brutal man, but he'd been one of the first into Eleyne's chamber to see the carnage and my own hands. He watched me closely, plagued by wounds of his own, weary of riding and defeat. It helped to talk to a woman, even me.

"You know the Saxons then?"

"I know them."

"Five days we rode that forest track, back and forth looking for them. Nothing but birds. We knew where some of them were, miles back already marking out

fields behind sharpened stakes like a pack of hedgehogs. The sixth day, riding back, the trees were full of 'em. No room for maneuver or charge. Dragged off the horses and slaughtered. Cut down with arrows. They didn't come out to fight until our horse was down to half. Charge them, they'd give way just to trap you on those goddamned stakes."

The Cornish were not at Badon; they didn't know what Saxons could do to cavalry with a wooden stake.

"They'll be on Badon next," the knight predicted gloomily. "Nothing to stop 'em. Hell." He threw up the whole thing. Life was short, he'd done what was expected of him. But for me when the King came—

"I'd be about seeing the monk, Lady. Put it all in order, you know. You must not expect . . ."

"No. Thank you. Come in, Lucullus."

The ambassador entered, ready for travel. He displayed his seal of safe conduct to the knight. "The King, as you know, is a close friend of mine. I regret I'm not able to greet him when he comes. Duty, sir. The Emperor of Byzantium is a demanding master." Lucullus rested a jeweled kid gauntlet on the knight's mailed shoulder. "But tell him I will not part from Britain without embracing my friend."

The knight retreated a bit from the scented aura of Lucullus. "I will tell him."

"This too: I am sensible of his grief."

"Y'mean Alun," blurted the tactless fellow.

"It may be inconsolable, but not incomprehensible to men of feeling who mourn with him. He'll understand until I return. Guenevere, farewell."

"I think it is indeed that, Lucullus."

"Perhaps not."

"I've been advised to put my life in order."

His epicene manner sobered a little. "After too short an acquaintance, Lady. My dear, I must tell you. Arthur indeed married well. May I embrace you?"

His lips against my ear, Lucullus whispered, "Any message for Icel?"

"Tell Gunnar he can claim my inheritance."

"I will. Lady, farewell." Lucullus paused in the doorway, turning again to the knight. "This woman is known like her husband as far as Constantinople. Tell the King,

for whatever weight it carries, that she should not die. Or if she must, then with dignity."

As the sun rose higher on the long day waiting for Constantine, the fog thinned, driven by a freshet of breeze. All about the villa the exhausted squadron slept while it could or crept about seeing to horses suffering like themselves. They reminded me of Bedivere, dogged and hopeless, fighting for ten years and no end in sight. With the fog went the peasants. Long adept at avoiding soldiers, they melted away before light, even Huw and his family, to hide in the nearby forest. I couldn't blame them, save that someone had stolen my horse, saddle and all.

"You won't be needing it," my guard predicted. "Been a long road for you, Guenevere, but I think you've reached the end. And what an end." He grimaced. "That poor bastard, Sawel . . . think you were a flaming Pict, that's their style."

"It was an execution. Constantine would have done the same. How does Eleyne?"

"The same; just sits there by them, moaning." He put it all, the hopelessness, moral and personal disgust, into his last word as he left me. *"God."*

Through the day and into the night, the men watched for their king with well-founded anxiety. They were few and worn and not that far from Gareth's combrogi. They ate near their saddled horses, looking west more than east. At evening they asked a mass of Brother Coel and posted pickets. At midnight there was still no sign of Constantine, nor by next day's light, but now there was another problem. Lancelot and Galahalt must be buried soon. Eleyne wouldn't hear of it. No persuasion, the summer's heat, the need for decent and speedy interment, no matter how delicately urged, would budge her from their side. She responded not at all, Lancelot's cold fingers clutched in hers—clumsily for the bandages wrapped about her limp right hand by the compassionate Coel. She would not hear them. In the end they lifted her with gentle force and carried her from the chamber.

I asked the squadron commander for a moment with Lancelot while Brother Coel gave extreme unction to father and son alike.

"Right then, a moment," my guard was told. "But watch her."

I stood back a little distance from the bed as Coel administered his office. He did it carefully, the Latin precise as a muffled drum beat against the heavy summer night around us.

My poor darling, I remember when Arthur told you to find a Grail for all of us and sent you home to Eleyne. I pity her. That's all I can feel now, not a tear left for any of us. Was it my weakness in taking you or yours in never letting go of me that brought us to this? My dear Lancelot, speed to heaven and leave ambiguity to me. You never had the shoulders to bear a sin.

Coel was finished. I knelt by the bed to smooth the hair over the creased brow. His skin was mottled with weather and age, the wrinkles deep where the breastbone met his neck. I unbuckled the top strap of his ring mail and laid the small bunch of pimpernel against his breast.

I am so sorry for all of us, my sweet lover. This time of ours was an island in itself—not really part of what was or what's to come. But the people tell such lyrical lies about us. They've already made us into what they need, and who's to say they aren't the wise? Thank you for loving me when I needed it.

As for Galahalt, like his uncle Geraint, he'd always charged death straight on. He died a martyr and couldn't have gone happier. He needed no duty in hypocritical tears from me.

When it was light a rusty shovel or two were found in the stable. The graves were dug within the atrium. Out of deference to Eleyne, I didn't stand at the graveside but watched from my chamber door with the ubiquitous Cornish guard beside me. Eleyne seemed shrunken, dazed. She twisted her hands and her lips moved continually throughout Brother Coel's prayers. At the end the monk spoke to her; she barely turned her head to see who addressed her—then, like a dreamer, Eleyne reached to the shovelful of earth held out by a knight and dropped a handful into the open graves.

She moved not at all while the graves were being filled. Only when the knight-commander dispersed his men did Eleyne raise her head.

"Captain!" She did not ask; she'd never asked in her

life. "You will give me two of your best knights to escort me home to Astolat."

The Cornishmen shuffled about, embarrassed. They owed nothing to Dyfneint, none of them wanted to go, not even sure the King would want them to.

"For I have duties and have been too long from my court. Astolat is my home, you see, and my holy charge. There alone resides Grace in Britain. I do not for that reason please to travel overmuch."

The knight-commander glanced about at his men and spoke respectfully to Eleyne, removing his flowered helmet. "If the King, when he comes, will give us leave—"

"The knights you select must be only those of proven virtue. I would leave betimes. See to it."

He tried with little success to explain his position. Eleyne bided in superior silence for a time, then cut him short. "Where are they? Have I not given an order? I would be away. My family is waiting."

Someone on the edge of the group muttered, "Jesus!" and turned away. Then one man in torn ring mail nudged a companion and they moved to the commander for brief conference. He let out his breath with a heave of his shoulders: let it be then.

Eleyne did not move until the knights were mounted, her own horse waiting and she felt her cloak with the worn cloth of gold edging draped about her by Brother Coel. When he offered her a leg up to the stirrup, she placed the heel of her boot on his palm as she'd done all her life to those who didn't matter. She did not rein the horse; it merely took a few steps after the other two, wandering.

"Why are we waiting?" Eleyne demanded of the walls and nothing. One of her escort took the reins and led Eleyne's horse toward the gate where she woke for an instant from whatever dream she drifted in, twisted in the saddle, looking for me—found me.

"*Guenevere.*"

Her escort halted. Eleyne sat rigid, fixing me with her hate before it lost all focus. "Guenevere . . ."

That was all. The dream enfolded her again. I think mercifully she forgot me before too long. She did not like to travel far from Astolat and its Grace. And her family was waiting.

By the sundial in the atrium, that was just before noon. Constantine came late that night.

"You have this night to confess and be shriven by your anarchistic little monk. And you'll sign a letter of succession. I don't care what you signed for Emrys, you'll repudiate that. Why didn't you stay dead and save me the trouble?"

The lamps did not light the triclinium very well, only softened the grime of neglect. Constantine wandered from his chair to the table, continually refilling his wine cup, spilling, pacing about, unable to settle or bring his full attention to anything for long.

The King of Britain was unshaven and unkempt, much leaner and gristlier now. His shoulders hunched with habitual tension. Sprawled about the villa, the lacerated remnant of his cavalry and foot licked the wounds from Trent and wondered where they went from here. One heard the same word rise up everywhere like smoke: Badon. There were no Catuvellauni on it now, nothing to keep the Saxons off. The hill that lost them seven thousand men against Arthur and Maelgwyn, the key to the south and west, was theirs for the walking in. And God knows, Saxons could walk. In actual distance they were only forty miles from this villa.

Beyond his inability to relax, Constantine could not get very drunk, hard as he tried. Thirty-five now, he was even more the winter wolf than Emrys. A long time on the hunt, unable to shed his wariness. Sometimes his voice weakened and broke or his eyes glistened with tears. He rambled, repeated himself, asked the same questions twice.

"Lucullus will come back, he said? Good. That is good. A man has few consolations. I've had . . . personal losses. Trent. My best friend. Close to him like my Uncle Marcus. You wouldn't know such loss, Guenevere. But how many of them you have to answer for. Yes, you may sit down. Guard!"

His guard appeared in the shadowed entrance. "My Lord?"

"Where's the writ?"

"Sir?"

"You fool, the writ! I sent for it."

"Not while I've been here, sir. What writ?"

"Oh." Constantine dropped into the chair again, cup and jug dangling loose from his hands. "In my chamber. On the table. Fetch it here. Bedivere it was . . . Bedivere and Gareth. Gareth held the old man's arms and Bedivere put the knife in him. And you said well done."

So I did and for reasons much the same as his. Nothing but power could be considered then. Power must first be grasped. Lord, what a bleak thought: we were all ghosts now, walking old ramparts out of dull habit, reaching out of a reason only dimly remembered for a right we couldn't name. Ghosts. In the last days of my rule, I was no different, only more efficient, than this gone-to-earth king hunched in his chair. And he could be me ten years ago, hunted out of Witrin, falling down to gasp for breath in the ruins of Aquae Sulis for one too-brief space before running on with the hounds on his heels.

I was to die and no happier about that than anyone would be, just older and easier resigned. Let be then; don't maunder at me with stale accusations. Let me sign your silly writ as I signed his, let me pray, confess, go to bed and in the morning, let the sword be keen.

"Brother Coel was on pilgrimage to Ynnis Witrin. There's no reason to harm him."

"What? Oh, the monk." Constantine started out of his inner torment as if just reminded of my presence. He drained the cup, spilling it down his chin and beard, poured it full again. "I don't give a damn about him. He won't sway them any more than you did."

"You'd be astonished at what peasants can do."

"Our plebeian heroes." He raised his cup in sardonic homage. "Reminding us of humanity from below the salt? Rubbish."

"I've seen it happen."

"Yes, Eleyne wrote me of your conversion. You weary old platitude: uplifted through suffering and humility. You? The lion sermonizes on the evils of meat. Folk meetings . . . old woman, I've read Cicero and the rest of them as well. Give power to one of those bleating sheep, you think he'll be a Brutus crying Up the Republic? He's no different from us, just hungrier and more brutal. And he can't read, but he can see the purple in our cloaks, the fine horses we ride, the jewels that shone in Guenevere's

crown. Why not *his* wife's as well? He'll grab for all the gaudy toys and snatch at more. Because he'll not have enough, never enough. In a year he'll have the habit of power, in two the addiction. And all must *see* his power. He'll put up his wife and whores like holly at Yule time—look what I've got!—and fight to keep it all for the mere sake of it all, and ten *times* more brutal than the lot of us. Because our plebe knows nothing of proportion, only that the stick's in his hand, like a bully boy playing king-of-the-hill. Government by the people? What bloody people? Who has he to mirror but us, and how many times could we afford mercy?"

He drank, wiping his mouth on the back of his hand. "And what has he to wait for, in his overdressed peril, but another bully to challenge him for the hill? I think the expression was Arthur's: business as usual. I wouldn't have ascribed naïveté to you. It must be age."

The writ was brought with stylus and ink. But that I recanted calling Constantine usurper and repudiated any rights of Emrys', it merely named the present king my true successor by right of possession in the hope of the Church's favor (and that of the people, of course). The last pale gasp of SPQR.

"They'll bend as we push them," Constantine muttered, his mind clearly elsewhere. He must have loved this Alun. "Sign it."

"Why not? Neither of you will win."

"Sign it, date it and you can go back to your monk."

"Here. May it well become you. If you're finished with me, I'd like to go."

"Almost." Constantine lolled in his chair, red-rimmed eyes unfocused. Not sodden, he couldn't drink enough for that respite. And perhaps only one man, miles away, could understand his loss or find the words to soothe it. But from me, Constantine would have full measure.

"Kneel to me, Guenevere."

"Oh, really. I wouldn't have put smallness among your sins. It must be age."

"Kneel!"

With a glance at the guard, himself mutely embarrassed at the demeaned sight of his lord, I knelt before Constantine. "I ask one boon of you, King of Britain."

Whatever pleasure he took in the humbled sight of me,

it was not enough to salve the misery clamped behind the hand over his mouth. "You ask for mercy?"

"Only to know one thing. All of it, Constantine, all ten years of it. Was it worth such a large candle?"

"*Yes.*" My question was just another barb in the wound of him, but he faced it as he faced all the others. There was no other choice for him now. "Yes, it was worth it. Because it's my hill."

"Since my last confession it has been three months. More."

By the fat lamp in my chamber, the door opened for the guard at a discreet distance along the portico, I made my confession to Brother Coel, the last of my sins murmuring with the rest of the night sounds. My ledgers might not balance well, but all was recorded now.

Ego absolve te in nomini Patri et Fili . . .

His office done, Coel became just my friend again, sharing my last meal at the broken table. Inconsistent to the end, Constantine decreed that I must lose my head in the morning, then sent a jar of decent wine, good wheaten bread and soup from his cook. He couldn't end me with quite Eleyne's detachment.

Summer nights are short in my country. The light that leaves the sky so briefly after the long twilight returns shortly after three and broadens gradually to day again. I slept only an hour or so, waking by habit before first light.

"You've barely slept at all," Coel said.

"English habit. Seems wasteful to sleep when there's light to see at all. But you may if you need."

"I'll watch with you, Lady."

"Thank you." Coel was good company, never reticent in speaking his mind, his obdurate views of the world burred out in his Brigante brogue, crisp as the black hair curling about his ears. There are fair Britons like myself and the dark like Coel. They are the older ones—Brigantes, hill tribes, Picts—and their right to Britain older than ours.

"So you were in love with me once."

Coel grinned. "Utterly."

"Repent that last of all. It's charming and good taste in the bargain." I poured the last of the wine into our cups.

"I taught good taste to Arthur. But I've often wondered whom I would have married if he'd not come north. Someone insignificant, I suppose. Peredur was too ill to last. Father needed a strong hand in Eburacum."

"It's inconceivable that you would marry anyone else," Coel asserted fervently. "You were born to put your hand with his on the reins of Britain."

"So I was. Arthur needed some time to realize that."

Just then the guard tapped politely and nodded in. "Getting light, Lady. The men are stirring."

"Yes. Thank you."

"He knew it, Guenevere. There was something he dictated to me there at the end." Coel pinched his eyes between thumb and forefinger. "What was it he said? Something simple; he had a talent for simplicity . . ."

"Along with fine artists and a few of the gods."

"What was it? Oh, that's irritating. I'll try and try and it'll elude me, but I won't think of anything else until it's remembered."

"Soon, let's hope." Clear and sharp in the morning air, over the muted whinnying of waking horses, I heard the zang-zang of a whetstone on iron.

Coel brightened suddenly. "Ah! I remember. You know the King's way of putting things, few words but no more needed. He said—most kings only have wives, but that he had a queen."

He said that at the end? Of me? "Truly, Coel?"

"I wrote it in his reminiscences. It is in the rolls at Avalon."

Well then. Through all the musical lies, someone might remember a bit of truth after all. "You must remember, Coel: through all our troubles and differences, we loved each other very much. But ruling is more than a right of birth. It's a difficult profession."

"The King said as much."

"An instinct developed over long years into a talent. Law and government are a profession." I inclined my head through the open door across the atrium to Constantine, just emerging from his chamber, rubbing at the dark pouches under his eyes. "If you doubt it, observe the amateurs."

A small knot of Cornish knights gathered about Constantine. One of them offered him a drink. Quite light

enough now to see all their faces. I gave my purse to Brother Coel.

"The people will come out of the forest when you call them. They trust you. Take them to Ynnis Witrin. And never stop trying to teach them or make them think, it's needed. I'm too late, but you're not."

Again the guard ducked his head in at the door. "Coming, Lady."

Coel knelt quickly and kissed my hand. "By God, it's a poor monk I am and me still in love with you."

"And I still woman enough to love the notion." I ruffled his curly hair to hide my rising fear. "I'll want you by me, Coel. You wouldn't think it, but I'm awfully squeamish now and then."

"I'll be that close, Lady."

The footsteps came on across the atrium cobbles, halted. "Bring her out."

Early August morning scented with heather and honeysuckle. I heard the birds singing as the escort led me out the broken gate around the west wall of the villa where an old stump used for chopping firewood had been brought from the stable and set conveniently by the fresh-dug grave. A burly Cornish knight waited by the stump, the honed longsword cradled in his arms. He handed Constantine a cloth which the king began to fold.

"Do you mind?" I said. "A moment. I've always loved summer mornings."

Constantine went on folding the cloth. "Let's get on with it."

"For the love of *God*, man, be you King or not!" Coel made no effort to conceal his disgust and outrage. "A moment? A lifetime. I should not be praying this good Queen to heaven."

"British monks." Constantine rolled his eyes to that heaven, my last sight before the cloth hid the morning from me. "You'd think they were senators. This old woman's taken too long to die as it is."

"You were always a clod, Constantine. Not a glimmer of style. Take my hand, Brother Coel." I felt his fingers curl around mine, then someone forced me to my knees—

What happened then was rather confused: a distant shout of warning, then Constantine roaring an order, feet

thudding about me, a cry from Coel—exuberant in view
of the occasion—and then I was dumped brusquely into
the open grave *Jesus God I'm not dead I can't be dead why
am I still so fright—* Jarred by the fall, I scrabbled to my
knees, hearing the rising rumble in the earth, the shouting men, the high scream of horses, and Coel at my ear,
jubilant.

"Are you hurt?"

"No, but what—?"

"Judgment Day!" he exulted, fumbling at the blind-
fold. "Oh, but see the *beauty* of it."

He was too excited to untie the knot. I simply yanked
the cloth down about my neck to see the Cornish knights
and their soldiers scattering frantically to horse, to
cover, anywhere to escape that flying wedge of horse hurtling at them from the cover of the forest. Before I recognized the leading shields, I saw Huw galloping my own
horse on their flank, screaming loud as the Cornishmen.
And behind them, at the edge of the trees, Lowri and
Mabli leaping up and down among my people, flailing
their arms in excitement. No time to see much more, all
a blur, but I recognized the sunburst on Gareth's shield
and the lean man who rode beside him, and Emrys himself at the wedge's point.

Quite forgetting me, my executioner was chasing his
own frightened horse. Constantine snapped commands
from the saddle, trying for some order before that swift
combrogi blade descended. I hauled myself out of the
grave and started to run for Emrys before I heard Constantine's high curse and the horse pounding behind me,
but there was a friend in sight.

"Bedivere! To me, Bedivere!"

His horse veered and plunged toward me as Coel
shouted, "Guenevere, mind out!"

I dodged aside, heard the whistle of the sword as it
missed me close, and Constantine was carried by sheer
momentum toward Bedivere. They met at full charge,
blades screaming together.

"Aunt!"

Emrys short-reined his horse so hard it went down on
its haunches, wheeled and shot toward me. He thrust out
his arm; behind me the shock of the combrogi wedge hitting the Cornish shook the ground. I reached frantically

for Emrys' hand. Disengaged from Bedivere, Constantine whirled to kill me. I missed Emrys' hand, but he hooked the blind still knotted about my throat and dragged me by the neck for a choking ten yards, drawing his sword left-handed to ward against Constantine.

Horses and dust roiled about me. Were I not strangling it might have been funny, like clumsy boys trying to wrest a ball from each other. Emrys lost his hold and dropped me—thank God—and someone's horse knocked me flat and wheezing for breath. As I rose groggily, someone else grabbed the neck of my garment and dragged me a few yards before Bedivere closed and forced him to drop me.

"Lady!" Gareth now, darting in, reaching for me, but his stiffened old fingers lost their grip as Constantine shot by, bent low in the saddle, hooked my waist and galloped away toward the Cornish lines to drop me where I'd started, next to my own grave. I lay on my bruised belly, panting, looking up through horses' legs. Then we all heard the horn—deep, imperative and of a remembered timbre.

"Kill her. Kill her now!"

But no one noted Constantine, every eye riveted on a rise just north of the villa. "What in the name of all the bloody angels is *that*?" Someone whistled.

No time for conjecture. With a deep *wush*! a thick storm of arrows lofted up, up, hovered and came down. Well-placed shafts, flown not to kill but to warn. The few riders from either side still straggling between the two forces, scattered for their lines as the flight sank into the ground between us. On the point of charging us, Emrys and Gareth paused, hands still raised, astonished as the Cornish.

"Up, Lady."

"Coel, what—?"

Like all the others he stared at the hilltop, bare a few moments ago but now alive with archers and in the rapid process of becoming a fort. Men on foot, two to a pole, were bristling the hill with sharpened stakes. More men appeared behind them and more and more. In little longer than it takes to write it, there was a horseshoe defense of palings along the hilltop as the men behind

took up their positions and two horsemen rode down from them toward our interrupted mayhem.

Coel quite forgot decorum in his surprise. "I'll be damned! Saxons! And Lucullus with them."

I recognized Lucullus before his helmeted companion. Constantine paced his horse forward a few yards. "To me, Lucullus!"

"Don't anyone move, I entreat you." Lucullus raised his voice to all. "I want to live to see home again." The prudent ambassador saluted Emrys and Constantine alike, riding directly between the lethal lines before turning toward us.

"Hold off, all of you. This may be averted."

Emrys called to him. "I don't see how, Lucullus."

"It's my office," Lucullus returned, casual as possible under the circumstances. "Don't run me down, I beseech you. And no harm to the Queen or they won't miss again."

"Gall," Coel admired, "and doesn't he have it all?"

Constantine glared at me, then up at the ranks of ready bowmen. We were easily within their range. Lucullus trotted to Constantine's off side and gripped his arm in greeting. "Well met, and with joyous news—if the King of Britain will accept it."

His husky companion dismounted and removed the cowling helmet as he strode to me, ignoring the Cornishmen around him.

"Gunnar. Oh—"

"*Hvordan har, Gwenda?*"

"*Ach, har de got nu, min egen elskede.* My God, man, I heard of Trent. Are you all right?"

"Are you? Lucullus told me, and we were close enough to do something about it. His English is only fair; tell the Welsh King I'd speak to him in peace. Tell him and the Gott-damned combrogi if anyone moves, my men will pepper the field."

I did. They would. "For God's love, don't anyone move."

"I read your will." Gunnar grinned. "Are you surprised I came?"

"Not half so surprised as you, I'll hazard."

"Oh, you know Mother. Just said she knew all along

you were one of them. Tell the Welsh King of my rights as your heir, Gwenda."

"Constantine, this is my former master whom you may have met on Trent. Thegn Gunnar Eanboldson."

"I've seen the barbarian," Constantine admitted. "What does he here?"

"His affairs are his," said Gunnar. "Mine are mine."

And that affair a revelation to Constantine: to inform the Welshman of the subject will signed by me. From the will, precisely itemized, Constantine learned with incredulity and then growing horror at the ramifications, that Gunnar laid legal claim to all that I left him as the last of my line. The personal property of my family since the governorship of Agricola, to wit:

Item: the palace at Eburacum.

Item: one thousand acres of arable, fallow and under plow, nearly ten full English hides, leased in tenantage to Parisi and Brigantes, all specifically located.

Item: the fifth part of all export profit from city trade in wool and lead.

Item: various smaller dwellings within and without the city, all built and maintained by my family.

Item: various personal treasures late looted from Camelot by pernicious war waged by Cornish, Silure and Demetae to the estimate of eighteen hundred pounds English silver or six hundred imperial aurei . . .

A tidy sum. Among the "late looted" treasures was one I could not resist appending for pure spleen: the imperial sword of Britain, our last link with Rome.

"You have that much effrontery?" Constantine wondered. "Even the sword?"

A classic sight in opposites—Constantine glaring in naked disbelief, Gunnar placidly sure of his own rights.

"Rights!" Constantine almost choked on it. "Does this barbarian think I'll give him half a city and six hundred pieces of gold?"

"Yes," said Gunnar when I'd relayed it. "I think he will. The same way he gave us Trent. Tell him that, Gwenda. I'll go for Eburacum because it's worth it to me, to my son, my family and every man who follows me."

Constantine stared at the parchment that held perhaps another decade of war if he denied it.

"Although there can be no question of inheritance

while the Queen lives," Lucullus suggested in his silken manner. "I believe Thegn Gunnar has a compromise."

"No."

"At least hear him."

"No release for Guenevere. I can't afford it."

"My friend, a word." Lucullus leaned out of the saddle, close to Constantine. "You know I might have been crowned instead of Arthur had it been my wish. How much better him than me, how much better you, but how close our aims: prosperity and imperial trade. That empire has sent me to deal with all princes—Gunnar's as well as you. We are benevolent but not sentimental. We will deal with those we think viable. And I would have you one of them, dear friend. Listen to his terms. He has Alun. Alive."

The animosity visibly wilted out of Constantine. His friend quietly offered him life. He wanted it as much as he wanted mine. "Alun . . ."

"Gwenda?" Gunnar advanced with his hand up and open, placed it on the King's saddlehorn. "Tell him he's lucky Lucullus reached my camp when he did."

Gunnar's other hand lifted to the hilltop, to the figure flanked by hulking Teutons.

"A bit nervous but in impeccable condition," Lucullus verified. "Be reasonable, my lord. The sun shines again. Alun for Guenevere, that's his offer."

"Hold, you men. Emrys, hold your men. I will do nothing." Constantine wanted to give in, I saw it. All that made his driven life bearable was waiting and perishable on that hill, no further from death than Gunnar's signal. But Constantine surprised me, still that much of a king.

"But not free to Emrys. Not free in Britain. Banished. To sail with you, Lucullus."

I breathed a little easier. "And an escort to the ship. Combrogi, not Cornish, if you don't mind."

"That's Emrys' affair. You are never to return on pain of death. I banish you for life, Guenevere."

For life . . . for life. So long it was. "So be it."

"And you here proclaim me as your successor."

"You have it in writing."

Constantine jerked his head at Emrys. "So does he."

We all waited, Gunnar impassive, the insects hovering

about, Emrys a drawn bow in front of his men, the English taut on their hill. As might be expected, the combrogi were in far better position for attack. Constantine's men were already pummeled and demoralized by these same damned English.

"I will proclaim to all. To yours, to Emrys and especially to them." I pointed to the peasants who'd crept closer, curious at the static outcome of all this.

Still Constantine wanted more assurance. "Lucullus, will you turn over your safe conduct and the hope of any future ones in pledge she sails with you?"

The ambassador rummaged in his saddle purse and passed the seal to his friend. "To Constantinople. On the word of the Empire and my future welcome in Britain."

"Done." Constantine gripped Gunnar's hand with brief distaste and let it drop. "Give me my knight, Saxon."

At Gunnar's sign, the Teutons stood away from their hostage, who started to walk down the hill, uncertain at first, then with grateful haste. Constantine walked his horse forward to meet him. I felt Gunnar's arm go about my waist.

"I should never have freed you. If I'd known who you were—"

"You'd have sold me to that charming man there."

Enough truth there to give Gunnar pause. "Yes. Not that I don't love you."

"Of course, darling. Just a matter of good business."

"You are hlafdian," Gunnar murmured with deep admiration. "Mother and Nilse would be proud to bring you the cup in our hall. Meanwhile, I have your will." Gunnar tucked it away, a whole future in his pocket. "Let me know when I may collect. Where is this city you go to?"

"The end of the world. Constantinople." I tasted the far inconceivability in the sound. "My God, Lucullus, I'm an exile again. Whatever shall I do in Constantinople?"

Lucullus turned from the reunion of the king and his knight to beam at me. "Improve it, Lady."

"You'll need a horse." Gunnar hooked his dangling reins into my grasp. "He's Welsh anyway."

"British, damn you. Don't you ever listen to me? British!" Up on tiptoe, I squeezed Gunnar's neck in my embrace. "Kiss the family for me, dear."

"When I see them. There's another march first."

"Where?"

"To Badon," said Gunnar with immense satisfaction. "We're going to jam those stakes deep in the ground and hold it forever. This king had better get used to us. Because I'm going to sit on that plowing hill and Eadward after me and his son after that. Tell him."

"I think he knows." I stroked Gunnar's beautiful beard. "Kiss me again? It's a long way, and you do it so well."

"*Farvel, skat.*" When he went between the lines toward his own men, Elfgifu's son bent thriftily to collect the fallen arrows.

"Constantine! Emrys! Let us stand before the people. Brother Coel, let the folk come closer. There will be a proclamation. Guenevere's last word to her people."

My final problem in that bee-droning summer morning. Emrys had a writ from me, so did Constantine. For that matter, so did Gunnar. And those people like Huw and Mabli gathered about Coel had nothing but my trust. They deserved a good word to remember. I mounted and beckoned Constantine to join me, Emrys as well, in the center of their forces. They met there like swords on guard.

"My Lord."

"My Lord."

"No treachery," Emrys warned. "Gareth will attack."

"And none from you, princeling. I'll do for you myself."

"Each of you nearest your own men," I suggested. "No, we face *this* way, toward the people. You remember them?"

I stood in the stirrups, my arms raised. "People of Britain! Hear me. I have given my word with assurances to leave Britain forever."

Halfway up the hill, his arms full of arrows, Gunnar stopped to listen.

"Is that true, Aunt?" Emrys asked.

"Yes, and don't pretend you're sorry. You're as strong a prince as I could make you, but this must be. People! I am constrained to publish the name of my successor in Britain, pending the choice of Holy Church and the tribes assembled. Here is Constantine of Cornwall. Will you, the people, cry *gwledig* to him? And here is Emrys

Pendragon of the blood of Arthur. Let you cry gwledig to him, if it please you."

"Guenevere, get *on* with it," Constantine hissed out of the side of his mouth. "I could kill you right here."

"And die with me. People!" My arm swooped to Gunnar standing on the hillside. "And there, whether you know it or not, is another successor of mine, one who at least knows the earth as you do. For you are my successors as well. No—this King and this pretender will not let you exercise the right, nor will you be worthy of it until you know how. But never forget your right to do so. Tell it to your children's children that they remember as well. Kings go down with the sun. You remain."

Emrys shook his head. "Aunt, what in hell are you doing?"

"I've given you what I can." Constantine barely contained himself. "Don't be ambiguous. Say it, woman."

I had to laugh at the sight of them. "Look at the two of you: one word from either and you'd end it all right here. And your people and the English couldn't care less. Last round of king-of-the-hill. Dear Nephew, I must proclaim this tragedy of a man as King. Constantine, look on Emrys and know he'll never let you rest with it."

"Damned right I won't. You didn't."

"And so it goes on. May it well become you both. All right, Cornishman, here's your due. People—"

"Aunt, don't!"

"Do what you will, both of you. I hereby proclaim Constantine of Cornwall as my choice to succeed in Britain. But let him hear your voice to remind him it will not be silenced. *Who shall carry the sword of Britain?*"

There was Coel's voice first, then others, Lowri and Huw, Mabli and the rest behind them: not king but queen. Gwladys.

"Gwladys!"

Propelled by their fervor, the people edged forward, Coel in the lead with the high cross. "Guenevere! Guenevere!"

And as they chanted, the litany deepened with male voices from the hill, English voices—

"Gunver! Gunver!"

"Gwladys!"

And even, I fancied, a voice or two among the combrogi, swelling the whole into a tide.

"GUENEVERE! GWLADYS!"

Emrys and Constantine could do nothing but endure it. "This changes nothing," my successor graciously pointed out. "Nothing."

"Not now, but at least you've heard their voice. By God's Eyes, a few more of them, I could still best the lot of you. And make no mistake, there will be more of them."

Constantine started to laugh. "Oh, but—"

"But—on to exile. It's all yours now. King-of-the-hill and ravening challenger. Fight over it, children—but do wait until I'm off the field. Mother wants to enjoy her obscurity."

"Goodbye, Aunt." Emrys extended his gauntlet to me. He swallowed hard, not accepting it, never able to accept it, but with more innate grace than Constantine. "God keep you."

"And you, Emrys. May you never be so sick of it all as I am now."

The wagons were tugged into line behind Lucullus, Coel and me. Coel set his cross in the lance socket of his saddle and gave the signal to move.

"And my escort, Lucullus?"

On the field, the two forces were still poised head-on, the English merely waiting. "Evidently not," Lucullus concluded.

"Let us go, then."

When we crested the first hill to the south, half a mile from the villa, Huw shouted, pointing back to the armed field. I recognized the shields of the riders galloping toward us from the combrogi ranks. Gareth, Bedivere, Bors and Ifan. For a dismal moment I wondered if Emrys had given order for my death. Not beyond possibility. These four, two young, two old, had no more future than he now: accept it or fight.

I crossed myself. "Stand away from me, all of you. I'm enough to die if that's the way of it."

But Huw knew the shields. "Not them, Lady. Didn't I near kill your horse to reach them? And while the Prince debated, it was them"—he flourished his arm toward the four—"who gave him the choice to lead them or stay be-

hind. The Gryffyn and the mac Diurmuid. Oh, did they blister the royal ear, and themselves halfway to horse in speaking it. Nae, Lady. Not them."

The four combrogi slowed to a canter as they neared us and drew abreast a few paces away.

"Well, my Lords. Are you my escort or only in a way of speaking? I'm glad he sent friends."

"Ah, don't be wet," Bedivere growled.

"Age has not impaired my hearing yet. It seemed down on the field that I heard several sweet and well-known voices cry Gwladys."

"Me, mum." Bors removed his helmet. "And proud to sing it out. Little good that it does."

"No less than me," said Ifan. "Your escort to Severn, Lady."

"And me." Gareth paced forward of his men. "I told the Prince, did he not come with us, I'd never ride in his service again."

An old man now, Gareth was breathing hard from his gallop and the hot sun. I saw how stiffly his gnarled fingers grasped the reins. "We heard you would be wanting escort," he said. "The Prince himself asked the four of us. Not that much asking was needed."

That was generosity. Emrys' four most experienced captains. There was grace left in Britain after all. Not Eleyne's sort, but warmer.

"I am grateful, my lords. And you, Bedivere? Did I hear your voice among them?"

The lean old man stepped down and hooked his helmet over the saddlehorn. He drew his sword, cradling it in both hands and went to his knee at my stirrup, offering up the sword in the gesture of fealty as he'd once sworn it to Arthur.

"Gwladys," said Bedivere.

I laid my hand across the sword hilt. "Thank you, Lord Bedivere. Please take me to ship—and God knows where after that. Lucullus, I have much to thank you for."

He dismissed it with his opulent modesty. "The empire needs such a treasure."

"Beloved Lucullus, my knight of the disguised blessings."

"Beloved exile." He bowed from the waist. "Shall we get on?"

Mabli began the carol as the wagons moved after us, her parents and the others joining in.

> For he'll a-go Midsummer night
> In horns and all green leaves bedight,
> And I will love my lord a-right—

"Look!"

The lovely song tore on the jagged edge of Lowri's horror as she pointed back to the field. Emrys and Constantine were no longer poised. The lethal wedge of the combrogi, an arrow with a prince at its head, shot forward against the waiting Cornish.

"Jesus." Bedivere took it all in with one fierce, pitying curse. "The boy had to do it. He had to try."

From our hill we saw the rush of them, the imminent collision frozen in time—the flying wedge, the answer already spurring forward, lances dropping to the ready. And beyond them on the other rise, that man with the farmer's stance waiting with his archers for the shock and clash, waiting for the dust to clear, certain as his mother of the outcome.

"That's the end, Gareth," Bedivere said—low, passionate, not wanting to look at it ever again. "I'm done. Didn't I say it to Arthur at Badon, *done* with it. I'll break my sword. On the quay I'll do it when the Queen's aboard, break the bloody thing in two and drop the pieces into Severn. Christ be my witness, I'm through."

"Come, Bedwyr." Once again I bent to caress his bony cheek, purpled with broken veins. "It's no part of us any more. Mabli, start the dear song again."

On the field we could see nothing now but the merciful dust that veiled them all. Under the song new-risen from my people, the war horns were too far and faint to hear.

X

Once Upon a Time

At Constantinople, the Imperial Court of Justinian
Fifth day, Kalends of Augustus, Anno Domini 538.
To MALGO, King of the West Britons, Greetings
    and long life.

My generous lord, you have my gratitude and my
prayers. Because my eyes are quite useless now, the
Emperor Justinian himself usurped the pleasure of
reading your letter to me and his scribe of writing
these joyful thanks. With your gracious permission, I will return to Britain.

I should like to dwell at Ynnis Witrin near the
tomb of my royal husband Artorius, beside whom I
would lie when it please God to call me.

I will not truly see home again. That must remain
an impoverished figure of speech as I can barely
perceive the brightest colors now, and Britain for
me was always a place of dazzling hues—swaths of
red and yellow and lavender, and the most startling
green one does not find anywhere else. There was
sometimes an improbable quality about the morning or evening light, as if substance and reality
were an illusion. Color is much in my mind in late
years, keenly remembered if no longer seen.

But I ramble, an old woman's indulgence. Your Majesty will forgive it, I trust, and take once again my deepest thanks.

Guenevere of Eburacum

At Constantinople, the Imperium
JUSTINIAN, Emperor, to MALGO, King of the West Britons—

My lord, we thank you for your generous dispensation anent Lady Guenevere of Eburacum who has served our forums of law as wisely as once she ruled in Britain. As earnest of our reciprocal good will, the courier bearing these presents will transmit to you as well our new trade schedules, substantially revised in favor of British lead, tin and your incomparable wool.

(The formal letter ends here over Justinian's seal. Eastern historians have cited the following postscript, although unsigned, as surely written in the Emperor's own hand on an attached papyrus. It is headed with the usual design of a rose to signify its confidential nature—Ed.)

My lord, let there be someone to meet her. Although in reasonable health, she will be eighty-seven soon and almost blind. Yet never have I known, even in youth, a mind so agile or so quick to touch the heart and spirit of law. She has illuminated much for me in my revision of jurisprudence and tells me the work keeps her young. I must believe her; there is little about Guenevere not touched with the fabulous. Why, my grandfather remembered stories of this woman and her husband. Legends, actually. I don't believe the half of them. But I shall miss her, Malgo.

Please forgive the error of my scriptorium in addressing you earlier as King of Wales. I understand it's a Saxon term. Guenevere herself corrected the scribes. . . .

. . . God, did I correct them! They never made that mistake again, be sure of it. Oh, sir, the English are good people, some of the best, but *they're* the foreigners . . . were the foreigners. Now they're damned well us, aren't they? I saw it coming thirty years ago, and I wasn't young then.

The breeze is marvelous. I'll be able to smell the land soon. Just have to keep my chest wrapped. No one should live to my age, it's presumptuous. My God, I've outlived everything. All my friends, my enemies—lot of right bastards they were, too—even my times. Likely find Britain itself leaning on a stick, blind and arthritic and falling apart like me. It's a different country now, worse off than ever. No notion of history or perspective or even good government. This lachrymose monk, this Gildas—now there's a mollusc for you. Very little good he has to say about his own country and very little he knows of it, either. Doesn't even mention Arthur, not a *word* of me, and we did as much as Ambrosius. More, by God's Eyes.

. . . No, not tired, just a little giddy. I should like to get lyrical drunk or make love. Oh, there's boasting! The mere contemplation of either would immolate what's left of me. But I just realized it again—isn't it grand, sir? I'm coming *home*.

The sailors tell me we'll anchor at Fowey soon to take on water. Will you call me when we're close? No, young sir, I do *not* see well at all. Otherwise I shouldn't need you to tell me. There, no offense. Are you going forward? Let me hold the child. Go along, she and I will keep each other company. . . .

Well, child. Your cheeky young da tells me he's a minstrel from Massilia. We have a few minstrels in Britain . . . had a few. We called them bards, and they were near to being holy men. I knew one of them when I was young as your father: not that holy but one of the best. Everyone knew Trystan of Castle Dore. You've heard the name? Let's see, how did your father begin that last tale—'Once upon a time' . . . like most things Gaulish, not much sense but graceful.

Well, then, once upon a time there was a minstrel knight named Trystan who loved a princess named Yseult . . . you've heard it? Interesting. I knew he trav-

eled much, but—then have you heard the story of the Holy Grail and how it was found by none other than my own brother, Peredur?

Percival? Oh, please, not that again. That is what the English persist in calling him, and they have their own way of doing things, quite arbitrary at times. But Peredur it was who found the Grail . . . you've heard that too. I see.

(Forward child. Always loved them but I wonder if I ever really *liked* them as much as flowers. All right, you precocious little—I'll spin a tale to curl up your toes.)

Girl, do you know how you feel when you wake in the dark? When your mum and da aren't there, and you can feel the dark like a living thing creeping closer and closer . . . standing over your bed, bending down by your ear, reaching out black arms to get you?

Aye, frightening it is. Imagine years of such darkness with no morning. Picture a land under such a curse, black moonless night filled with evil faeries slipping through the dark to steal little girls who interrupt too much.

In this nighted land, under a spell that even Rome couldn't break, a princess waited in the darkest tower for a worthy prince to rescue her. And one day such a prince came. He didn't look a prince at all, just a common soldier. But he knew the magic to fight the evil spell. His men were a magic of their own, with horses so swift the ground couldn't hold them, and so they flew! They soared over the land with great torches of light and hope to push back the dark and bring the long-missed morning.

And when the dark was whisked away, the soldier came to the new-lighted tower at Eburacum for his princess—

Mark! Is that your father calling? Is it the land? Yes, *yes*. I can smell the flowers. Here, girl, give me my stick. Take my hand. Lead me to the rail. Tell me what you see. It's summer . . . oh, it must be dazzling.

The cliffs come all asudden up from the sea, black and brown and chalk. White where the sea batters against them. And up above on the downs, it's a very special kind of green, isn't it? And yellow with ragwort, purple with heather and foxglove. . . .

The red? Oh, my dear, that's pimpernel. Scarlet pimpernel, my land grows them everywhere. I wore pimpernel in my hair the day I was married, for my husband came on swiftly and there wasn't time to gather anything else—

What? Oh, bother the silly story! Of course they got married and became a great king and queen, lived long and were very happy. It was once upon a time, wasn't it?

Tell me about the flowers, child.

Born in New York City, PARKE GODWIN was raised all over, drifted through a variety of places, schools and careers, including the army, government, theater, research, the staff of *Sports Afield* and as a short-order cook before writing his first novel, *Darker Places*, in 1971. He first attracted attention in the SF/fantasy field with *The Masters of Solitude* (1978), written with Marvin Kaye, and followed in 1982 by *Wintermind*. In that same year he won the World Fantasy Award for his novella "The Fire When It Comes," which has since been optioned for film production.

Beloved Exile is the second volume in a triptych of Roman Britain which began with *Firelord*, the story of Arthur. It became a finalist for the World Fantasy Award in 1981. The concluding volume, *The Last Rainbow*, will be published by Bantam Books in 1985.

Godwin's friends call him Pete. His chief delight is drinking coffee and wasting time, or wandering the beaches at Cape Cod. He loves dogs and Prokofiev, cooking, rapping, jogging, collecting obscure sound-track records. He tolerates children and cats (if tethered) and conservatives (if muzzled), enjoys relaxing on the Staten Island ferry, sailing nowhere in particular, or at his favorite restaurant, R. J. Scotty's. Following investigation, he was found to be completely uninvolved in the mystery death of Warren G. Harding.

WEST
of
EDEN

Harry Harrison

From a master of imaginative storytelling comes an epic tale of the world as it might have been, a world where the age of dinosaurs never ended, and their descendants clash with a clan of humans in a tragic war for survival. . . .

"An astonishing piece of work." —Joe Haldemann

"A big novel in every sense . . ."
—*Washington Post Book World*

"Brilliant." —Phillip Jose Farmer

"Epic science fantasy." —*Playboy*

"The best Harrison ever—and that's going some."
—Jerry Pournelle

"I commend this rich and rewarding novel to those who know and love Heinlein, Asimov, Herbert and Clarke; they will find no less than what those masters provide here." —Barry N. Malzberg

"This is the way they used to write them, high adventure with lots of thought-provoking meat."
—Thomas N. Scortia